Commercializing Successful Biomedical Technologies

Successful product design and development require the ability to take a concept and translate the technology into useful, patentable, commercial products.

For scientists and engineers, this book demystifies the commercialization process, guiding the reader through each practical stage, describing key issues including market analysis, product development, intellectual property and regulatory constraints.

- A robust product development plan is provided though a step-by-step model, from concept to regulated, commercially viable product.
- Key business issues are highlighted, taking into account critical business aspects, such as budgetary impact, time constraints, and quality control in the development cycle.
- Case studies and contributions from industry are included for a practical perspective.
- Learning points and exercises reinforce the most important concepts and strengthen understanding.

Written in a concise manner, this book will be the indispensable guide for professionals and entrepreneurs in biomedical technology development. With the increasing need for students to be fluent in such business skills, this book is an ideal accompaniment to a capstone design course in engineering and biotechnology.

Foreword written by **Frank L. Douglas Ph.D., M.D.** *Former Executive Vice President, member of Board of Management and Chief Scientific Officer of Aventis Pharmaceutical, Former Professor of the Practice and Executive Director of the MIT Center for Biomedical Innovation and Partner at Pure Tech Ventures.*

Shreefal S. Mehta is Vice President of Business and Corporate Development, Cytopia Inc., and Clinical Associate Professor of Biotechnology Management and Biomedical Engineering, Rensselaer Polytechnic Institute. He was CEO and co-founder of Myomatrix Therapeutics, a cardiovascular pharmaceutical startup and recipient of the "40 under 40" award for rising business leaders in New York. He has been a reviewer for the NSF Biotechnology Commercialization SBIR Review panel.

Additional resources, including sample syllabus, suggested reading and website resources can be found at www.commercializingbiotech.com.

Commercializing Successful Biomedical Technologies

Basic Principles for the Development of Drugs, Diagnostics and Devices

SHREEFAL S. MEHTA

Vice President of Business and Corporate Development, Cytopia

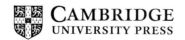

CAMBRIDGE UNIVERSITY PRESS

CAMBRIDGE UNIVERSITY PRESS
Cambridge, New York, Melbourne, Madrid, Cape Town,
Singapore, São Paulo, Delhi, Tokyo, Mexico City

Cambridge University Press
The Edinburgh Building, Cambridge CB2 8RU, UK

Published in the United States of America by Cambridge University Press, New York

www.cambridge.org
Information on this title: www.cambridge.org/9780521870986

First published 2008
Third printing 2009
First paperback edition 2011

A catalogue record for this publication is available from the British Library

ISBN 978-0-521-87098-6 Hardback
ISBN 978-0-521-20585-6 Paperback

Cambridge University Press has no responsibility for the persistence or
accuracy of URLs for external or third-party internet websites referred to in
this publication, and does not guarantee that any content on such websites is,
or will remain, accurate or appropriate. Information regarding prices, travel
timetables, and other factual information given in this work is correct at
the time of first printing but Cambridge University Press does not guarantee
the accuracy of such information thereafter.

www.commercializingbiotech.com

To Gauri, whose continuing support and encouragement, whose patience and willingness to shoulder my share of parenting when necessary, and more, made the completion of this book possible. Without your help, there would have been no book.

Contents

Foreword

The deciphering of the human genome at the dawn of our twenty-first century not only fueled expectation of an increase in speed of developing therapies for many diseases but also exploded some cherished myths. Among the myths exploded was the belief that there were about 100 000 genes in the human genome and that this would lead to thousands of new 'targets' (receptors, enzymes, transporters, ion channels, etc.) for the discovery of new drugs. Although still somewhat in question, the number of genes in the human genome is felt to be about 30 000, thus dampening considerably some of the initial euphoria over the anticipated results of this outstanding achievement: the deciphering of the human genome. Another disappointing projection is that the number of druggable targets will only increase some threefold, from about 550 to 1500. Nonetheless, this incredible achievement, enabled by many technologies associated with genome sequencing, has fueled additional technologies, such as proteomics and metabolomics, for the innovation of new drugs and diagnostics.

The dawn of this century has also seen an increase in awareness of the importance of unwanted side effects in marketed drugs and safety issues in device usage. This debate has not only captured the attention of the public, as some widely used drugs, such as Vioxx and Pergolide, have been removed from the market, but also that of the Congress. Members of Congress have questioned whether there should be an agency separate from the Food and Drug Administration (FDA) to assess and monitor the safety of marketed drugs and devices.

In addition to the discussion of benefit and risk of new therapies, the cost of drugs is an increasingly popular topic of debate, along with the overall rapid rise of healthcare costs. The cost for major medical coverage has increased 124 percent above the consumer price index (CPI) every year since 1957. Meanwhile, the fully loaded cost of bringing a new drug to the market is over a billion dollars and only about one third of these drugs make more than $300 000 in sales per year.

Another challenge facing the industry, as the first decade of the twenty-first century ends, is the number of innovative drugs that will lose patent status and be converted to generics. Although this is good news for the consumer, it will be a challenge for the companies who innovated many of these drugs. For example, between 2004 and 2012, the top 15 pharmaceutical companies will see 95 of their drugs converted to generics. Thus in this first decade, these companies will lose billions of dollars in revenues.

It should be noted that manufacturing in devices and drugs has also had its challenges. Manufacturing problems at Chiron led to a potential shortage of flu vaccines in 2004 and manufacturing problems at Schering Plough led to significant loss of sales for their introduction of Clarinex. In fact, the FDA has had only modest success with their Process and Analytical Technology (PAT) initiative in their attempts to improve good manufacturing processes in the companies. Thirty-two serious Class 1 device recalls in the first six months of 2007 and 56 class I recalls in all of 2006 show that quality assurance and other manufacturing issues in the device industry continue. Thus, manufacturing remains an area for significant improvement and cost reduction in the industry.

Where then are the opportunities?

The first two decades of the twenty-first century will undoubtedly see the fulfillment of the hopes that genomic-based technologies, predictive modeling, automation, and miniaturization will revolutionize the way drugs are discovered, manufactured, and marketed. Two streams of importance will be the ability to identify that subset of patients that will best respond to a therapy and those patients who are likely to experience unwanted effects from that therapy. This will be the coming of age of "stratified medicine." Presently, Herceptin, for the treatment of a subset of breast cancers, is the best example. In this example, patients whose breast cancer is found to have HER2/neu receptors respond better to a regimen including Herceptin than to other regimens. Thus the diagnosis of the type of cancer and best therapy for that person are linked by a diagnostic. To be sure, not every therapy will lend itself to this unique constellation of diagnostic enabling therapy, as it is clear that at least three specific criteria will be necessary for this to occur. These criteria include the presence of: differential biological mechanisms, many treatment options, and a biological marker or diagnostic. The biological marker might be genomic-based, clinical observation, or imaging (M. R. Trusheim, E. R. Berndt, F. L. Douglas; Strategic and economic implications of stratified medicine, *Nature Reviews Drug Discovery*, April, 2007).

Another opportunity will be the combination of devices and therapy. A good example of this is the drug-eluting stent for the treatment of occluded coronary arteries. Other applications wait in areas such as diabetes, with the measurement of glucose accompanied by the release of the appropriate amount of insulin from an indwelling insulin reservoir. Other examples exist in cardiology and rheumatology, where measurement of arrhythmia or acute changes in an analyte by indwelling devices can lead to an appropriate release of drug to normalize the condition.

When stratified medicine becomes a standard part of the approach to healthcare, changes in the manner of commercialization will occur. It is quite likely that new commercialization paradigms that focus on specialists as opposed to the general practitioners will be associated with this approach. The supply chain issues will also be affected and perhaps there will be more opportunities for "just-in-time" type approaches in the biopharmaceutical industry. The PAT initiative of the FDA may very well benefit this area.

A final area of progress will be in organizations and this is an arena where Dr Mehta's book will make a major contribution. Because of the complexity and the long times (8–15 years) involved with bringing a biomedical product (drugs, novel devices) from idea to market, few employees enter the industry with an appreciation of the pre-clinical, clinical, manufacturing, commercial and regulatory issues, and expertise needed to achieve this noble task of making novel medicines and devices accessible to patients. Dr Mehta's book not only introduces the reader to the nomenclature and issues but, through problem discussions, he gives the reader (student or industry employee) a sense of the complexity, the creativity as well as the regulatory requirements that must be satisfied to achieve the task. This book should improve the public's understanding of the challenge of innovating devices and drugs and thus improve the dialogue of benefit and risk decisions associated with the approval and marketing of devices and drugs.

Frank L Douglas Ph.D., M.D.
Former Executive Vice President, member of Board of Management and Chief Scientific Officer of Aventis Pharmaceutical, Former Professor of the Practice and Executive Director of the MIT Center for Biomedical Innovation and Partner at Pure Tech Ventures.

Preface

This book will help readers draw a roadmap of the process of taking a biomedical invention and creating a product that can pass regulatory approval to be successfully commercialized. The regulated products included in this context are drugs (both small molecules and biologics), medical devices, diagnostics, and their combination products, as defined by the Food and Drug Administration (FDA) – the regulatory agency that is responsible for overseeing the world's single largest healthcare market, the United States. The term "biomedical technologies" refers to the collective technologies underlying these FDA-regulated products: biotechnology, various engineering technologies, chemistry and materials science, etc.

The book highlights key issues that might help improve chances of success through the complete commercialization process for biomedical technologies and products. This text started as an expansion of a series of lectures given to students at the Lally School of Management and Technology, Rensselaer Polytechnic Institute in Troy, NY as part of a class called "Commercializing biomedical technology." However, going beyond the classroom in writing this book, information has been taken from many sources and experienced people from industry have contributed to add current and practical information to various segments of the book.

This book could be used to bring science and engineering students together with business and law students, and show them the benefits of approaching this complex process as a team. Many of these students have found the information useful in job interviews and in planning careers in the biotech industry and its service sectors.

This book has a practical perspective, so that current scientists, engineers and managers in the industry can apply these concepts, issues, and exercises within the context of their job functions in the industry. What's more, aspiring entrepreneurs may seek to apply these concepts to their invention or idea; walking through all the steps and exercises to create a sound commercialization plan that can form the basis for a business plan for a new venture (see figure).

Business models and financial plans vary with the economic or personal context and the goals of the founders. However, any business model, to be successful, must come from an understanding of the complete commercialization path for the regulated product. The linear roadmap shows the components that must be assessed to build a sound commercialization plan, but the processes are all carried out in parallel, with shifting emphasis on each component as one proceeds down the plan. The sequence of components is mirrored in the sequence of chapters in the

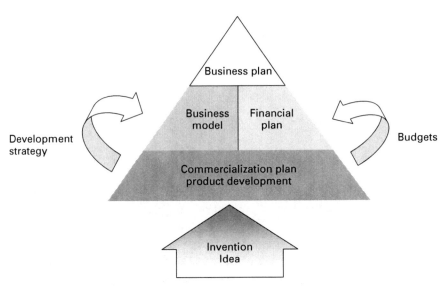

First you have to understand how your idea will be developed into a product and reach the paying customers; then you can choose one of many successful business models in the biomedical industry and prepare a business or financial plan to execute that development strategy.

Components of a product commercialization plan and roadmap

Plan	Position	Patent	Product	Pass!	Production	Profits
Industry context	**Market research**	**Intelluctual property rights**	**New product development (NPD)**	**Regulatory plan**	**Manufacture**	**Reimbursement**
Technology positioning and strategy, corporate portfolio strategy, industrial value chain context	Market need, Specific indication of interest, market size and segments, product characteristics	Intellectual property management and licensing strategy, Patent content for market protection, Business models	Stage gate new product testing and development plan, budget, Gannt chart	Regulatory strategy – working with FDA towards approval	Production planning	Coverage, Coding, Payment, Distribution, Marketing and sales planning

Roadmap to create a commercialization plan. The linear stages shown here reflect the layout of the book.

book. The arrows below the components in the roadmap illustrate the fact that all these components must be kept in mind to achieve a successful commercial and product development plan.

The process of doing science and also the process of building commercial entities can be represented as a linear thought process, but the practice of both is a

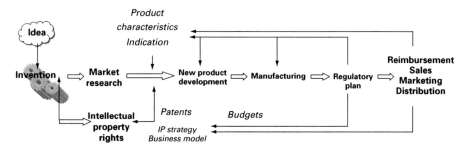

Successful development of new biomedical products for a competitive and regulated marketplace requires a full and thorough understanding of specific issues in the full value chain, discussed in the book. As feedback from various areas is defined for the specific product concept, the commercialization and product development plan will be revised (indicated by thinner feedback arrows above).

path-dependent, iterative process, where learning and understanding grow by doing each experiment or building each step of a commercialization plan. The schematic (above) illustrates, with arrows, the process of feedback between the various components of a commercialization process. As an example, the regulatory process influences the product development plan and also defines the markets accessed by the product. Likewise, access to intellectual property rights influences the direction of development and access to specific markets. Thus, iterative feedback from evaluating the specific regulatory pathways or intellectual property rights might require reconfiguration of the product characteristics or might require choosing a different application from that conceived during original invention.

The process for planning new product development might, for instance, follow the steps:

Idea – invention – market research – intellectual property search – define product and indications of interest – plan the key product development steps – check on regulatory strategy – revise product development plan and characteristics – check on reimbursement strategy – revise product characteristics and product development plan.

The result will be a comprehensive product development and commercialization plan with a timeline and budget. The exercises at the end of the chapters will help guide the reader through these steps.

While the original multidisciplinary (scientists, engineers, management, and other humanities students) course continues as a graduate-level course, much of the developed material has been incorporated into the Biomedical Engineering undergraduate capstone design course at Rensselaer Polytechnic Institute (RPI) as part of the core curriculum, hopefully creating a more conscious and self-aware breed of product development scientist and engineer.

Finally, it is my hope that better thinking and planning in the development of regulated products will help improve the efficiency, success, and quality of biomedical technology commercialization, increasing the number of innovative products that can be delivered to help people.

Acknowledgements

The contributions and suggestions of friends and colleagues who shared their time, their insights from years of industry experience, their editorial suggestions, and specific case studies, have significantly improved this book. I would particularly like to recognize the formative early discussions and exchanges with my colleague Dr Jan Stegemann during the creation of the eponymous class that we co-taught at Rensselaer Polytechnic Institute (RPI).

Contributors and reviewers

Jim Greenwood, President of Biotechnology Industry Organization, USA

Christoph Hergersberg, Global Head of Bioscience Technology, GE

Mark Leahy, President of Medical Device Manufacturers Association, USA

Andrew Marshall, Editor, *Nature Biotechnology*

Parashar Patel, Vice President of Health Economics and Reimbursement, Boston Scientific; and past Deputy Director of Hospital and Ambulatory Payment Group, Centers for Medicare and Medicaid Services

Kim Popovits, Chief Operating Officer and President, Genomic Health

Tony Rao, Principal, Stantec

Dan Recinella, Vice President of Product Development, Angiodynamics Inc.

Phil Roberts, Head of Process Development, Nektar Therapeutics

Lawrence Roth, Vice President of Product and Business Development, Percardia Inc.

Randall Rupp, Sr., Vice President of Manufacturing, Regeneron

Robert Schaffer, Partner, Darby and Darby PC

Jayson Slotnick, Director of Medicare Reimbursement and Economic Policy at the Biotechnology Industry Organization (BIO)

Jo Ellen Slurzberg, Vice President of Reimbursement and Health Policy, Almyra, Inc. and Chair of Medical Device Manufacturers Association Reimbursement Task Force

Mitchell Sugarman (and colleagues), Director of Health Economics, Policy, and Payment, Medtronics

Lawrence Zisman, Vice President of Cardiovascular Research, Cytopia Inc.

Reviewers

Jori Frahler, Director of Federal Affairs, Medical Device Manufacturers Association

Mary Pendergast, Principal, Pendergast Consulting and past Assistant Commissioner of FDA

Hanson Gifford, Founder and CEO, The Foundry Inc.

Tanvi Mehta, freelance editor

1 The biomedical drug, diagnostic, and devices industries and their markets

Plan	Position	Patent	Product	Pass!	Production	Profits
Industry context	Market research	Intellectual property rights	New product development (NPD)	Regulatory plan	Manufacture	Reimbursement

Roadmap of a product commercialization plan. Stage 1

Learning points:

- Description of types of FDA-regulated products covered in this book,
- Understand the technological base and application for each product type,
- Description of functions and processes involved in commercialization activities for each product type,
- Analysis of industry sector competitiveness by value chain model and Porter's five forces analysis,
- Understand the technology trajectories for the biomedical industry.

1.1 The healthcare industry

The healthcare industry and the markets for healthcare services and biomedical products have one significant difference from the rest of the free-market industries in the US – the healthcare market is heavily regulated. But several other differences are also notable. For example, while purchasing a retail item or a service in a competitive market, the user is the primary customer and makes the purchasing decision, the user is given all appropriate requested information on the product, and the user is then the payer. In the healthcare marketplace, the user (patient) usually does not make the purchasing decision (the provider and other intermediary institutions, such as pharmacy benefit managers make that decision), the patient does not get all the information (the provider typically gets the detailed briefing and information packages) and the patient is not the payer (the patient usually does not know the true price of services and products; the payer is the insurance company or government). This marketplace is highly regulated, starting from the early product development stages to the preparation and dissemination of marketing information, and including the flow of payments, goods, and information. The government is also the largest single payer organization in the healthcare industry and, thus, politics influence payment policies and procedures in the industry. Laws and policies enacted by the legislative bodies play a very important role in shaping the healthcare marketplace. Manufacturers or product developers, therefore, need to pay attention to laws and policies as changes could affect their product development process. In fact, as noted here in Box 1.1 by the heads of two major biomedical technology company associations, companies must be proactive in monitoring and interacting with legislators (elected representatives) in government and with regulatory agencies. The manufacturers must monitor changes in policy that impact the market and take an active role to educate and inform the drafting of such policy and regulation. Any commercialization plan for a new biomedical technology must be carried out mindful of the context of this regulated and politically charged healthcare marketplace.

The rest of this chapter discusses the various product development sectors involved in the larger healthcare industry and highlights methods to analyze and understand better the functional structures from a product development perspective.

1.2   Biomedical technology – definition and scope; applications

This book covers regulated biomedical products that go through the FDA (Food and Drug Administration, USA) for marketing approval, including therapeutic or prophylactic drugs (the term includes small molecule and biologic drugs), diagnostics, and devices. The term **biomedical technology companies** will be used to refer to companies whose products need FDA approval to get to market. The "technologies" include engineering and various sciences, including natural (e.g., life sciences or biology) and applied sciences (e.g., materials science).

Proceeding through these first few chapters, it will become apparent that the terms "biotechnology" and "device" have blurred boundaries today, as an increasing number of leading medical device companies are incorporating biological therapeutics such as cells, DNA, or proteins, and pharmaceutical companies are increasingly tying their products to diagnostic or delivery devices. Such products, codependent or intermingled with other technologies are called combination products. Some examples of combination products are the drug Herceptin (used to treat breast cancer), which has to be prescribed based on a diagnostic test for the gene HER2, drug-eluting stents, bioresorbable sponges with growth factors, skin grafts containing live cells embedded in a matrix and insulin pumps with glucose monitors. The following sections in this chapter define specific product areas in greater detail.

Box 1.1 Policy matters

Building a successful biotechnology company is a risky business. The science is challenging, the endeavor is expensive, and the time horizons from discovery to sales revenue are long. Drugs often fail in clinical trials and investors can be fickle.

But even the most skilled research and development teams backed with the brightest management and supported with hundreds of millions of investment dollars can fail in a policy environment that is not conducive to success.

If patent law doesn't adequately protect intellectual property; if the FDA takes too long or demands unrealistic submissions; if CMS refuses to adequately reimburse; if Congress inadequately funds the NIH or the FDA or imposes irrational requirements on drug approvals; if state, federal, or foreign governments impose price controls or ban technologies, the most competent biotech enterprises cannot succeed.

Every biotech company employee must add his or her voice to our effort. The future depends upon our success.

James C. Greenwood
President and CEO
Biotechnology Industry Organization (BIO)

The importance of medical technology companies engaging in the policy debate and dialogue in Washington, DC has never been greater.

Although most start-up companies are primarily concerned with raising money or moving products towards commercialization, the decisions made by policy makers in Washington often have a greater impact on a company's ability to succeed in the long term. For example, in the past year alone, MDMA and its member companies worked on issues impacting intellectual property, FDA regulations, CMS reimbursement, and barriers to market access.

In the past, advocacy efforts were primarily discussed and driven by large companies. However, increasingly, small to mid-size companies are joining associations and organizations in Washington to ensure that their voice is heard on critical issues. Furthermore, there is a growing appreciation in Washington that the majority of innovation is developed by smaller companies. Therefore, the health of the industry requires policies that foster innovation and competition, not hinder it.

Mark B. Leahey
Executive Director
Medical Device Manufacturers Association

1.3   Drugs and biotechnology – definition and scope

Today, drugs are developed from one of two distinct technological platforms –

(1) Synthetic organic molecules – *small molecules* (the preferred term used here) made de novo by synthetic chemistry processes or naturally occurring compounds, which have been isolated or re-synthesized in the lab. These are interchangeably called small molecules, drugs, or pharmaceuticals. Oligonucleotide-based drugs (RNA or DNA; composed of nucleic acids) made using synthetic processes are also included in this classification of small molecule drugs as they have more in common with small molecule drugs than the large molecule biologic proteins.

(2) Biological molecules made by living organisms – using cells or other living organisms to produce therapeutic proteins or biological molecules. These are interchangeably called drugs, biotech drugs, biopharmaceuticals, large-molecule drugs or *biologics* (the preferred term used here).

Therefore, the term *drugs* includes both biologics and small molecule pharmaceuticals. The US Food and Drug Administration defines a drug rather broadly as a substance (other than food) recognized by an official pharmacopoeia or formulary, that is intended for use in the diagnosis, cure, mitigation, treatment, or prevention of disease, and that is intended to affect the structure or any function of the body.

The term *biotechnology industry* was intended to refer to the biologics segment of the drug industry, where core life sciences technologies (and living organisms) are used to make products. However, the term biotechnology industry is currently often used to refer to small or start-up pharmaceutical firms that are developing drugs (whether small molecules or biologics), as most of them are founded based on key inventions in the life sciences. It is important to note that biotechnology companies also develop products for other (non-health related) applications and industries (see Box 1.2). The definition of biotechnology is, in fact, "the use of cellular and molecular processes to solve problems or make products."

Among the therapies produced by biological production processes (produced in cells or bacteria), the various classes of biotech human therapeutics (biologics) being developed for a large variety of diseases are:

Vaccines, another class of human therapeutics and prophylactics, are produced in biological systems, such as chicken eggs, or engineered cell lines.

Biologic drugs are based on large-molecular proteins or complex biological molecules, such as growth hormones, enzymes, etc. Examples are insulin, growth hormone, enzymes, and immunoglobulins. Erythropoietin (sold as Epogen and other brand names) is a blockbuster drug, with over $10 billion of sales in 2005. These biological drugs are most efficiently produced by cells or within other living organisms. Biopharmaceutical companies use bioreactors where cells, engineered to produce a specific type of protein, are grown in large

Box 1.2 Diverse applications of biotechnology

While "biotechnology" in this text focuses on life-sciences-based products commercialized in the healthcare industries (needing FDA approval), it is important to remember that many other applications of biotechnology also have great commercial value. In the popular media, the term "biotechnology industry" is used loosely to refer to activities that may be based on a range of technologies unrelated to the life sciences, such as laboratory equipment manufacture, device manufacture, lab automation, reagent production, and synthetic chemistry with small molecules. Therefore, it is always important to understand the specific context in which the term biotechnology is being used.

The use of biotechnology processes at the organism, cellular, and molecular level has many diverse applications, some of which are described briefly below but not covered any further in this book (e.g., even though biotechnology food products are regulated, they are not in the same market and approval paths as other biomedical products discussed here). A common technology base of tools and processes for manipulation and analysis of cells, DNA, and proteins ties all these diverse applications together across these different industries.

Healthcare

This is discussed in the main text.

Environmental biotechnology

Engineered microbes and enzymes can efficiently clean up pollution, and the application of the life sciences to this process is called bioremediation. Environmental applications also include biobleaching, biodesulfurization (removal of sulfur from oil and gas), biofiltration, biopulping, etc.

Industrial biotechnology

Engineered microbes and enzymes can be used as highly efficient components in many industrial chemical synthesis processes. Various industrial applications of biotechnology include the efficient use of enzymes to convert sugars to ethanol (transportation fuel), to make polymers such as polylactic acid (PLA) for consumer plastics production, and to improve processes in the production of fine chemicals, bulk chemicals, and commodity chemicals. Currently efforts are underway to convert cellulose to sugars (and ethanol) on a large scale, thus harnessing biomass that would otherwise be discarded as waste products of food and grain processing.

Agriculture

Biotechnology has been used to engineer new plant and crop varieties that are pathogen-resistant or have greater yield, or add new nutritional benefits to

---

Box 1.2 (cont.)

existing crops. Some specific applications are in the development of new genetically modified plant and seed varieties, improved processing of grain products and the development of biofertilizers. Basic biotechnologies are also used to improve livestock for food production and to provide new treatments for veterinary medicine. Genetically modified foods are already in widespread use in the US food supply. Agricultural biotechnology is arguably the oldest continuing application of life sciences and includes the manipulation of plants and micro-organisms to enhance yield, add new characteristics, such as increased nutrition or taste, and reduce the use of toxic pesticides or fertilizers; these are all key goals of biotechnology in agriculture and in the food-processing industry.

---

quantities. The proteins are then purified and most are formulated for intravenous delivery.

A *monoclonal antibody (mAb)*, a particularly significant type of biologic drug, is a highly specific, purified antibody (protein) that is derived from only one clone of cells and recognizes only one antigen. Monoclonal antibodies (one class of biologics) are an ideally targeted therapy that will only affect the specific protein target against which this antibody is made. The current wave of biologics is driven by mAbs: e.g., Johnson & Johnson's Remicade (infliximab), Roche/Genentech's Avastin (bevacizumab) and Herceptin (trastuzumab) and Rituxan/MabThera (rituximab), Bristol-Myers Squibb's Erbitux (cetuximab) and Abbott's Humira (adalimumab). With 18 mAb products already on the market (as of June 2006) and over 70 in clinical trials, billions of dollars of revenue are projected to be generated by these mAb therapies in the next decade. Like most biologics, mAbs cannot be given orally (they are degraded by digestive enzymes) and hence are infused intravenously. New drug-delivery technologies are also being developed to allow oral administration.

Cell based therapies and tissue engineering – for tissue and organ replacement or functional augmentation. The market for regenerative medicine worldwide is in the billions of dollars, primarily using autologous cells. Gene therapy holds many promises but has been hampered by limitations in delivery vehicles and side effects in some patients. In particular, cell-based therapies are attracting a great deal of attention because of the promise shown by stem cells (embryonic and adult) to become truly regenerative therapies.

Nucleic acids therapy is a particularly interesting, emerging class of drugs that uses synthetic production processes.

Nucleic acid therapies include gene therapy, which is the introduction of specific genes appropriately into the body to enable tissues to produce proteins currently lacking or malfunctioning in the diseased state. Many different gene therapies are being developed, with antisense therapeutics being the first approved in the US. Among other nucleic acid technologies, such as ribozymes, antisense oligonucleotides, and triplex and chimeric endonucleases, siRNA (short interfering RNA, ribonucleic acid molecules) has tremendous current commercial and scientific interest, as seen by the awarding of the 2006 Nobel Prize for Medicine to the discoverers of gene silencing by double-stranded RNA (Andrew Fire and Craig Mello) and Merck's acquisition of siRNA Therapeutics for over US $1 billion in December 2006. Short interfering RNA interferes with gene expression and uses the cell's own mechanism to control the production of specific proteins.

The biotechnology and biologics segment of the pharmaceutical industry is only 25–30 years old and has seen its revenues grow at an average of 16% per year over the last decade, to reach over $48 billion in global revenues in 2004 (data from Ernst and Young *Annual Biotechnology Industry Reports*). For the sake of comparison, it is worth noting that small molecule drugs had global sales of over $400 billion in 2004 (data from annual reports, IMS Health). Although still a small segment of the overall pharmaceutical industry, the growth rate and strong product pipeline of biologic drugs has attracted interest from investors and from the traditional pharmaceutical companies themselves. In particular, the recent biotech impact on the pharmaceutical industry has led to the industry naming itself the "biopharmaceutical industry," as more large pharmaceutical firms (e.g., Johnson & Johnson, Novartis, Wyeth) adopt biotechnology manufacturing platforms to make drugs. The drug industry thus includes not only large conglomerates with tens of thousands of employees in globally distributed offices, but also includes many small start-up companies formed out of university inventions in the life sciences. Smaller and mid-sized companies are increasingly seeking out niche markets to commercialize their innovations, building focused sales forces and taking their own products to market (for more discussion on business models in the biotechnology sector, see Section 3.9).

The interest in the biotechnology sector lies in the future impact of this technology, as more and more biologic drugs appear, with over 350 biotechnology drugs in the clinical development pipeline in 2004, for a variety of human diseases. An indicator of this rising wave of biologic drugs is that for the first time in 2004, over half of the new drugs approved by the US FDA were biotechnology-based drugs. Another component of the interest in biotechnology (life sciences as a more general science platform) today is in the promise of forthcoming discoveries that will lead to an even better understanding of normal and pathological (disease) processes in the human body, as discussed later in this chapter. The hope is that discoveries will be followed in time with new therapies that will cure disease instead of merely offering palliative treatment or temporary symptomatic relief.

It is important to mention that a significant portion of the biotechnology industry is composed of companies that provide services or make non-regulated products, such as research tools, reagents, bioinformatics programs or services, biomaterials, etc., that are sold to the drug or diagnostic companies or to the research community in general. The business models, product development cycles, financial, and investment profiles of these companies are quite different from most of the companies discussed in this book. An example of a large company of this type is Invitrogen.

1.4   Devices and diagnostics – definition and scope

1.4.1   Medical devices industry

Devices are defined by the US FDA as an instrument, apparatus, implement, machine, contrivance, implant, in vitro reagent, ..., which does not achieve any of its primary intended purposes through chemical action within or on the body of man or other animals, and which is not dependent upon being metabolized for the achievement of any of its primary intended purposes. Medical device companies use traditional materials like metals or ceramic and advanced materials like composites to produce devices that work by providing mechanical or physical (not chemical) support and interaction with the human body. Some of these devices are implanted (defibrillators), some are non-invasive (EKG monitors) and others are called minimally invasive (catheters). These companies have shorter product cycles and thus are more dynamic in product introductions than biotechnology companies.

Medical device products can be classified by two distinct types of markets – commodity products and innovative medical device products. The former are typically made by large mature companies, such as Johnson and Johnson, Becton Dickson, Welch Allyn, and feature a broad portfolio of commonly used products sold to clinics and hospitals. These products have a long life cycle in the market and their development is marked by incremental innovations that do not change the product mix, merely adding specific features to the design. Profit margins for these products are typically low as customers have high price sensitivity.

On the other hand, innovative medical products such as implantable devices, minimally invasive surgical devices, and new imaging devices are made by both large and small companies, such as Medtronic, Guidant (now part of Boston Scientific and Abbott), Bard, Stryker, and many others. These innovative devices have a short product life cycle, with the next generation entering advanced development even as the first generation enters the market. Innovative medical devices command high profit margins by delivering greater life-saving benefits directly to the patient, but also require high investment in research and development (R&D) for continued improvement and incorporation of new technologies. The medical device industry's gross revenues for 2005 in the US were greater than $80 billion. The industry is composed of a few large players, which hold market access and brand name, and many small companies, which have found niche markets in the device industry. The industry sales, broken into the various therapeutic and clinical areas, are summarized in Figure 1.1. Orthopedics and cardiovascular are the two largest device market areas, but others are growing too, as the population demographics shift.

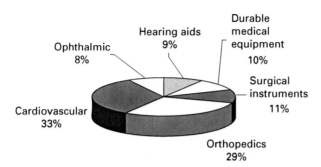

Figure 1.1 US medical device sales by clinical category ($ 63.9 billion, 2004). Data from Frost and Sullivan, as reported in Standard & Poor's Industry Survey. For current data and graph, visit www.commercializingbiotech.com.

1.4.2 Diagnostics – IVD industry

The diagnostics market is segmented broadly into the in vitro diagnostics (IVD; in vitro means in the test tube, in the laboratory, or outside the organism) and in vivo diagnostics businesses (in vivo means within a living organism). In vivo diagnostics is a specialty market, with the key players being large instrument manufacturers of imaging or instrumentation technology (GE, Philips, Siemens). Examples of in vivo diagnostics are blood pressure screening, MRI, thermometry, and ultrasound, X-ray, and computed tomography (CT) scanning.

This book will focus mainly on *in vitro diagnostics (IVD)*. The imaging machines that make up the bulk of in vivo diagnostic products are made and sold by a handful of large companies and represent a specialized market segment of the device and diagnostics industry. Additionally, the development, sales cycles, and regulatory issues (e.g., radiation issues) are quite different from most of the products discussed here. However, it is important to keep in mind that most of these large companies, GE, Siemens and Philips, have announced initiatives in molecular imaging diagnostics (which will be regulated as imaging agents or drugs). Thus, this exclusion (from the book) is on the basis of a specialty market segment, not an exclusion of specific companies.

In vitro diagnostic products are largely regulated as devices by the US FDA. There are two types of IVD products: devices (analyzers for samples like blood, serum, urine, tissue, etc.) and reagents (chemicals used to mark or recognize specific components in the samples). All devices and reagents perform tests on samples taken from the body and the applications can be divided into five broad types of IVD testing:

(1) *General clinical chemistry* – measurements of base compounds in the body, e.g., blood chemistry, cholesterol tests, serum iron tests, fasting glucose tests, urinalysis, etc.
(2) *Immunochemistry* – matching antibody–antigen pairs to indicate the presence or level of a protein, e.g., testing for allergen reactions, prostate-specific antigen (PSA) tests, HIV antibody tests, etc.

(3) *Hematology and cytology* – the study of blood, blood producing organs, and blood cells – e.g., CD4 cell counts, complete blood count, preoperative coagulation tests, etc.

(4) *Microbiology and infectious disease* – detection of disease-causing agents, e.g., streptococcal testing, urine culture or bacterial urine testing, West Nile virus blood screening.

(5) *Molecular, nucleic acid tests (NAT), and proteomic and metabolomic testing* – the study of DNA and RNA to detect genetic sequences that may indicate presence or susceptibility to disease, e.g. HER2/neu overexpression testing in breast cancer, fluorescence in situ hybridization (FISH) tests for prenatal abnormality testing, HIV viral load assays, etc.

In vitro diagnostics companies are primarily one of three types:

(1) Large pharma with diagnostic divisions,
(2) Diagnostic companies, which focus on the manufacture, distribution, and marketing of diagnostic test kits (reagents) and devices,
(3) Biotechnology (smaller start-up) companies, which focus on the discovery of technology devices and reagents for novel diagnostic methods or tests for specific diseases (e.g., a marker for cervical cancer).

In vitro diagnostics is a mature market (estimated US$28.6 billion world-wide in sales in 2005) with the highest volume being clinical tests using immunoassays and simple blood tests. More than 20 billion blood tests are performed annually world-wide. However, a rapidly growing segment of IVD markets is in vitro molecular diagnostics or nucleic acid testing (NAT), which analyzes DNA or RNA from a patient to identify a disease or the predisposition of a disease. These nucleic acid tests also have applications in the area of in vivo diagnostics in the emerging molecular imaging techniques and in the development of pharmaceuticals. Biotechnology processes are used to make NAT diagnostic reagents, such as nucleic acid probes.

The industry is fragmented, with larger companies like Quintiles, LabCorp, Covance, Roche, Johnson & Johnson, Abbott, Bayer, and others dominating market access, along with large independent companies such as Bio-Rad, Guerbert, bioMerieux, and Idexx. In terms of lab service revenues, the largest market share, of about 60%, is captured by hospital labs, while independent labs (also called reference labs) hold about 30% of the market share and physician offices cover the rest. Most small private companies either find a niche or get acquired as they are typically unable to attain the market reach of the big players to sustain growth.

1.5   Industry analysis

There are many ways to analyze an industry, with some of the more common methods discussed here. The questions addressed in the following sections are:

Where are the biomedical industry clusters and what are their key characteristics?

How can you understand rivalry and rise above the competition ? Porter's five forces analysis gives us a method to look at industry rivalry through forces exerted by suppliers, buyers, substitute products, barriers to entry, and intrinsic industry rivalry. These five forces govern competitive advantage in an industry.

What are the elements that make up the industrial system – the value chain – the context for putting form and function together in industry evaluation?

The NAICS (North American Industrial Classification System) codes for the biomedical industry are listed and discussed in Appendix 1.1. These codes can be used to access various economic databases, e.g. labor and trade databases can usually be sorted by NAICS codes (also known previously as SIC – Standard Industrial Classification – codes) or by region or state.

1.6 Biomedical industry clusters

1.6.1 Biopharmaceutical and biotechnology concentration in clusters

The growth of the biotechnology industry (mostly biologics-driven drug and diagnostic companies, but in this section, also non-regulated products, such as research tools) has taken place in specific areas in the world, usually driven by the creation of new intellectual property at universities. Thus, it is no surprise that the *most active* industry clusters in the USA are located around highly active research universities. Some characteristics of three of the top US clusters are described in Table 1.1. The three most active biotechnology clusters with companies and commercialization activities in the USA account for about 27% of total NIH extramural grants given to the top 100 cities or regions in 2000.

Table 1.1 Some selected characteristics of the three most active US biotechnology clusters

Key Characteristics	San Diego and San Jose-San Francisco California	Boston–Worcester Massachusetts	Raleigh–Durham– Chapel Hill North Carolina
Medical research activity of total NIH funding given to top 100 cities (2000)	11.8%	12.2%	4.0%
Number of top-twenty medical research universities	4	3	1
Venture capital 1995–2001 (% of of total)	46.5%	19.7%	3.9%
Number of life scientists (1998)	4520	4980	910
Pharmaceutical biotech research alliances until 2001($ million)	$5476	$5060	$225

Note: data from National Science Foundation and National Institutes of Health websites and reports and DeVol *et al.* (2004)

Table 1.2 Global biotechnology clusters with number of private and public companies

Biotech region	Company type					
	Public	%	Private	%	Total	%
USA	**329**	23%	**1086**	77%	**1415**	100%
%	49%		31%		34%	
California						365
Massachusetts						250
North Carolina						85
Maryland						75
New Jersey						63
Canada	**81**	18%	**378**	82%	**459**	100%
%	12%		11%		11%	
Ontario						143
Quebec						134
British Columbia						74
Europe	**122**	8%	**1491**	92%	**1613**	100%
%	18%		42%		38%	
UK 49				Germany		355
Germany 13				UK		274
Sweden 13				France		177
Asia-Pacific (including Australia and New Zealand)	**139**	19%	**577**	81%	**716**	100%
%	21%		16%		17%	
Total	**671**	16%	**3532**	84%	**4203**	100%
%	100%		100%		100%	

Data source: Ernst and Young (2006)

Note: California includes San Francisco, San Diego, and Los Angeles/Orange County (in decreasing order of total number of public companies present)

The global biotechnology industry and size of clusters in the top five US regions and the top three Canadian and European regions are shown in Table 1.2. Industry cluster sizes are quantified by the number of companies in a region. In Europe, the UK cluster is by far the largest and most mature, but France, Germany, and Sweden also have sizeable clusters.

The growth of biotechnology-based companies in the Asia Pacific region in various countries like India, China, Brazil, Taiwan, Korea, Australia, New Zealand, Malaysia, Thailand, Singapore, Vietnam, and Japan is notable, with increasing interest being drawn to the large market potential in these areas. These regions are also bringing their intellectual property rights and regulatory regimes up to global standards, making it more attractive for US or European companies to consider these areas for investment and partnership.

Table 1.3 Top states with medical device companies in the US

State	Number of medical device companies
California	2217
New York	895
New Jersey	784
Massachusetts	764
Florida	748
Pennsylvania	722
Illinois	717
Texas	513
Ohio	504
Minnesota	411

Data from Courtney Harris, Home Base, U.S.A.,
published online December 2003 at www.devicelink.com.

1.6.2   Biomedical device clusters

The top USA states, ranked by number of medical device companies, are listed in Table 1.3.

1.7   Competitive analysis of an industry or sector with Porter's five forces model

In Michael Porter's five forces model of industry analysis (Porter, 1985), the five dominant forces of supplier power, barriers to entry, buyer power, threat of substitutes, and industry rivalry can be analyzed to understand the best way to gain competitive advantage in that industry. This method is a commonly used strategic planning and analysis tool and is summarized briefly here:

For a given industry, analyze various inputs to determine:

Supplier power How much influence does a supplier have in the industry and how is it exerted? Is there a need to consider a strategy that includes the supplier as a partner?

Buyer power How much influence does an individual buyer have in the industry and how is it exerted? What is the price sensitivity among various buyer groups? Is there a need to consider a strategy that includes the buyer as a partner?

Threat of substitutes Is there a switching cost to switch to a rival's products and what are the trade-offs and comparisons between alternatives and substitutes?

Barriers to entry If a particular barrier to entry (patents, large investment, specialized knowledge) is identified, how can you cross it and then keep it up to slow down competitors?

Industry rivalry What are the exit barriers, product differences, brand power, growth rate in industry, fixed costs among firms, concentration of firms in market share, etc.?

By going through each point and addressing the general and specific issues in that area, a picture of the industry can emerge, giving a direction for development of competitive advantage in the industry. A summary analysis for each product type (device, drug, diagnostic) is presented here. These analyses serve as general overviews for the industry. A specific analysis around an innovative product allows one to focus strategic attention and resources on the primary basis of competition and the specific competitive advantage in the product market of interest.

1.7.1   Competitiveness summary for the pharmaceutical industry

Suppliers to the pharmaceutical companies are typically chemical manufacturers and switching costs are low, hence suppliers have low power in this industry. The drug industry is facing challenges as buyer power increases over time. State and federal governments (buyers) are also placing tremendous pricing pressure on the larger pharmaceutical industry. Substitute products are typically generics; generics manufacturers enter markets when a patent expires but have recently been using legal mechanisms to enter markets before anticipated patent expiration, reducing profits of innovator companies. Hence, substitute power is high in this industry. The long and expensive product development cycle is a barrier to entry and leads to multiple risk-sharing and profit-sharing alliances between biopharmaceutical firms and larger pharmaceutical companies and between smaller firms. Merger and acquisition activity in this sector continues, with larger players capturing development pipelines and market share. The competition within the industry is fierce and follow-on products to a new innovation emerge rapidly (18 months or less). Hence, industry rivalry is a strong (high) competitive force. The pharmaceutical industry is, thus, under tremendous pressures from many interfaces (forces). The increased sophistication of contracted research houses could give rise to a stabilizing factor, serving to reduce the cost and time for development. Even with a few large players, smaller firms can still survive through innovation and intellectual property capture; niche drugs can allow smaller companies to address focused markets. Small innovative companies will continue to play a role in this industry as generators of new technology and translators of innovation from academia to industry.

Biologic drug companies (the biotechnology industry) face similar pressures from various forces (as compared with the overall pharmaceutical industry), with a few key differences – the supplier power is medium as specialized techniques need to be developed and maintained up-to-date for production of biologics, and the power of substitutes (generics) is rather low at this point owing to a poorly defined regulatory path forward for biogenerics, but is not likely to remain low in the future. Barriers to entry are high, requiring investment in specialized production facilities and analysis techniques that can be quite complex. Overall, the biotechnology segment of the drug market has a higher hurdle for competition and launching innovative products is the primary means to gain and maintain competitive advantage.

Porter's five forces analysis can also be carried out at the company level, from the perspective of either a large pharmaceutical company or from the perspective of a small biotechnology company; not focused around a specific product, but focused around the company. Each of these perspectives will probably yield different conclusions as the context of analysis changes.

1.7.2 Competitiveness summary for the biomedical devices industry

Owing to the diversity of firms and technologies in the device industry, a general analysis is presented here, largely assuming innovative, implanted devices.

Buyer power tends to be medium, since larger purchases by hospitals or group purchasing organizations can be offset by individual physician preferences at a hospital. Buyer power is very high in the case of commodity products (such as syringes). For new innovative products, the manufacturer may have substantial negotiating power, owing to the limited market monopoly the patent provides. Device firms typically take relatively common parts and materials and transform them with knowledge to provide extensive added value. Consequently, supplier importance and power is generally relatively low. The multi-year, multimillion dollar process to take a product to market through FDA approval creates a barrier to entry in the industry, but the path through FDA approval can be relatively short (as with generic drugs) in many instances. Patent protection reduces competition for many new products and a first-mover advantage has been noted in many medical device markets. Consequently, a firm that is first to market or temporarily controls a market using patent protection is well placed to dominate the market with brand recognition once the patent expires and competitors are able to enter the market. However, there has been a tendency for established products to become commodities in the device industry. These commodity product markets are highly competitive, low-margin markets with a focus on reducing manufacturing costs.

1.7.3 Competitiveness summary for the diagnostics market

The diverse nature of this product type also forces a generalized review and analysis of this section of the industry. Thus more qualitative discussion is presented here of various issues in the diagnostics industry.

The customers (buyers; hospitals, central labs, and clinics) have been gaining bargaining power over the last few decades, owing to the formation of hospital buying groups and large HMOs that use the power of scale to choose specific tests and reimbursement levels. Buyer power is medium to high in the diagnostics segment of the biomedical industry.

Supplier power is medium to low, depending on the type of reagent (monoclonal antibodies are specialized products; basic chemical reagents are not) or device used.

Several large players in the IVD industry have established technology platform standards and control distribution channels. For example, Bayer/Chiron are market leaders in blood testing and Roche controls a large part of the nucleic acid testing (NAT) markets owing to its proprietary position and established standard base of the PCR technology. A smaller company, like Gen-Probe, a leading developer of nucleic acid tests, has had to establish distribution and sales collaborations with Chiron, bioMérieux, and Bayer. Companies that have diversified product menus and strong commercialization infrastructure (channel access and established technology platforms) are positioned for the long term to capitalize on the opportunities in the diagnostics markets. Competition is intense at the market level and is focused on cost in the clinical diagnostics area. Industry rivalry is high, and barriers to entry into the traditional markets (central labs or physician clinic labs) for a young company are high, as market access is controlled by a few standard-setting large firms. However, in the NAT market segment, patent rights on innovative tests allow smaller companies to establish themselves. A lowering of the regulatory bar also lowers the barrier to entry and these firms can start earning early revenues by selling their tests for "research use only" as specific reagents directly to the clinical laboratories. The emergence of NAT tests puts emphasis on innovative content in the IVD markets. In particular, about half (49%) of the industry is composed of small companies, with less than 20 employees. Another 17% have less than 100 employees.[1] Smaller firms are usually focused on specific disease areas or even on single diseases, but larger companies have a diverse portfolio.

Manufacturers of device platforms (devices that analyze specimens) also command significant margins in this industry, giving rise to strong marketing power for established platforms on which multiple different assays can be run.

The majority of IVD tests are used in reference labs (national centers with high volume), centralized labs in hospitals or nursing homes (accounting for 60% of IVD industry revenue), or in physician practice labs. Access to these customers requires building a sales force or partnering with the larger firms to gain access to markets, limiting paths for successful commercialization of IVD tests. Innovative proprietary tests, which are based on the many emerging insights and discoveries into the human genome and proteome, will always command a premium and interest in the market, but could take time to reach commercial success.

Significant barriers to widespread adoption of NAT exist – lock-in by specific test platforms, reimbursement issues (Chapter 7), changing regulations, education and awareness of the clinical utility of a test, the inability to interpret test data fully, and the fact that (in some cases) gene patents hinder adoption of the tests by routine clinical laboratories and also prevent competitive development, which would be good for increased market development. Unclear or changing regulatory environments and reimbursement practices that create disincentives for innovation,

---

[1] Data from US Census Bureau. *In-Vitro Diagnostic Substance Manufacturing: 2002*, 2002 Economic Census, December 2004. Available from www.census.gov.

particularly for the new NAT tests, remain as key impediments to successful commercialization of new IVD tests. Acceptance of a new test by a few leading academic research clinical centers may be rapid, but adoption in the larger volume markets typically takes time. However, new tests that result in improved outcomes in diseases such as cancer should see substantial market pull (demand by market forces) and these market hurdles could be overcome as more biomarkers are clinically validated and familiarity with NAT testing grows through the new tests that are being launched. (See Box 1.3)

1.8   Industrial value chains

The value chain of an industry or product offers another way to understand the dynamics of the industry and to understand relationships between its component companies. In particular, the value chain can be used to assess the capabilities of the company and see its dynamic fit and growth opportunities within the industry. A value chain is a high-level model of the various steps involved in converting raw materials to finished products that are used by customers, as shown in Figure 1.2 and in the description below. The individual product development stages are discussed in greater detail in Chapter 4.

As a product moves from basic R&D to market, each step increases the value of the work in progress, with the product reaching maximum value when it is finally sold in the marketplace to the end user. A value chain schematic can be used to describe the steps in the development process and also to give an overview of the entire process of taking a concept to market. A supply chain, a common term in many industries, is a part of the overall value chain. The supply chain model focuses on activities that get raw materials and components into a manufacturing operation smoothly and economically. The value chain is a broader concept, looking at every step from raw materials to the eventual end users and their experience with the product. The goal is to deliver maximum value to the end user for the least possible cost and to analyze the specific functions of the company and define strategic advantages. Supply chain management is, therefore, a subset of the value chain analysis.

The value chain concept is useful in analyzing the specific activities that the organization performs in the context of the entire industry value chain, and in understanding how the organization can use technology better in specific areas, or reduce costs, or reconfigure operations to add value. The value chain analysis can also help in business model analysis, wherein a specific organization's business model can be analyzed by virtue of its current and planned location in the value chain.

The following general descriptions represent some typical value chains in the various segments of the biotechnology industry, acknowledging that there can be specific products and developments that take radically different routes. For example, some companies can license technologies at one point in the value chain and sell them at another point, capturing the incremental value represented by that

---

Box 1.3 A competitive analysis for a novel medical device using Porter's five forces

Porter's five forces analysis can also be applied at a product level, as shown in this example.

The product is a vena cava filter. This is a metal filter placed in the large vein near the heart to block an embolus (blood clot) from going to the brain or lungs where it could cause death. The following analysis identifies the key competitive forces in this market, using porter's five forces model.

Supplier power   Supplier bargaining power is a weak competitive force as the device companies are taking up commodity materials and adding high value processing to make the filters.

Buyer power   Buyer bargaining power is a strong competitive force with high impact in this industry, owing to the small number of decision makers (physicians) at each purchasing hospital. Therefore, the firms all compete to get the attention of these physicians and the buyers can exert significant force in the sales process. Buyers will become more powerful as the type and number of filters increases.

Substitute products   Substitute products are a weak force, as the only other option to the filter is a blood-thinning drug. Many people cannot take blood thinners for long periods of time and in fact blood thinners are a complementary product. There are no other known innovations in development at this time. Competition from substitutes is likely to be very low.

Barriers to entry (or new entrants)   New entrants are a weak force in this industry, as brand recognition, limited access to decision makers (physicians), and high regulatory requirements and long development times, combined with high development costs, keep new entrants away.

Rivalry   Rivalry among competitors is very strong as each competitor fights for market share in a mature market that has seen no significant growth. A combination of innovation in product and aggressive sales methods is used to compete for market share. High profit margins are possible with innovative products and rivalry will increase in the future.

Summary

The main competitive forces in the vena cava filter market are, thus, rivalry among competitors and buyer influence on purchasing decision. Rivalry is likely to grow and gaining competitive advantage will continue to hinge on product innovations that show significant clinical utility and positive clinical outcome.

Note: another type of analysis that can be used at the company or product level is the SWOT – strength, weaknesses, opportunities, and threats–framework. This and other analysis frameworks are useful for thinking through product development characteristics (cheaper or more differentiated), marketing tactics, or corporate strategy around a particular product innovation or for setting a higher-level organizational strategy.

Input value chain

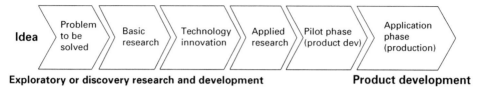

Exploratory or discovery research and development   **Product development**

Output value chain

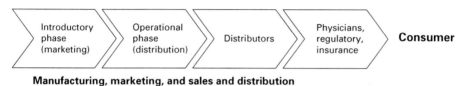

Manufacturing, marketing, and sales and distribution

Figure 1.2   Typical biomedical industry value chain.

intermediate development step. Another important point to remember is that although a linear path and growth in value is represented here, new product development (NPD) is seldom a straight-through path. As discussed in the Preface, there is a detailed interaction between functional groups during NPD, which typically will lead to iteration in planning, testing, and development.

Exploratory research and development (R&D)

Research and development usually begins with a broad concept of the problem to be solved (e.g., cancer, a new AIDS vaccine, or a disease driven by a particular known mechanism). Basic biological research and technology innovation go hand in hand, with new technologies giving rise to novel insights into biology, which in turn lead to new tools. These new innovations lead the way to a possible product idea, and applied research tests the feasibility and scope of the innovation. Serendipity often has a significant role to play in this period of exploratory research, but as the saying often goes: "The harder I work, the luckier I get." Organizational functions include performing and managing basic R&D, prototype testing, and concept testing. In biomedical organizations this can range from discovery efforts to animal testing for proof of concept or feasibility studies.

Product development

Prototype development or advanced feasibility testing is usually the next step, and larger scale human clinical trials follow. A formalized product development process is usually introduced shortly after the first feasibility test is positive. Manufacturing and marketing functions are involved early in the product development stage. Important issues here are definition of product characteristics and the specific input from intellectual property, regulatory, finance, marketing, and reimbursement divisions or functions.

Manufacturing, marketing, and sales

These final stages of commercialization can easily become the most challenging. In the early stage, the technology, direction of research, etc., were still under company control; at this stage, outside regulatory agencies, payers, users, and others dictate procedures and processes, and standards have to be followed. Reimbursement of the product through third-party payers adds a level of complexity to the regulated biotechnology and medical device industry, when compared with other commercial manufacturing industries.

1.8.1   Drug development process

The drug-development value chain shown in Figure 1.3 (and discussed in greater detail in Chapter 4) begins with a discovery project. The project is typically initiated by discovery of a target's key involvement in a disease. The target is usually a protein, an enzyme, or a receptor in a cell or tissue that has been discovered to play a central role in the development of a disease or its symptoms. The drug can be a synthetic chemical small molecule that binds to the target and inhibits or activates its function or it can be a biological molecule that replaces a missing or defective enzyme or protein. A large part of the effort in pre-clinical research work is to verify the validity of the target (to verify that interventions aimed at the target will have the desired effect on the system) and to develop a molecule that can become a drug compound. This pre-clinical research stage then ends when the two key milestones

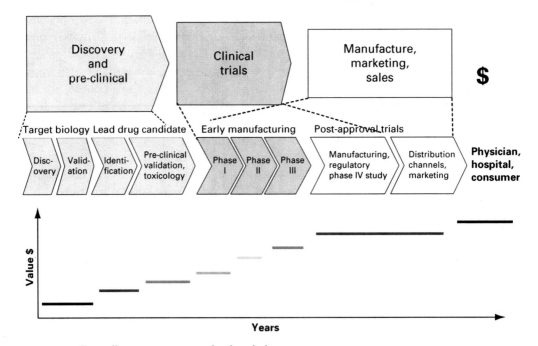

Figure 1.3   Drug discovery process and value chain.

or gates (see Chapter 4) are passed: (1) validation of a therapeutic effect of the drug in animal models of the human disease and (2) satisfactory clearance of formal toxicology and other (absorption, distribution, metabolism, and excretion profiles, other in vivo behavior) testing.

The clinical trial process is carried out in specific development steps, phase I–IV clinical trials, each with specific goals.

Phase I   Toxicity and behavior of drug in humans (pharmacokinetics and pharmacodynamics),
Phase II   Establish that the drug works to treat the disease (efficacy, dosage),
Phase III   Establish efficacy in larger population (statistical validity of drug effects),

Once the clinical trials are complete, the results are analyzed and submitted to the FDA for approval to market the drug. The review by the FDA can take up to two years.

Phase IV   Post-marketing surveillance (usually required by the FDA after approval, to further validate efficacy or safety with longer term or broader population exposure to the drug) or may be conducted to expand use of the drug to new indications or diseases or a different population (e.g., children).

This entire process can take from 12 to 16 years and hundreds of millions of dollars. The process itself has a high failure rate in chemical compound development (slightly lower for biologics), with only an estimated 1% of compounds that enter early pre-clinical screening successfully becoming drugs for a given disease. The current average cost is $800 million, which includes the cost of failures dropped at various stages of development and the cost of lost returns on alternate investments that could have been made with that capital (DiMasi *et al.*, 2003).

Examining the industry's functional segments through this value-chain perspective reveals a view of the industry's structure. Some companies focus on the supply of specialty raw materials, others specialize in design layouts and engineering design, still others may only do contract manufacturing work for regulated products, while some work on value-added distribution services. Some areas of the value chain – discovery research, for example – are very fragmented, while others have high barriers to entry and thus see few large players – manufacturing of biologics, for example. Quantifying various outcome measures (e.g., profit margins, return on investment, etc.) of these companies' operations in various segments of the value chain would allow one to understand the highest value-added component of the value chain and the dynamics of each process that involve multiple stakeholders. For example, economic development agencies could choose segments of the value chain to invest in, and aspiring entrepreneurs can lay out better expectations of returns for companies with similar business models. An example for the biotechnology industry is shown in Figure 1.4 with a caveat that although this analysis is valid only for a handful of firms in the biotech industry (most companies are private and occupy niches in the value chain), it is certainly a good benchmark and indicator.

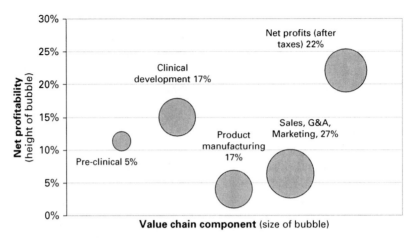

Figure 1.4   Profitability and share of value chain components (shown as bubbles) in the biotechnology drug development value chain. The area of the bubble indicates the % cost of that activity (label next to bubble) and the height represents the profit margin. See details in text.

The graph in Figure 1.4 is illustrative in nature and represents one possible method of analyzing the value chain and profitability along the value chain. The major component processes in the value chain – pre-clinical studies; clinical development; manufacturing; sales, general and administrative (G&A) and marketing; and final profits captured in the system – are shown as bubbles, respectively arranged from left to right in the figure. Therefore, the total value created = total revenues = (cost of each component process + profits) for a fully vertically integrated company. However, in this case, the *x*-axis is not a quantitative scale and only serves to lay out the value chain components in a progression. The area of each component process bubble relates to the costs incurred for that component, expressed as a percentage of the total cost of development. These component percentages were calculated from reported financial statements of a few fully integrated, representative biotechnology firms. Profit margins (averaged over a five-year period) within each functional process (pre-clinical, clinical, manufacturing, etc.) were obtained from financial statements from a few representative publicly traded firms that specialized in the specific segments of the value chain. The individual profitability figures within each component process are thus independent values that are not supposed to add up to the total net profit reported by the fully integrated firms. These profitability values were used to position the height of the bubbles, with the most profitable component process placed highest (along the *y*-axis). Both calculated terms, the percentages of the component processes (as part of the total value) and profit margins for each component process, are not expected to add up to the final figures (100% of value created or total contribution to net profit of 22%), as these value assignments are done for illustrative purposes rather than to generate strictly quantitative models.

This method of plotting value chain components works for industries in which the right type of data are available. Entrepreneurs can use this chart to

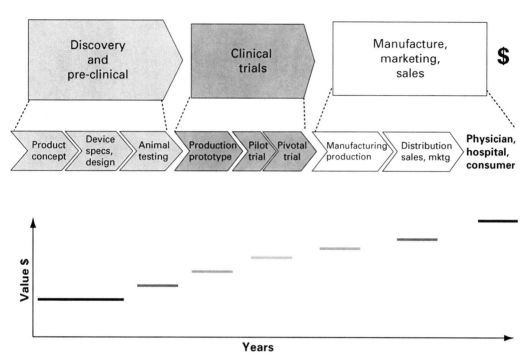

Figure 1.5   Biomedical device value chain.

assess quickly the best component of the value chain in which to build their
business models.

1.8.2   Biomedical device and diagnostic development process

The medical device and diagnostics industry value chain, represented schematically
in Figure 1.5, typically starts with an R&D project where a concept is developed
around some core innovative technology or biological or physiological insight.
A project team then develops a design, which is then used to make a prototype with
some iteration to the design process. For IVDs, assay development takes place at
this stage and a prototype assay protocol is developed. Prototype testing at this
stage is typically in vitro or laboratory testing. In IVDs, at this point, the test is
placed in the context of usage and a test principle is chosen (the technology platform for the specific assay is chosen). Feasibility testing for IVDs is typically done
in cells or in archived human clinical samples to which the company has access.
At this point, the IVD company can start to generate revenues by the sale of specific
reagents for "research use only" to a selected group of certified laboratories.

The final prototype is then refined for manufacturing processes (sometimes in
parallel with the design iterations). A refined prototype is then tested in animal
models or possibly on human beings, as appropriate. Human testing follows with
pilot and then pivotal clinical trials. New IVD tests are typically first validated
retrospectively in clinical trials and then more rigorously through prospective

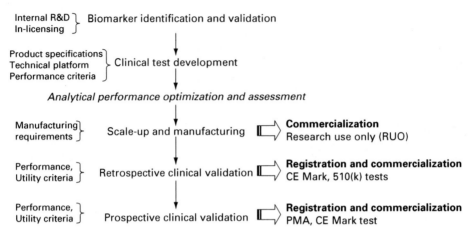

Figure 1.6   Diagnostics commercialization value chain.

clinical trials. The results are submitted to the FDA and on approval, the device can be distributed and marketed. This entire process can take from two to six years and from a few million to tens or hundreds of millions of dollars (time and costs vary widely owing to the diverse nature of products in this industry). Product development stages are discussed in greater detail in Chapter 4. The component profitability has not been analyzed here, because of the diverse nature of products and firms in the device and IVD industry. A specific value chain and pathway for development in the diagnostics industry is shown in Figure 1.6. Diagnostics offer several intermediate steps for commercialization, as the industry has a large market for non-regulated supplies – hence the value chain for diagnostics is shown in a different format here.

1.9   Technology trends in biomedical device and drug development

In depth information in an area builds momentum as multiple iterations improve understanding of a phenomenon or a technology, ultimately leading to better tools and new applications and products. These new applications, tools, or products eventually lead to new information that enters the cycle shown in Figure 1.7. The spark of curiosity of humans and the intensified, globally competitive research activities of this century are the drivers for innovations, new technologies, and applications entering the market.

1.9.1   Drug development technology trends

Technology has played an important part in drug development and discovery over the years, either by opening new pathways for better treatments or by speeding up the process of developing drugs. Most early drugs were derived as extracts from natural sources. The components of these extracts, when purified, were identified and synthesized using chemical synthesis methods to yield a reproducible

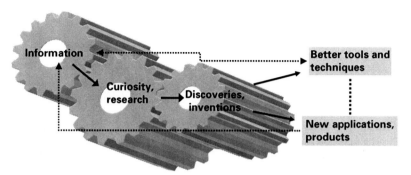

Figure 1.7   Technologies link curiosity, discoveries, and new applications in a cycle of innovation.

compound. Drug technologies have seen a big change in the methods of production with the advent of biotech drugs (biologics).

These biotech drugs, typically proteins that are enzymes or antibodies (monoclonal antibodies), are produced using genetically engineered living cells. The biotech industry started off with two basic technologies in 1975, recombinant DNA (rDNA) and monoclonal antibody (mAB) production from hybridomas, and has now accumulated several breakthroughs in its technology platforms, leading to an ever-increasing range of applications, going beyond basic manufacturing techniques to enhance the entire supply chain in drug and diagnostic development (Figure 1.8 and Figure 1.9). Figure 1.8 overlays the actual revenue figures for the biotechnology drugs-based segment of the pharmaceutical industry with a few selected technology milestones. These technology and commercial milestones are meant to be representative and not comprehensive.

The next set of emerging technologies includes stem cells, tissue engineering, gene therapy, siRNA, and in silico biology. This new generation of human therapeutics will probably require the development of new production technologies.

Additionally, advanced material technologies will also influence the pharmaceutical sector throughout the production value chain, from R&D and drug discovery to manufacturing and packaging. New emerging applications, which include nanostructured polymers (dendrimers) for advanced drug delivery, analytical life sciences instrumentation, biochips, membranes, bioreactor design, coatings, and fine chemicals, will all affect the future development of new classes and types of drugs.

However, in spite of a steep increase in total industry investment in R&D over the last decade (grown to $40 billion in 2005; data from PhRMA), there has been no increase in filing or approval of new small molecule drugs. The issue of cost-effectively building a business of new products is looming large for many companies, as their blockbuster products are going off-patent or revenues are falling to generic competition. One possible explanation for the lack of increase in new product submissions is that the explosion of information and new targets, with a paucity of historical data, has led to a net loss of productivity, even though individual technologies promise better productivity (Figure 1.9). Both IT systems integration and data integration issues have increased the computational intensity used in drug companies. Pharmaceutical companies are still working on the integration of a large number of new technologies and

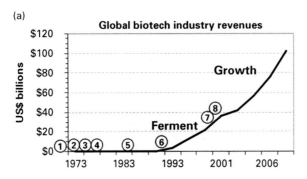

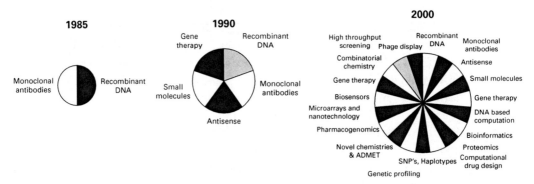

(b)

	Key growth steps for industry
(1)	1953 – DNA structure solved by Crick and Watson
(2)	1973 – Cohen and Boyer perfect recombinant DNA techniques 1975 – Kohler and Milstein produce mABs from hybridomas
(3)	1976 – Genentech founded – first commercial life sciences company
(4)	1980 – Diamond vs. Chakrabarty – Supreme court case approves principle of patenting genetically modified organisms
(5)	1983 – PCR technique is developed
(6)	1990 – The International Human Genome Project is launched
(7)	1998 – RNA interference phenomenon published
(8)	2000 – Human Genome Project 1st draft completed – genomics and technology stock markets spike and fall

Figure 1.8   Technical milestones in biotech industry development.

Figure 1.9   Technologies used in the drug discovery and development industry are increasing and the process is more complex (data adapted from Alta Partners slide presentation, 2004).

methods that have emerged over the last decade and have been individually shown to have great promise in discovering targets or drugs that can lead to a cure for diseases. It is possible that the expected outcome of these new insights will not emerge in the form of real curative medications for some years hence. However, the increasing number of targeted therapies (e.g., monoclonal antibodies and drugs that target specific cell signaling mechanisms) and therapies that require pre-selection of patients using genomic diagnostics make it clear that an era of new medicine is emerging (see Foreword).

1.9.2 Medical device and diagnostics technology trends

Medical products rely on technologies such as metallurgy, materials science, electronics and microelectronics, and precision machining. A general technology trend has been that of increased miniaturization of devices over time. Additionally, there is a trend towards greater functionality and intelligent sensing embedded in a single device leading to interactions with the device once it has been implanted.

Another emerging generation of devices has materials that are biologically active and serve to enhance the therapeutic effect of the device. These emerging combination devices are being developed with many mixed types of materials and technologies, such as electronics and microfluidics, cell encapsulation (material + biologic), metals with protein coatings, and tissue-engineered scaffolding biodegradable materials. This combination of technologies, which blurs boundaries between traditional science and engineering disciplines (truly multi-disciplinary technologies), holds great promise for improved devices that are increasingly integrated into our body function with minimal disruption and maximal benefit. The diversity of devices (sizes, applications, material types) precludes a succinct summary of technologies and market trends for medical devices.

Technology development in the traditional IVD (traditional blood analysis clinical diagnostics) market has slowed, with continuing incremental innovation in automation and simplification of existing IVD tests, and a focus on increased throughput, automation, and cost reduction. However, the accelerating technology developments (Figure 1.10) are in the nucleic acid testing (NAT) or DNA based genomic diagnostics market. These enabling technologies include genetic sequencing, polymerase chain reaction (PCR) technologies, and DNA microarray devices, and are leading to new discoveries linking human genetic code and disease.

1.9.3 Emerging technologies and materials in the nucleic acid diagnostics field

- *Alternative amplification technologies* – new techniques for copying genetic material for increased sensitivity or speed of testing (compared with PCR) are being developed.
- *Bio-chips and lab-on-a chip* – DNA, protein, glycosaccharides, and lipid array chips with multiple probes arrayed on a chip can provide large amounts of information from a single sample. Microfluidic technology and micro-electromechanical system (MEM) technologies combined with standardized semiconductor industry

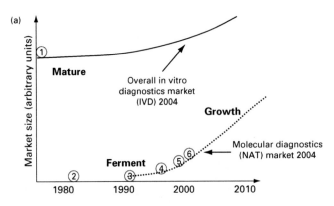

(a)

(b)

1960s and earlier	① Discovery of various biomarkers and diagnostic tests linked to disease or pathogens. Immunoassays developed
1980's to 1990's	Pharma companies buy and sell diagnostics companies; consolidation into large players.
1983	② Polymerase chain reaction (PCR) technology, which uses heat and Taq polymerase enzyme to make multiple copies of a DNA sequence, is conceived and rapidly becomes a major tool in biotechnology research and product development world-wide.
1991	③ Microarray products launched.
1997	④ FDA approves analyte specific reagents (ASR) to be sold to authorized labs[a]
2000	⑤ Completion of human genome project.. Large scale sequencing, laboratory automation, microarray technologies increase commercial presence.
2002	⑥ Initiation of haplotype (SNPs) mapping project (HAPMAP project).
2003	FDA reviews guidelines for use of biomarkers in clinical trials.

a Manufacturers use this route to test a diagnostic in the clinic before going through FDA approval, by selling analyte specific reagents as a component to be added in to a test platform, creating a "home-brew" or specialized diagnostic test. By having the user add one ingredient that is not "packaged" in the test allows companies to sell a test (and clinicians to use it) as long as it is labeled, "For research purposes only."

Figure 1.10   Technology and market trends for IVD (in vitro diagnostics) with key milestones.

silicon-chip fabrication and opto-electronic technologies have made possible the creation of various versions of a "lab-on-a chip." Materials that have been used so far include silicon substrate, rubberized silicone, gallium nitride and other electronic-industry-based materials. Additionally, nanoscale materials (quantum dots, etc.) are being developed as markers and readouts for various assays. It is anticipated that these technologies will shift the industry from the current techniques of detection of single analytes to the large-scale, parallel testing of tens, hundreds, or, perhaps ultimately, thousands of genes or proteins in the same multi-analyte test. Together with increased automation, these new lab-on-a-chip devices could also shift the focus from central labs to testing at the patient's bedside.

- *Breath testing* – The first breath test for *Helicobacter pylori* (a bacterium that causes stomach ulcers) was approved by the FDA a few years ago and others are being developed, potentially to replace invasive and expensive procedures.
- *Other multi-probe technologies* – novel techniques, such as mass spectrometry, with simultaneous probes to identify a "molecular signature" that is indicative of disease, rather than a single molecule at a time.

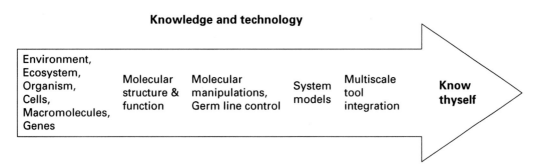

Figure 1.11   Convergence of knowledge base and various technologies towards personalized medicine.

1.10   Convergence of technologies in biotechnology

In the biotechnology industry, the level of information that is now available at the molecular level is increasing rapidly, and that knowledge is spreading rapidly at all scales of study of biotechnology processes.

As shown schematically in Figure 1.11, early observations many centuries ago were made at the phenotype level, usually for individual traits. Detailed observations, even though they may have been made at tissue level or greater detail, were either not well recorded or were not carried out with sufficient scientific controls in a rigorous and systematic manner. Emerging from the processes of European scientific inquiry, the reductionist approach to biology took shape, where individual elements were studied in isolation from their organisms or systems to determine the parameters of functional activity and interaction. For example, blood was first studied as a system, then at the level of isolated vessels, cells, and individual serum components to study how each changed and behaved in healthy or diseased states. Further reductionist approaches led to isolation of individual receptors on cell membranes, elaboration of intracellular signal transduction pathways, genes, and DNA codons. The goal was always to take this information and knowledge and put the individual pieces back together to be able to understand the complex organism and system – like a child with a box of gears trying to build the mechanism of a complex and delicate clock. However, this approach has seen limited success until the recent technological developments of computational speed and data storage and the development of algorithms that can combine disparate types of data.

By putting together computational simulations derived from this increased knowledge, the ultimate goal would be to develop a multiscale model of behavior of any given biological system. Knowing and predicting, at once, the activity of the organism and the molecular or cellular drivers of that particular state of activity (healthy or disease), will allow the true advent of personalized medicine, where a disease state is recognized, understood at the level of specific protein or gene dysfunction and a therapy developed for the individual that specifically treats the cause of the disease in that individual. This still remains many years away.

Thus, ultimately, the drive in basic biomedical research is driven by the dictum "know thyself" – towards a future where personalized medicine and individualized therapy are the norm, made possible by integrating technologies at various scales to achieve detailed knowledge of the inner workings of each individual. This is what each one of us would eventually like to have; a complete knowledge of conscious and unconscious, macroscopic and microscopic body processes that allow us to make the best decisions about our health.

To truly gain that broad and deep understanding, current research is examining the organism through a variety of different perspectives and techniques that include technologies more closely related to traditional engineering disciplines. For example, we are using robotics and informatics to analyze genetic coding differences among individuals. The increase in information and knowledge in biological sciences is now critically integrated with technological improvements in basic engineering disciplines and in physical sciences.

Additional convergence of technologies is seen across traditional industrial boundaries (depicted in Figure 1.12), when new tools developed for human medicine find applications in other areas and may in fact be enhanced in interactions with traditional engineering processes in other fields.

Applications of biotechnology that include considerable interaction with other emerging or advanced technologies, such as advanced materials and nanotechnology, include some of the following areas:

- Biomass renewable energies, e.g., biodiesel,
- Biosensors,
- Diagnostic medical devices,

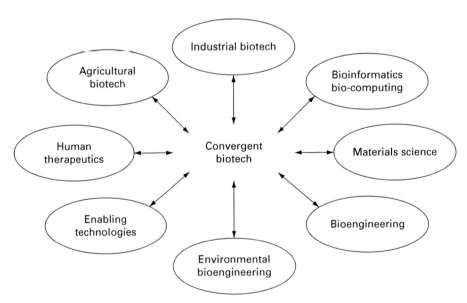

Figure 1.12   Technologies from various disciplines interact in biotechnology today (adapted from slide presentation at BIO 2004 Industrial Biotechnology).

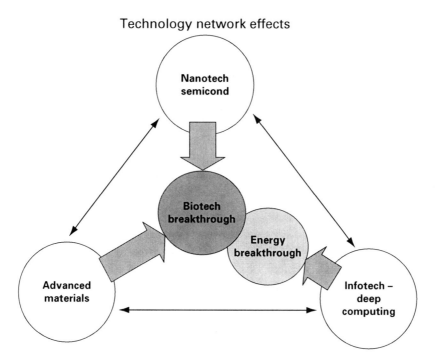

Technology network effects

Figure 1.13   Convergence across industries and interdisciplinary studies will result in breakthrough applications at the interfaces in the focus areas of energy and healthcare.

- Bioremediation,
- Digitization of healthcare information,
- Bioinformatics,
- Biotherapeutics,
- Biometrics,
- Biosecurity.

Continuing along this trend is an increase in multidisciplinary research and development, with advances in other disciplines impacting developments in energy and biotechnology. As represented in Figure 1.13, the integration of various emerging technologies in the energy and biotechnology industry makes it likely that breakthroughs in performance or reduction in cost, or both, will result.

1.11   Summary

This book focuses on products that are regulated by the US Food and Drug Agency. While the products covered here come from diverse technological backgrounds, all are applied to improve the human health condition by treatment, prophylaxis, or diagnosis. As the biomedical (drug, diagnostic, and device) industry is dependent on complex knowledge, high levels of risk capital, well trained personnel, and innovation as a basis for competitive advantage, most firms developing these products are clustered in areas where access to these characteristics is possible. The industry value-chain components in drugs, devices, and diagnostics have a significant number of elements in common. Analyzing a value chain can help in planning a business model or in optimizing operations across the company and industry. An overview of technology trends in each product area shows the increasing trend to convergence of technologies (multidisciplinary product development needed) and products, such as drug–diagnostic, device–drug, or device–diagnostic combinations.

Exercises

1.1 Map your technology or product idea on an S-curve (growth curve) for the overall industry and for your own technology platform. What unit will you choose for your y-axis (dollars in gross industry revenues; number of units sold, number of companies in sector, number of products – each choice of unit will give a different insight)? Are you close to maturity in that technology platform? Is the industry segment you are approaching growing rapidly or just taking off? How would you now qualify your product opportunity?

1.2 What new opportunities might arise if you look at the technology trajectories in other industries and their intersection with the biomedical technology industry segment of interest?

1.3 Can you plan for the next generation technology that might replace or threaten your product?

1.4 Analyze the components of the value chain for your industry (see figures in Section 1.7) and understand where your organization fits in currently and in the future. Who holds the largest component by cost in the value chain? Which component has the highest profitability?

1.5 Do you understand the functions, information, and materials from the other parts of the value chain that feed into the processes your organization performs? Is there a strong positioning statement for your organization? Are the investments now being made appropriate for maintaining the strategic advantage of the company?

1.6 Given the trends for biological research and development identified here, are there specific areas that you should consider investing in to gain competitive advantage in the future value chain?

References and additional reading

Bronzino, J. (ed.). *Biomedical Engineering Handbook*, CRC Press, 3rd edn., 2006.
Burns, L. (ed.). *The Health Care Value Chain*, Jossey-Bass, 2002.
Burns, L. (ed.). *The Business of Healthcare Innovation*, Cambridge University Press, 2005.

Chiesa, V. and Chiaroni, D. *Industrial Clusters in Biotechnology*, Imperial College Press, 2004.

Collins, S. W. *The Race to Commercialize Biotechnology*, Routledge, 2004.

DeVol, R., Wong, P., Ki, J., Bedroussian, A., and Koepp, R. *America's Biotech and Life Science Clusters*, Milken Institute, 2004. Available at www.milkeninstitute.org/pdf/biotech_clusters.pdf.

DiMasi, J. A., Hansen, R. W., and Grabowski, H. G. The price of innovation: new estimates of drug development costs, *Journal of Health Economics*, **22**, 151–185, 2003.

Ernst and Young. *Beyond Borders: Global Biotechnology Report*, Ernst and Young, 2006.

Estrin, N. F. *The Medical Device Industry: Science, Technology, and Regulation in a Competitive Environment*, Marcel Dekker, 1990.

Hartford, C. T. *The Worldwide Market for In Vitro Diagnostic Tests*, Kalorama Information, 2002.

Kayser, O. and Müller, R. H. (eds.). *Pharmaceutical Biotechnology: Drug Discovery and Clinical Applications*, John Wiley & Sons, 2004.

McKelvey, M. D., Rickne, A., and Laage-Hellman, J. (eds.). *The Economic Dynamics of Modern Biotechnology*, Edward Elgar Publishing, 2004.

Moore, J. E. and Zouridakis, G. (eds.). *Biomedical Technology and Devices Handbook*, CRC Press, 2004.

Porter, M. *Competitive Advantage: Creating and Sustaining Superior Performance*, The Free Press, 1985.

Ratledge, C. and Kristiansen, B. (eds.). *Basic Biotechnology*, Cambridge University Press, 2nd edn., 2001.

Roco, M. C. and Bainbridge, W. S. (eds.). *Converging Technologies for Improving Human Performance*, Springer, 2004.

Sasson, A. *Medical Biotechnology*, United Nations University Press, 2006.

Useful websites

www.bio.org – *Biotechnology Industry Organization*
www.phrma.org – *Pharmaceutical Research and Manufacturers Association*
www.medicaldevices.org – *Medical Device Manufacturers Association (mostly small to mid-sized device and diagnostics companies)*
www.advamed.org – *Advanced Medical Technology Association (large medical device manufacturers' advocacy and lobbying association)*
www.devicelink.com – *Medical Device Link (trade publication)*
www.biomaterials.org – *Society for Biomaterials*

Appendix 1.1 Industry classification system for government and other databases

An industrial classification system is useful for researchers to look into larger government databases and gather industry level information, as companies that work in specific sectors are recognized and classified by standard codes, known as the NAICS (North American Industrial Classification System). A four-digit code identifies a high-level industry sector and further digits break down activities within the sector. Companies involved in biotechnology and biopharmaceutical companies are classified as follows (2002 NAICS codes):

Human and animal therapeutics and diagnostics – including biopharmaceutical (drug) companies; also includes tool developers – genomics, bioinformatics, proteomics companies, and companies developing advanced materials for human therapeutics:

NAICS 325411	Medicinal and botanical manufacturing
NAICS 325412	Pharmaceutical preparation manufacturing
NAICS 325413	In vitro diagnostic substance manufacturing
NAICS 325414	Biological product (except diagnostic) manufacturing
NAICS 541710	Research and development in the physical, engineering, and life sciences

Agriculture, aquaculture, animal health and food – includes seed and livestock development:

NAICS 3253	Pesticide, fertilizer, and other agricultural chemical manufacturing
NAICS 32519	Other basic organic chemical manufacturing
NAICS 11511, 11521	Support activities for crop and animal production
NAICS 112	Animal production; raise animals for the sale of animals or animal products
NAICS 5417	Research and development in the physical, engineering, and life sciences

Industrial and agriculture derived processing – including chemical manufacturing companies:

NAICS 32519	Other basic organic chemical manufacturing
NAICS 32531, 32532	Pesticide, fertilizer, and other agricultural chemical manufacturing

Environmental remediation – including utilities, petroleum industry:

NAICS 5629   Waste management and remediation services

Device and diagnostic company industrial classification:
The federal government NAICS system lists most subsectors of medical devices under the category "miscellaneous manufacturing." The following NAICS code groupings are relevant to the industry:

334510	Electromedical devices and equipment
334517	Irradiation apparatus
339112	Surgical and medical instruments
339113	Surgical appliances and supplies

339114 Dental equipment and supplies
339115 Ophthalmic goods

Relevant 2002 NAICS codes for the diagnostic (IVD) industry sector are:

325413 In vitro diagnostic substance manufacturing
621511 Medical laboratories
325413 Diagnostic reagents

While these industrial classifications are of use in collecting data on various trade or labor parameters, the data have to be carefully examined as most companies are self-nominated into these categories. Some companies fall into more than one classification. However, these classifications are used to compile data for policy direction and impact, for government investments in regions, and for economic development analysis.

2 Markets of interest and market research steps

Plan	Position	Patent	Product	Pass!	Production	Profits
Industry context	Market research	Intellectual property rights	New product development (NPD)	Regulatory plan	Manufacture	Reimbursement

Roadmap of a product commercialization plan. Stage 2

Learning points:

- Goals and methods of market research,
- Market segmentation; estimate the market size for the new biomedical products,
- Assess general drivers and hurdles that help or hinder market growth,
- Define the product concept and market positioning,
- Identify the various stakeholders in the patient referral chain and the impact of the new biomedical technology on them,
- Assess economic impact and adoption hurdles for the new biomedical product in the context of the referral chain,
- Use market research to help new product development planning and product characteristics.

2.1 Introduction

Many great technologies fail to make it to market or fail to achieve a profitable return. While most product ideas or new ventures start with a technological innovation or biological insight, product development plans must begin and end with the market and commercial issues in mind. Biomedical product development first starts with defining a set of ideal product characteristics based on positioning the product in its specific market application. To balance various ideal product characteristics for a successful product, good market research and analysis of the needs and economics of the markets is imperative. For entrepreneurs, market research is also used to define the market potential of their innovation and is an important step towards writing a convincing business plan.

Market research methods are used to achieve one or more of the following goals:

- To identify and segment markets for technology,
- To identify new product opportunities,

- To define the required product characteristics from an understanding of market needs and context,
- To understand the competition,
- To project sales revenues and profits and appropriate pricing.

How large is the market for this idea or innovation? This is typically the first market question that new product development projects have to answer in an entrepreneurial new venture or within a large company. This is a sweeping question that covers several questions – what is the need in the market that has been identified as the target for this product, how well does the product meet that need, is the competition going to eat your lunch, do the product patents provide enough protection against competition and for how long? These and other issues make it difficult to answer, "What is the size of the market?" with a great deal of accuracy. I have yet to see a market forecast for a new technology that proved to be exactly true (sometimes underestimated, usually overestimated). Steps to develop a market size estimate are described in Section 2.2.3.

The following sections briefly discuss the various methodologies used to address the above questions and then provide guidelines on processes to define key indications of interest and potential competitors.

2.2 General market research methodology

Market research information is either primary or secondary information. Primary information is collected by the researcher through first-hand experience or interaction with the source of information and is usually collected through experiments (experiential), observation, or surveys. Secondary information is collected from data recorded by someone else and is obtained by reviewing and analyzing reports and published information.

2.2.1 Reports, projections, and historical data

Information on past events is used to suggest future trends, but must be assessed carefully (see example in Box 2.1). Past records of product sales, characteristics of successful products and specific market segments are useful for technologies or products that are similar to the innovation in consideration. However, if the new innovation is radically different in usage, application, or outcome from historical products, using secondary data can be rather unsatisfactory. In this case, data that would be useful include historical data on treatment of the disease, growth rates of procedures or costs of existing treatments, or data on past rates of incidence and prevalence of the disease.

2.2.2 Experimental

Testing a prototype is the most reliable way to get assessments from possible customers (see example in Box 2.2). For many biotechnology innovations, making

---

Box 2.1 Using historical data to project sales revenues

A newly designed catheter that has an easier hookup into veins for delivery of fluids into the body can be evaluated by looking at sales of intravenous (IV) catheters in general. Assuming that usage of this new catheter will be spread evenly over all current patient segments, obtain the total market size and sales for catheters from available historical data (check financial statements of a public company whose main products are catheters; look for market data in company's SEC filings or their presentations, check proceedings of trade conferences; look for economic data, etc.) and then assume that the rate of market growth follows the trajectory of the last few years. Check whether the market is near saturation. You now know the total size of the market and the rate of growth of this particular market. You may also want to check these financial statements to see if historical data showing increase in sales over time with the launch of a major new catheter brand can be separated out, giving even better comparable data for your new product's projected revenue growth. For a new drug product, financial data for a drug that is sold to treat the same disease, with a similar mechanism of action (inhibits the same enzyme or blocks the same receptor on the cell), could be used as a benchmark to collect potential market size or growth rate estimates.

Box 2.2 Focus groups and prototypes for market research

Before launching a new type of syringe, a focused group of representative users (nurse, physician's aide, emergency worker, physician) would be used to test prototypes of the syringe in a human-like tissue model and give their feedback. Similarly, for a new diagnostic assay platform (e.g., one based on microfluidics) one could place a working prototype in a general lab to be used in parallel with established methods. One would then get user feedback on features that they like or don't like about the prototype device or on functional elements such as speed, reproducibility, true costs of usage, etc. Drugs or implantable devices can be prototype tested in animal models of human disease or in laboratory constructs to test specific features or characteristics.

---

a prototype (early clinical or animal testing) is a very expensive process and is typically not a commonly used route for conducting market research. However, there are some product characteristics that can be assessed with this method, such as ergonomic design parameters, color of drug or device, packaging preferences based on experimental usage patterns of prototype, etc.

2.2.3   Observational

Observational methods could involve visiting and observing physicians and patients in the healthcare setting appropriate to the innovation of interest.

Observation methods are useful in collecting data if specific questions and protocols are set up beforehand and comfort and privacy of patients is addressed. Observation of the course of treatment from diagnosis to amelioration of the problem will provide a rich context to gage the real needs of the market, the actual behavior of patients (e.g., compliance issues, where patients frequently forget or neglect to take medication can significantly affect revenue projections) and the potential for adoption in the application context of interest. Observational methods can also include the collection of data from a focus group. A focus group can be formed from a sample of healthcare participants taken aside in a space where they are given situations and are closely observed (sometimes by unseen observers), to understand the true context of first usage of an innovative product. Professional market research firms are usually contracted for this type of research.

This method is best used with a product that has high interactivity with the stakeholders or where a particular method of use is really important for obtaining benefit from the product – e.g., the surgical technique used to implant an artificial knee joint or the compliance of patients with their heart failure medication over a month.

2.2.4 Survey

Survey methods involve posing a number of questions to the stakeholders in the markets of interest – these stakeholders could range from nurses to cleaning staff to doctors and surgeons to hospital administration. Surveys on insurance companies, pharmacy benefits managers, and other organizations can also be run. Most typically, this methodology would be used to ask specific questions that need verification. An example would be better identification of a price point for a drug with known efficacy and side effects when advantages are compared with existing therapies in a survey. Any one of several textbooks on survey design and statistical analysis of surveys will help construct a good survey that will yield valid results; an important point is to check the validity of the data received in response to a question by asking the same questions in different ways throughout the survey.

Typical response rates for direct mail surveys, telephone surveys, and personal interviews are 2–10%, 25–60%, and 70–100% respectively. Web and email surveys have a higher response rate, of 30–50%, and the added benefit of significantly lower cost per response than phone, mail, or personal interview methods.

2.2.5 Primary sources of information in biomedical market research

- Physicians and lead user groups (leaders in advisory board put together by company),
- Local hospital, nursing home, clinic, dentist's office,
- HMOs, insurance companies.

2.2.6   Secondary sources of information

- Public sources;
  - Reports by government agencies, www.census.gov, physician associations website – e.g., the American Heart Association has an annual statistics databook on various diseases,
  - The National Center for Health Statistics (www.cdc.gov/nchs) has a wealth of information on disease incidence and prevalence in the USA. The National Hospital Discharge Survey (www.cdc.gov/nchs/about/major/hdasd/listpubs. htm) gives detailed numbers of admissions for each disease and numbers of each major surgical procedure performed in the USA,
  - Internet search engines (Google, Yahoo, or other search engines).
- Commercial sources;
  - Industry and trade associations, equity research firm reports, company financial reports, or securities filings.
- Educational and peer-reviewed publication sources;
  - Lexis-Nexis, PubMed; check introductory sections of scientific papers as they typically review the literature or discuss disease prevalence or incidence.

2.3   Sizing and segmenting the markets (a stepwise approach)

This section will describe market scope and size; it is useful to get a first estimate of context of application space. The questions to be asked at this stage are of the following nature: Is your technology entering a global $100 million market, a $1 billion market, or a $10 million market? And is that market mature or growing or shrinking? Are there specific geographic areas that are growing or shrinking?

A good rule of thumb is to place the innovative (potential) product in the context of the overall market size and growth rate for a particular application space. For example, the size of the global cancer therapeutics market is known relatively well, but the market for a specific therapy is harder to estimate; however one can estimate that an effective therapy will grow at least as fast as the overall market or a similar class of chemotherapeutics that are already on the market. Tables 2.1 to 2.4 give an indication of upper or lower bounds of overall market sizes to provide a quick context for this query.

2.3.1   Market size segmented by application

There are three main categories of FDA-regulated human medical products, primarily divided by intrinsic differences in methods of use, product characteristics and distinct development processes.

(1) Drugs, including both pharmaceutical drugs (small molecules, chemicals) and biotechnology drugs (biological molecules),
(2) Medical devices,
(3) In vitro diagnostics (IVD).

Table 2.1 Major market segments of world-wide pharmaceutical sales. For current data and graph, visit www.commercializingbiotech.com.

Therapeutic areas	World market share
Cardiovascular	20%
Central nervous system	18%
Alimentary, metabolism	14%
Respiratory	9%
Anti-infectives	8%
Musculo-skeletal	6%
Genito-urinary	5%
Cytostatics	5%
Total US market	US $266 billion (2005)
Total world market[a]	US $565 billion (2005)

Data from IMS retail drug market report for 2005.
[a] Figures are from sales for the calendar year 2005, in selected countries around the world (only audited data included). The total global pharma market is estimated at US $605 billion from other reports.

Table 2.2 Major therapy segments of world-wide medical device sales. For current data and graph, visit www.commercializingbiotech.com.

Therapeutic areas	World market share
Cardiovascular	41%
Orthopedics	24%
Urology	12%
Neurology	9%
Digestive disease	8%
Peripheral vascular	6%
Total US market	US $ 35 billion
Total world market (for therapeutic areas listed above only)	US $ 75 billion

Note: data from Standard and Poor (2004). Data are projected sales in 2005 and do not include medical supplies and consumables market (approx. >US $100 billion industry). Data collected from company reports and Standard and Poor's estimates.

Within these product categories, the markets can be segmented by the therapeutic application space that they treat.

2.3.2 Market size segmented by geography for drugs, devices, and IVD

The United States is by far the largest single geographic market for most products, somewhat disproportionately to its population rank. The other large geographic

Table 2.3 Major market segments of world-wide in vitro diagnostics (FIVD) sales. For current data and graph, visit www.commercializingbiotech.com.

Application segments	World-wide sales, 2005 estimate
Clinical chemistry	42%
Infectious diseases	14%
Immune diseases	6%
Hematology	5%
Endocrine testing	4%
Cancer	4%
Blood processing	4%
Coagulation	3%
Blood grouping and typing	2%
Other	16%
Total	US $28 billion

Data from Kalorama Information (2004).

Table 2.4 Drugs, devices, and IVD revenues segmented by nation or region. For current data and graph, visit www.commercializingbiotech.com. Also see Figure 1.1 for segmentation by therapy area.

	North America	Europe (Western)	Japan	China, India	South and Central America	Australia, NZ, Pacific rim	Total world-wide US$ millions
Drugs[a]	52%	25% (top 5 countries only)	17% (incl. hospital sales)		4% Latin America	2% (AUS, NZ)	~360 850[a]
Devices[b]	40–50%	23%	9%	~9%	~12%	~3%	~175 000
IVD[c]	41%	31%	11%	NA	NA	NA	~21 500[c]
Population[d]	328 million	360 million	127 million	2.4 billion	518 million	32 million	6.4 billion people

[a] from IMS drug retail report Jul 2005
[b] from Standard and Poor's Industry survey 2005 and Epsicom Business Intelligence 2004
[c] from Datamonitor report for 2001
[d] population from http://www.geohive.com
NA – not available or estimates not reliable

medical markets are Western Europe, Japan, Brazil, China, and India, followed by other geographic areas, such as South and Central America and the Pacific rim countries.

2.3.3 How big is the market for my technology or innovation?

Step 1: In the context of the larger market, start by segmenting the market. For example, if your innovation is a new drug that can treat headaches, you can segment the market by several variables, including age, price sensitivity,

Table 2.5 Market segmentation example. The heart failure market for a new heart failure drug that is indicated for treatment of Class III and Class IV patients could be significantly less than the total number of heart failure patients, once the percentage of targeted patients who are actually taking their medication (compliant population) is considered.

Congestive heart failure (CHF)	Chronic patient population United States	
Category	Fiscal year 1998	Fiscal year 1999
Total prevalence	7 902 225	8 044 465
Percent diagnosed	60.0%	60.0%
Total diagnosed population	4 741 335	4 826 679
Percent drug treated	80.5%	81.0%
Total drug-treated population	3 815 826	3 907 818
Percent compliant	75.3%	75.6%
Total compliant population	2 873 317	2 954 358
Percent in NYHA Class III and IV	50%	50%
Total Class III and IV compliant population	1 436 658	1 477 179

Note: New York Heart Association (NYHA) classification of chronic heart failure patients is based on severity of disease; Class III and IV are the two most severe. Population data from IMS Health, US Census, and medical publications.

chronic vs. acute, and degree of pain (migraines vs. mild headaches). As another example, the heart failure market can be segmented by geography, race, and disease status (Class I–IV heart failure; see example in Table 2.5, for a drug that is developed specifically for treating patients with severe heart disease). With more information about the characteristics of the innovative therapy, the market could be further segmented by background medication (e.g., for the heart failure market, the number of patients on beta blockers at time of eligibility to receive innovative therapy) or other factors. Several available databases (commercial subscriptions needed) will provide the number of prescriptions per day written for each of these segments, giving the current size of the specific market segments of interest. Pricing the innovation at this stage may not be too reliable, as the final price will depend on many parameters that are not yet known, including the specific outcome of clinical trials.

Step 2: How much of the market can I hope to capture and how soon? Predicting the future is difficult, but historical trends and market shares for other products and similar companies in the industry segment can give an acceptable benchmark for market share projections. It is best to state all assumptions clearly when presenting these projections. Evaluations of the competition are particularly relevant in producing relevant projections. Specifically, issues of market acceptance, reimbursement, and hurdles to growth of the market need to be carefully dissected and analyzed, requiring experience, a wealth of data and time.

Step 3: Also consider possible scenarios with sensitivity analysis on key assumptions – how sensitive is the projection to changes in assumptions and which parameters are the key ones? This can also lead to a scenario planning

---

Box 2.3 Impact of incorrect market prediction
How inadequacies in market prediction got a biotech success into trouble

Adapted from Weintraub (2001).

Immunex had a major success on their hands with the FDA approval of their blockbuster drug in November 1998. Their biologic, Enbrel, was approved for rheumatoid arthritis and sales in 2000 almost doubled from $367 million in 1999 to $652 million, the highest rise amongst all previously launched biologics. But in 2001, Immunex could not manufacture enough quantities of the drug, leaving thousands of patients on waiting lists and creating opportunities for competitors. Only 7.5% of the 1 million patients who might have benefited from Enbrel could get the drug.

Immunex's initial sales estimates projected the market as the 25% of rheumatoid arthritis patients who failed traditional therapies and when the FDA approved the drug for children in April, 1999, and then as a first-line treatment and preventive for early-stage patients in June 2000, Immunex was not prepared for the rapid increase in demand.

Immunex retrofitted a factory to produce more Enbrel and used contractors and partners to build or buy capacity. However, Immunex shares were down to around $15 each (May 2001), from a 52-week high of $56. "The pressure is on," says CEO Edward V. Fritzky as he grabs his gut, "and I feel it."

---

exercise, which is an important discussion to have with the involvement of decision-making managers. One must consider upside and downside scenarios in sales projections and make adequate preparations for both extremes, or the results can be equally disastrous (see Box 2.3).

Step 4: Run some benchmark checks. Check the output of the projections in context of the larger market size and historical growth rate. How have other innovations or product launches fared historically in this market? Run a quick check through the list of drivers and hurdles listed in the section below to see how the market projections might be helped or hindered by these factors.

2.4   Drivers and hurdles

A quick list of growth drivers or hurdles that could foster or impede future market growth, development, launch, or acceptance of FDA regulated products is given here. This is a useful list to run checks and balances for any marketing research output and also for an overall product commercialization plan. Stepping down this list, each topic is used to raise questions against the commercialization plan or projected markets for the products.

2.4.1 Drivers

Demographics

For example, an aging population bodes well for continued growth in most disease areas; an increasing urban population in the world also means that diseases linked with urban areas will continue to have a strong market need.

Growth trajectory and history

For example, revenue growth rates in innovative medical devices have historically been higher than in commodity medical technology products; also emerging areas, such as molecular diagnostics, have a potentially higher rate of growth than established clinical diagnostics.

High levels of investment in biotech – government and venture capital

For example, areas of biodefense research and nanobiotechnology research are receiving high amounts of funding in the USA, whereas certain European and developing nations are attracting investment in biotechnology manufacturing facilities with taxes and grants.

Basic research leading to innovations and new products

In the USA, National Institutes of Health funding trends often dictate future emergence of new products – e.g., increased funding for cancer research 15–20 years ago has now resulted in a broad and deep pipeline of new anti-cancer therapeutics. The current NIH roadmap is another example of a concerted effort, focused on improving drug development processes. As another example, the recent increase in biodefense funding in the US portends that newer anti-infectious disease therapies, including vaccines, rapid-response diagnostics and biosensor applications and products will emerge in a few years.

Approvals and streamlined FDA processes

Prioritization of specific disease areas by the FDA shortens product development times, increasing economic attractiveness. For example, many cancer drugs that show good efficacy are given priority review. Typical drug review times vary from 16–24 months.

New laws and regulations (e.g., orphan drug act, bioterrorism act, pediatric extension)

Just as regulatory acts can change market attractiveness, the legislative bodies in many countries play a major role in affecting market conditions for specific areas and it is advisable to stay alert to any legislation in medical areas, such as the Medicare Modernization Act of 2005, which extends Medicare coverage to prescription drugs. Also the Orphan Drug Act of 1983 gave special benefits to drugs for small populations, including grants and market exclusivity on approval. The IVD industry has been affected by changing regulations both in reimbursement (government laboratory reimbursement fee schedules) and regulatory guidelines for new products.

2.4.2   Hurdles

Food and Drug Administration regulatory delays and inconsistency

For example, drug development includes a review period of about 18–24 months between submission of final data from clinical studies and possible approval by the FDA. The FDA has usually always tried to balance the risk–benefit ratio while making approval decisions, but the weights are inconsistent among therapeutic areas and may vary, depending on the current leadership at the FDA.

Increasing buyer power

As HMOs, pharmacy benefit providers, and other buying collectives increase in scale, their purchasing power and ability to negotiate discounts and enforce price ceilings becomes greater, decreasing the profitability of manufacturers in the medical device and drug industry.

HMOs, Medicare, insurance

The price that an innovative medical device or drug receives in the marketplace is set by a complex process and manufacturers must work closely with insurance companies to make sure they get a fair price.

Pricing pressures

An increasing cost burden of healthcare on companies and individuals, political and social perceptions, inefficient payment and oversight in national healthcare systems, and rapidly increasing prices of certain innovative products all contribute to feedback on pricing pressures. These pressures are exerted at various points in the value chain in a multi-party payer system such as the USA. Awareness of issues surrounding pricing pressures will help ensure a sound product-positioning strategy.

Generic competition

Patent lifetimes and patent rights vary in countries and country-specific rules and regulations must be considered when planning global launch and commercialization strategies.

Pipeline of blockbuster products

Companies that aim for blockbuster products could lose opportunities for delivering niche products to smaller markets that could prove to be more profitable. The scale of large pharmaceutical and device companies forces them to continue to develop products that meet the needs of larger populations.

Development costs and low success rate

In the drug industry, innovative products face a seemingly impossible hurdle – the high cost of development ($800 million estimated) along with a high failure rate – 1 compound out of 10000 that enter screening makes it through to commercial launch. Sound business models reduce the risk by including commercialization strategies that have several product lines or multiple partnerships and diversified early stage revenue streams. Some companies have a harvest-as-you go strategy, with early revenues from animal health products or sales in non-regulated markets.

2.5 The referral chain – developing market context and understanding customer needs

Project funding decisions are based on many factors, a key one of which is the size of the market. Once the project is funded to begin development, market research is used to understand the context of product application. With this context, appropriate product characteristics can be selected and weighed against each other. Any successful product fills someone's need – either implicit or explicit. *Understanding the context of that customer need is the key to developing a good market understanding* and a good product design, development, and sales plan.

The market research methods outlined earlier can be used to answer the following questions:

- What is the referral chain[1] for the disease? Identify steps of diagnosis and treatment through to resolution of the disease problem (Boxes 2.5 and 2.6 contain examples). How does your product affect the referral chain? *This information can help define the value proposition of the new biomedical product.*
- Define the value chains for product development, industry supply chain and patient care delivery – who are your customers (purchasing decision makers) and the stakeholders for the product? Who makes the payments back to your company for the product?
- What do patients need – what do caregivers need?
- How does the product meet their needs?
- How does the product get delivered to them?
- How much will they pay for your product based on alternatives or direct competitors?
- Are there issues with patient compliance or other customer acceptance issues (esthetics or ergonomics of product; price sensitivities, or other impediments in the purchasing process)?

2.5.1 Market context – insight into biology or disease pathology

What core element of a disease or medical problem is being addressed by this technology or product and what is the impact on the life of the patient (not just life span, but quality of life)?

---

[1] *Referral chain* is usually used to describe the movement of a patient's care from a primary care physician through referral to a specialist for further diagnosis or treatment. The term is used here to describe the patient's perspective and experience from the first realization of the problem through referrals and various diagnoses or treatments to some level of resolution.

> **Box 2.4** Segmenting the market – example of the artificial retina
>
> ## Case example of market context
>
> The innovative technology is an organic retinal implant that integrates with the neuronal circuitry and provides some visual perception to a blind person while releasing drugs to help retinal cells grow from stem cells. The implant eventually degrades, leaving behind a rejuvenated eye. Where is the market and what key problem is this technology solving? This technology seems to address two problems – providing sight for those who are blind and providing a stimulus for regeneration of a degenerated or damaged retina. Keeping a broad perspective while first stating the problem will help to reveal multiple potential markets. The next step is to define, as specifically as possible, the core benefit – there are different levels of "blindness" – is this going to help one who has been born blind, or one who is legally blind but still has some visual perception? Eventually, it is clear that this technology is intended for a specific type of blind person – one who has become blind due to a retinal problem, not due to a neuronal or cerebral problem. Thus, this product solves the problem of restoring vision to a person whose retinal cells (but not retinal neuronal cells) have been injured or damaged due to trauma or disease. However, for all regulatory product development, identify a specific grade or type of injury and perhaps age of patient based on pathology of the disease or trauma for maximum benefit, depending on more detailed knowledge of the technology and the science behind the product concept. One more step in thinking can help bring more insight – can the device adjust to any changes in size of the tissues surrounding the eye – if not, then we can only implant it in adult patients. Therefore, the context of usage becomes clearer – the implant device is indicated for adult patients with blindness caused by advanced retinopathy.

Answering this question can be an invigorating experience for the technologist and a trying experience for the non-scientific business executive, but it is a critical step that helps position the innovation in the right context. An exploration of market and technical context can explain the scope and potential of the innovation (see Box 2.4 for an example).

2.5.2   Market context – the referral chain

Evaluate all transactions that start with the patient's realization of a need and end with the fulfillment of that problem or need. This is the referral chain, within which the economic impact can be evaluated. For example, start with the diagnosis of a disease or health problem and step through all the transactions that occur until the end user or patient sees a final resolution of the problem (see Box 2.5).

> **Box 2.5** Referral chain; economics of new technology in market context
>
> ### Referral chain case example 1: wound healing
>
> A wound healing biotherapeutic is made of innovative living cell material that heals quickly without scars or pain. To treat minor skin wounds in daily life, a "band-aid" costing $0.50 or less is the common solution. In that context, introducing a new wound-healing innovation that heals the wound much quicker but has a limited shelf life (user has to go to pharmacy to buy product as it cannot be stocked at home) and a cost of $15.00 per wound will demand a shift in economic and usage context that may not be sustained by the market, despite any obvious benefits of the new innovation. "Price sensitivity" of the market is a term used to describe this issue. More market research, perhaps with focus groups, may be necessary to identify better the feasible applications and the segments of wounded people that would benefit from and thus use this innovative living-cell skin-healing material.
>
> ### Referral chain case example 2: organ transplants
>
> The innovation is a solution and complex apparatus for perfusion used to incubate an organ before implantation and extends the life of the transplanted organ. In the case of a heart transplant, if the innovative treatment improves long-term survival of the heart, but does not change the cost of the procedure itself, its significance may not be as clear to the surgeon as it introduces an extra step in the process. However, the entire cost of treatment over the life of the transplant patient is decreased as the transplanted organ and recipient will be healthier. With $750 000 to $1 million invested into each patient, the parties affected by this new process are the patients themselves, the insurance companies, the cardiologists who care for these patients, and society as a whole. The innovation must now be sold or marketed to a customer audience that includes not only physicians but also insurance companies. Thus, understanding the various parties involved in the referral chain as the patient passes from one physician to another gives a better understanding of which physician or other caregiver is affected by the innovative intervention. Marketing the treatment to the consumer may also have some influence on the surgeon's adoption of the apparatus in his or her practice.

Step 1: Determine the condition that drives the first interaction with medical care. Then follow the treatment choices available to the caregiver for that condition. If the treatment branches into various degrees of resolution (early resolution for mild disease), keep to the referral path (diagnosis and treatment path) that is of greatest importance to the innovative intervention.

Step 2: Identify the point of intervention with the innovative product and the cost of the intervention.

Step 3: Identify the altered referral path (diagnosis and treatment path) for the patient post-intervention until resolution.

Step 4: Document as far as possible the probable time to healing, savings in materials, and other savings in the entire economic system (e.g., reduction in lost time at work due to bedrest).

Step 5: Does the delivery of the innovative product give a specific benefit to any stakeholder to create an incentive for them to adopt or pay for this innovation? Identify and explain this benefit.

These steps will result in data that would be used to identify the key value proposition for the new product for multiple stakeholders and to define the economic benefit that can be used to convince payers to cover and pay for the product. See the example in Box 2.6.

2.5.3   What competitive or alternate products exist?

An assessment of competitive products must also include radically different technologies that are treating the same problem – for example, while evaluating competition for a new drug for headaches, consider all of the following alternatives that a patient might have – an ice bag on the head, rest or sleep, and medicines such as Tylenol, aspirin, etc. For a highly innovative product, consider the biology and pathology of the disease and consider the point of intervention of your product compared with the intervention points of other products. Box 2.7 covers some examples of competitive analysis.

2.5.4   Defining the end user

The status and role of the end consumer in the value chain (the patient) is very different in medical technology markets as compared with other industries. The end consumer is usually not a fully informed one and does not always have full choice in the marketplace. For example, an average patient receiving a hip replacement does not usually know which artificial hips are available or which one is best for him or her. In other cases, patients with high blood pressure do not know which drug and dosage is best for their particular situations and cannot thus exercise fully informed freedom of choice in the market. Additionally, many insured patients do not know the true cost of the treatments as they typically make only a co-payment with private insurance or, in some countries, a national health service program covers all costs (geographic context). There may also be constraints unknown to the patient, such as a limited formulary available, owing to insurer's decisions.

Is a large institution the primary purchaser of the product or are individual users or physician groups directly purchasing from you? Analysis of the market needs for

> **Box 2.6** Market stakeholders and adoption of new technology
>
> ## Referral chain case example 3: bone fracture
>
> Excerpted and adapted with permission from a class report written at the Lally School of Management and Technology, Rensselaer Polytechnic Institute by Peter Ryan, Brian Monthie, Aaron Germain, and Grant Cochran, Spring 2006.
>
> The innovation is a novel diagnostic technique that uses a non-invasive detection mechanism (ultrasound based) to assess the quality of bone material in a healing fracture. This device has been shown to detect changes in fracture healing with great sensitivity and accuracy. The device is being evaluated for use in early diagnosis of a non-union fracture. Current medical practice and insurance companies define the classification of a fracture as non-union after three months of standard fracture care have failed to heal a fracture. Therefore the referral chain is as shown in Figure 2.1.
>
> A common timeline for a simple fracture starts with the patient presenting the broken bone, let's say the wrist, to the emergency department. When a patient comes to the emergency room with wrist pain and evidence of a possibly broken wrist, the first step is to obtain X-rays of the injured area. If there is a broken wrist, the X-rays will be carefully reviewed to determine if the fractured bone is in proper position, and to assess the stability of the bone fragments. If the bone fragments are in proper position then the wrist will normally be placed in a cast. The patient will then see an orthopedic surgeon within the week to discuss the accident and to get an overall health update. In the case of a simple fracture the patient could be seen by a family doctor every 2 to 3 weeks. X-rays will be taken to monitor fracture healing and the cast may be removed if desired by the patient, or if the fracture has healed significantly. Around 12 weeks later, an

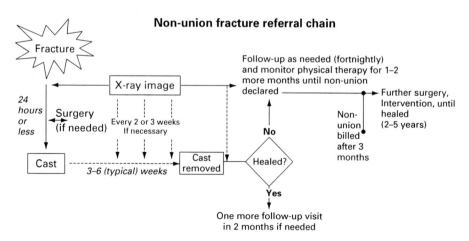

Figure 2.1 Referral chain (diagnosis and treatment pathway) for non-union fracture. The physician has to wait until three months post fracture to be able to establish diagnosis of a non-union fracture.

Box 2.6 (cont.)

additional X-ray image will be taken to determine if proper healing has occurred. At this time the patient may be permitted to ramp back up to normal activity. Non-unions are medically defined as fractures that do not show any clinical progress in healing over three consecutive months. "Clinical progress" is specifically radiographic. The American Academy of Orthopaedic Surgeons (AAOS) has this to say regarding non-union diagnosis:

To diagnose a non-union, the doctor uses imaging studies. Depending upon which bone is involved, these may include X-rays (radiographs), CT scans (computed tomography), and MRIs (magnetic resonance imaging). Imaging studies let the doctor see the broken bone and follow the progress of its healing. A non-union may be diagnosed if the doctor finds one or more of the following:
- Persistent pain at the fracture site,
- A persistent gap with no bone spanning the fracture site,
- No progress in bone healing when repeated imaging studies are compared over several months,
- Inadequate healing in a time period that is usually enough for normal healing.
Blood tests may also be used to investigate the non-union's cause. These could show infection or another medical condition which may slow bone healing, such as anemia or diabetes.

The cost of diagnosing a non-union is substantial. X-ray imaging is relatively inexpensive ($60) but an MRI or CT scan costs roughly $1200. The AAOS recommends several MRI and CT scans as well as X-rays for diagnosis. Thus, it may cost upwards of $5 000 just to diagnose the non-union. If it takes 6 months just to diagnose and possibly another 6 months to a year to treat this injury, the patient will probably suffer at his or her work and miss other important activities. Throughout the diagnosis process there is also a time strain on the physician who is not getting compensated any more than for a simple fracture even though several office visits are involved, as each fracture has a flat fee assigned to be paid. Once the case is diagnosed as a non-union this will allow the orthopedist to bill insurance additionally for the visits associated with the condition. Non-unions also adversely affect insurance companies because the treatment of these conditions commonly calls for costly procedures.

The tibia is the most common site of non-unions. Approximately 72 000 tibial non-unions occur every year in the USA. Some tibial cases respond well to non-operative treatments, such as bone growth stimulators, but most need additional surgery. In surgery, internal fixation using plates and screws or intramedullary nails are used to immobilize the fracture site (too much movement is a common cause of non-union and can result in the development of a mid-bone joint called a "pseudojoint") whereas bone autografts, allografts, and void fillers can fill in the gaps. Some surgeons favor the use of bone morphogenic proteins within the tibia to stimulate more growth. Each of these procedures would cost between 10 and 20 thousand dollars and is just a

Box 2.6 (cont.)

small portion of the total costs – a non-union could take from 24–36 months to heal. Three years of monthly office visits, physical therapy, etc., could add up to well over $50 000. Insurance companies and physicians thus have a significant financial incentive to have a non-union detected earlier and treated aggressively.

Benefits of intervention

The innovative diagnosis technology will be applied starting at 1 week after the fracture occurs and will be used to track the healing process of the bone tissue. It will be used to complement X-ray images, but its use should reduce the number of X-ray images that need to be taken. As the technology will be approved for early diagnosis (at 2 months instead of 3 months, for example) of non-unions, the opportunity for earlier surgical or other therapeutic intervention should significantly reduce the healing time for a non-union (due to earlier and more aggressive intervention). The stakeholders that have an incentive to adopt and pay for this treatment are the physician, who can now bill for the extra time taken to work with non-unions, and the insurance companies (payers), who will see financial benefits from lower costs required, owing to earlier healing and potentially less expensive intervention of the non-union. These benefits can be quantified with more data collected in actual clinical trials. Society benefits generally with earlier healing and reduced loss of productivity at work and the patient is happier to have an early resolution of the problem, which in the past (before this diagnostic innovation), would have taken much longer to resolve.

the former will include different considerations, such as the portfolio of the purchaser or the economics of the intermediate supply chain to final consumer.

Therefore, to understand the market for medical products, the researcher must address a broader spectrum of end users – the patient, the caregiver and the reimbursing institution – in market research.

2.5.5 Defining the indication

An *indication* for a drug or device refers to the use of that drug for treating a particular disease. For example, diabetes is an indication for insulin, or a severely arthritic knee joint is an indication for an artificial knee joint. Another way of stating this relationship is that (the product) insulin is indicated for the treatment of diabetes. *The identification of an indication is a key first step in formal product development of FDA-regulated technologies.* Another way to look at an indication is to identify the *target market segment*.

Box 2.7 Identifying and analyzing the competition

Competition case example 1: heart failure

An innovative drug treats the enlargement of the heart in congestive heart failure, by stopping progressive hypertrophy of the heart muscle cells (cardiomyocytes). Its competition will come from devices in development that can prevent the enlargement (i) by providing electrical stimulation to the heart muscle, (ii) by wrapping the heart in a custom-fitted tight glove-like device, or (iii) by providing a left ventricular heart assist device that can be implanted long-term to take the load off the heart and allow it to recover. Other possible competitors also include new and existing drugs that can help improve the heart function, allowing it to maintain size and function.

Competition case example 2: ultrasonic head check

(Excerpt with permission from a class report written in Spring 2006 at the Lally School of Management and Technology, Rensselaer Polytechnic Institute by Oscar Perez Prieto, Disha Ahuja, Sam Christy, and Linda Yin Chen.)

Background

The transcranial ultrasonic Head Check is a novel application of low-frequency ultrasonic waves for the detection of brain injury. The underlying concept behind this device is the use of ultrasonic waves to detect disruptions in the right–left symmetry of the normal brain after a contusion has occurred. The novelty of the device is in the application of its method and not in the technology per se. The main benefit of this method is the creation of an accurate and portable traumatic brain injury (TBI) detection device that detects trauma rapidly and on-site, leading to rapid triage and more success in treatment.

Medical indications

The transcranial ultrasonic "Head Check" device is a portable device that detects the shift of the midline of the brain or other central structures from the sagittal plane of the head in a human brain after contusion or whiplash effect has occurred.

Markets, competition, and applications

According to The Center for Disease Control, 1.5 million Americans suffer from traumatic brain injury annually. Of this number, 235 000 are hospitalized and 50 000 die as a result of their injuries. Some of the common types of brain injuries include contusion, whiplash-type injuries associated with the rapid acceleration

Box 2.7 (cont.)

and deceleration of the head can result in swelling of the brain. If the pressure within the skull is not relieved through surgery, cooling, or medication, the brain will gradually be pushed against the skull, causing the death of the patient. Studies have shown that accurate diagnosis within the "golden hour" after trauma can help in guiding further treatment with successful outcomes. Delayed diagnosis can lead to brain injury, lifetime disabilities or death. There is a need for early diagnosis in this indication and current market. Other emerging technologies that claim to offer similar benefits; that is, to provide information about hemorrhages in the brain within the "golden hour" are described below and advantage of the "Head Check" device is summarized in Figure 2.2

Glasgow Coma Scale (GCS)

This is the most widely used scoring system used in quantifying level of consciousness following traumatic brain injury and is based on a subjective

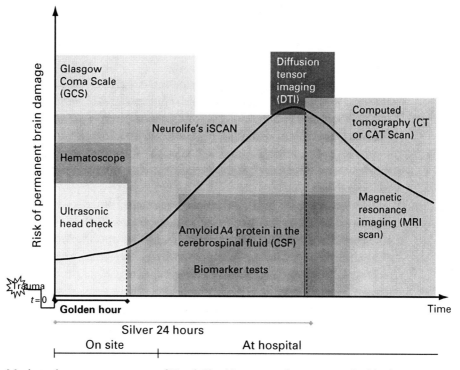

Figure 2.2   Market advantage assessment of Head Check's new product compared with alternate technologies.

Box 2.7 (cont.)

assessment of three aspects of the patient; eye opening, verbal response, and motor response.

NeuroLife's iSCAN

iScan uses fiber optics and proprietary software to measure changes in the eye's blood supply. Small changes in the blood supply to the eye correlate with brain pressure.

Hematoscope™

The hematoscope is a hand-held, non-invasive, near-infrared (NIR) based mobile imaging device to detect brain hematoma at the site of injury

Other technologies as CT, MRI, biomarker tests, and diffusion tensor imaging (DTI) can be considered complements rather than substitutes to the transcranial ultrasonic Head Check as they are meant to be used at the hospital setting. These complementary technologies are used after the golden hour as further assessment of the extent of the injury. The market value of the "Head Check" device is clearly in the early detection (in the first hour after trauma) of brain damage and must be sold to and used by emergency medical technicians who triage patients at the site of trauma.

For example, if a drug is being developed to treat heart failure disease, it could be indicated specifically for congestive heart failure class III, which defines the specific degree of symptoms that the disease has reached when the drug can be prescribed. If indicated for class I heart failure, there will be different criteria for regulatory approval, and the market size will change. A market segment is identified by various considerations, primarily commercial (market need) and regulatory considerations.

Another example, in breast cancer treatments, describes how the market gets segmented based on the specific indications under which the drug is developed or approved. Breast cancer is the general disease but specific forms and stages of the disease are indicated for use of approved drugs. Herceptin, as a single-agent drug, is indicated, "for the treatment of patients with metastatic breast cancer whose tumors over-express the HER2 protein and who have received one or more chemotherapy regimens for their metastatic disease." Or: "Arimidex is indicated for the treatment of advanced breast cancer in post-menopausal women with disease progression following tamoxifen therapy." Or: "Xeloda is indicated for the treatment of patients with metastatic breast cancer resistant to both paclitaxel and an anthracycline-containing chemotherapy regimen or resistant to paclitaxel and for whom further anthracycline therapy is not indicated." All three are breast cancer drugs but they address slightly different segments of the breast cancer market.

A device is also approved or cleared for a specific indication. Take for example, this approval for a balloon catheter:

This device is indicated for the dilatation of stenoses in coronary arteries for the purpose of improving myocardial perfusion in those circumstances where a high pressure balloon resistant lesion is encountered. In addition, the target lesion should possess the following characteristics: discrete ($\leq$15 mm in length) or tubular (10 to 20 mm in length) with a reference vessel diameter ranging from 2.0 mm to 4.0 mm; readily accessible to the device; light to moderate tortuosity of proximal vessel segment, non-angulated lesion segment ($<$45 degrees), smooth angiographic contour; and absence of angiographically-visible thrombus and/or calcification. (accessed at FDA search engine: www.accessdata.fda.gov/scripts/cdrh/cfdocs/cfPMA/pma.cfm)

Another balloon catheter was approved for the following:

... indicated for balloon dilatation for the stenotic portion of a coronary artery or bypass graft stenosis for the purpose of improving myocardial perfusion. The balloon dilatation catheter (balloon models 2.5 mm–4.0 mm) is also indicated for the post-delivery expansion of balloon expandable stents. (accessed at FDA search engine: www.accessdata.fda.gov/scripts/cdrh/cfdocs/cfPMA/pma.cfm)

The indication for the product, as worded by the FDA in their approval letter, restricts the marketing of the product to patients with that particular indication and can make claims to treating only that segment of the market. The wording of the indication is derived primarily from the results of studies designed to test the efficacy and safety of their products. In the above examples of cancer therapies, the drug developers cannot claim in any marketing message that their product can be useful for any other state of breast cancer other than that indicated in the approval letter.

Hence, it is important to define the population and specific benefit of the technology or innovation as best as possible in the early marketing research (Box 2.8 and 2.9). Marketing research can be used to identify the most beneficial,

---

Box 2.8 Referral chain, indication, and basis for competition for an insulin pump

As an example, consider the *referral chain and specific indication* for application of an insulin pump. A company decides that it has some new innovation in insulin pump design and fabrication and wishes to enter the market. A fully featured insulin pump that is technologically superior to its competitors seems like the best way to enter and capture the huge diabetes market. But a little research into the application referral chain will reveal a different picture, also indicating the segments in the market. Most diabetic patients do not immediately go to an insulin pump prescription after being diagnosed with diabetes. Most of the patients will be treated by their physicians first with oral medication or combination of various oral medications. Failing to respond to that, they will have insulin added to the oral medications and then combinations of daily insulin injections will be tried to control their disease before the doctor suggests

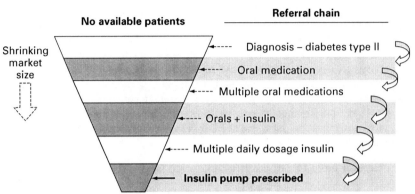

Context – diabetic patient

Final indication – diabetes Type II patients who are refractory to insulin or other medications

Figure 2.3   As the referral chain for the disease is identified, the market segments are defined and the true available market becomes clearer. Additionally, this market segmentation can help guide clinical trial design. For example, after initial approval in the last segment, a market expansion strategy might be planned to move up to the next largest market segment.

Box 2.8 (cont.)

an insulin pump. Finally, an insulin pump has few differentiators for increasing competition for this small group of patients. Even though the overall diabetic patient population is increasing, better oral medications will mean that fewer patients will reach a stage that is indicated for insulin pumps. Lastly, the fact that competition will increase in the insulin pump business means that eventually the competition will turn into a cost-based competition with commoditization of the insulin pumps. Therefore, a new entrant will be better suited to give more weight to cost of the pump than to features during product design, giving the product a better chance of success by the time it gets to market (see Figure 2.3).

---

and commercially attractive, potential application (market segment) of the product. A manufacturer must define this indication as early as possible in the development process to understand the market better and to guide product development with greatest efficiency. Two other factors (apart from market size) that are important considerations in selecting an indication are time to market (regulatory and developmental path) and competition. Section 4.7 discusses these two points in further detail.

Box 2.9 Market research for improved definition of opportunity

Contributed by Lawrence Roth, Vice President, Business development and operations at Percardia

Percardia Inc. was developing a unique system, VPASS™, for treating advanced coronary artery disease (CAD). In the early stages of CAD, patients are typically treated with drugs to improve heart function, reduce the risk of acute closure of a vessel from thrombus formation (resulting in a myocardial infarction or "heart attack") and to mitigate the pain (angina) associated with reduced blood flow. If medication is unable to provide relief of symptoms, physicians will attempt to restore blood flow to the heart by either catheter-based techniques (inserting a stent to prop open the obstruction) or surgery (creating a bypass around the obstruction with a vessel graft). The VPASS system is a catheter-based procedure that supplies blood to the heart by connecting the left ventricle (the heart's main pumping chamber) to the coronary vasculature with an implant placed directly in the heart muscle. It is intended to allow the interventional cardiologist to treat patients who are otherwise not amenable to current therapy; these patients are commonly referred to as having "refractory angina."

Although physicians were universal in agreeing that there is a strong unmet need for a therapy (such as VPASS) to treat refractory angina, literature-based estimates of the number of refractory angina patients varied from a low of 75 000 to a high of 800 000 patients annually. In addition, initial clinical evaluation of the VPASS system was proceeding much slower than anticipated, creating questions about the potential market. An accurate understanding of the market size and patient referral process was required, to develop an effective commercialization plan.

Finding that there were no commercially available research reports that analyzed the refractory angina patient population, Percardia contracted a firm to perform a semi-quantitative market research study. The firm combined primary research through direct physician interviews with secondary research through literature reviews to characterize the refractory angina patient population and to provide an understanding of the management and flow of this target patient. This research led to several key findings:

- The refractory angina market in the US consists of ~400 000 patients with an additional 45 000 patients diagnosed annually.
- Only those patients with the most debilitating symptoms (40% of the total or 160 000 patients) would be considered candidates for VPASS.
- Initial clinical studies should target physically active patients considered most likely to benefit (40% of candidates or ~64 000 patients).
- Significant long-term data would be required to expand the use of VPASS in patients with less debilitating symptoms.
- Additional indications were identified, providing a long-term pool of up to 750 000 potential patients.

> **Box 2.9** (cont.)
>
> • Primary care of refractory angina lies with either the clinical cardiologist or primary care physician while the cardiac surgeon and interventional cardiologist perform treatment.
> • Clinical trials and initial marketing efforts should focus on the clinical cardiologist as the clinician who will recommend VPASS.
>
> Understanding your market is critical to the development of a viable business plan. By identifying patient flow and market segmentation, Percardia was better prepared to design effective clinical studies and market launch plans.

2.6 Market research in the context of medical device design and development

Output from market research feeds into the medical device design and development processes through specific design parameters, where there is a constant balancing act between features and cost of the product (see Figure 2.4). Quality has to be maintained throughout this process, but data from market research can be used to assign weights to parameters for decision making between cost and features of a device. This is done formally through user or patient interviews, surveys, and internal engineering planning (see Chapter 4 for more details and examples of the use of market research in product development).

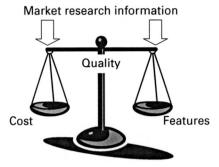

Figure 2.4   Market research data impact new device development by influencing choices between cost of product and features. In new drug development, market research information can steer the product towards more profitable indications, suggest a market expansion strategy, or help in choosing product characteristics, like oral or infused delivery.

Exercises

2.1   In simple terms, briefly describe the invention and summarize the significance of the underlying technology innovation.

2.2   Define clearly the specific market need or core problem that your technology addresses.

2.3   Identify the specific indication for your product and identify other potential indications for future development.

2.4   Also brainstorm to identify non-medical or non-regulated applications (animal health, other industries) for your technology (if so needed in the business and financial model, the product can be commercialized in a market where time to market may be shorter and revenues might help fund medical product development).

2.5   Describe the referral chain for the indication and the economic context (costs).

2.6   Describe the patient population and identify the payers (see Chapter 7).

2.7   Identify the purchaser, user, prescriber, and other stakeholders who are affected in the value chain (e.g., nurses who will see the patient each week for four-hour infusion of the drug).

2.8   Describe the benefit from the new product to each stakeholder or to the primary purchasing decision maker.

2.9   Describe the savings in the entire referral chain from the intervention made by the new product. This will also help define the actual economic value proposition for the insurers, payers, or purchasers.

2.10 Write, in one sentence, why your technology will be purchased over others and over current treatment options – in other words, define the value proposition for your technology or product for the chosen indication.

2.11 Identify competitors based on the specific problem that the new product or technology is addressing. Describe very briefly why a certain competing solution is a competing technology or product.

2.12 Classify alternatives and competition in a comparison table highlighting the advantage of your product, considering appropriate parameters – efficacy, safety, price, etc.

2.13 Collect specific value propositions that the stakeholders will value and translate those into product characteristics that would be appreciated by the stakeholders. Give more weight to the primary purchaser's perspectives. This list of preferred product characteristics will serve as input to a product design.

2.14 For a market research project follow these steps:

(a) Define the specific goals of the market research program. Examples include: (i) Define and segment markets to clarify reimbursement strategy; or (ii) Define potential market opportunity in order to drive investment decision; or (iii) Provide input on specific market needs for better defining desirable product characteristics.

(b) Decide on the extent of primary vs. secondary research to be carried out and make sure that adequate resources are available.

(c) Collect data and tabulate results without any bias entering the summary tabulation.

(d) Analyze the data and then present the specific output required – based on the defined goals of the market research project.

References and additional reading

Cohen, W. A. *The Marketing Plan*, 2nd edn., Wiley Press, 1998.

Kalorama Information. *The World-wide Market for In Vitro Diagnostic Tests*, 4th edn., Kalorama Information, 2004. Available from www.marketresearch.com.

Standard and Poor's. *Medical Device Industry Survey*, Standard and Poor's, 2004.

Ulrich, K. T. and Eppinger, S. D., *Product Design and Development*, 3rd edn., McGraw-Hill, Boston, MA, 2003. (Note – this book also has a practical section on working out client or customer needs through various steps of market research).

Weintraub, A. Biotech and the spoils of success, *Business Week*, August 13, 2001.

Useful websites

www.cdc.gov/nchs – *The National Center for Health Statistics for information on disease incidence and prevalence in the USA*

www.cdc.gov/nchs/about/major/hdasd/listpubs.htm – *The National Hospital Discharge Survey gives detailed numbers of admissions for each disease and numbers of each major surgical procedure that is performed in the USA.*

www.imshealth.com – *Prescription drug sales information reports*

http://rarediseases.about.com/ – *Orphan indications*

www.wrongdiagnosis.com/ – *Symptoms, disease description, and epidemiology*

www.hoovers.com – *Hoover's industry lists*

Navigate from www.lib.rpi.edu home page by clicking through Home > Research assistance > Course web pages > Lally School – *Resources webpage for market research*

3   Intellectual property, licensing, and business models

Plan	Position	Patent	Product	Pass!	Production	Profits
Industry context	Market research	Intellectual property rights	New product development (NPD)	Regulatory plan	Manufacture	Reimbursement

Roadmap of a product commercialization plan. Stage 3

The only thing that keeps us alive is brilliance. The only way to protect our brilliance is patents.

Edwin Land, founder of Polaroid

Ideas are to the Information Age what iron ore and other raw materials were to the Industrial Age – only you can't put a fence around ideas. The closest thing is a patent.

Thomas Field, Jr.

The patent system added the fuel of interest to the fire of genius.

Abraham Lincoln

Learning points:

- What are the different types of intellectual property and what is their purpose?
- What is a patent and how does one interpret a patent?
- What is patentable material ?
- What is the process of filing and obtaining a patent ?
- What are the different models used to manage or make money from patents by licensing?
- What are the key terms in a licensing or a technology transfer agreement?
- What is the value of a patent?
- What is a reasonable "royalty rate" and what other financial terms are there for licensing my patent?
- What are the damages I can claim if someone infringes my patent?
- What are the various business models around commercialization of biomedical technology patents or products?

3.1   Types of intellectual property

"Intellectual property" is the term used to describe a set of commercially valuable rights that result from formally codified inventions, literary or artistic works, or other representations of creative thought, or particular symbols of commerce. Intellectual property includes patents, trademarks, copyrights, and trade secrets. Patents are concerned with discoveries, inventions, methods, data, designs, or practical implementations of algorithms. Trademarks are concerned with symbols of good will in a business, such as brand names and logos. Copyrights are concerned with the unique artistic expression of an author or artist. A trade secret is "know-how" that is protected only so long as it actually remains a secret.

Intellectual property is increasingly viewed as an asset, a tradable piece of property. There is clearly some value attached to intellectual property, just as there is value attached to a physical asset such as land. However, just as land by itself usually has little economic value unless there is development, intellectual property or "IP" has value only when the underlying work is being developed and commercialized. In this book, we are primarily concerned with patents, which comprise a set of laws and legal documents that protect new and useful discoveries and inventions in most countries of the world. Specifically, each country has its own patent laws, which allow for the development and commercialization of innovative products. The perceived "market" value is based on the status of development of products, size of market, strength of particular intellectual property to block market access, and many other parameters. Thus, there is intrinsic value in registering and holding intellectual property.

What are the different types of registered intellectual property?

- Patents,
- Trademarks,
- Copyright,
- Trade secrets.

3.2   Patents and patent rights

Patents are a widely used form of intellectual property registration to capture the value of a discovery, invention, or innovation, and are particularly important in the commercialization of biomedical technologies. In exchange for disclosing an invention to the public, so that it can be made, used, and improved upon, the inventor or patent holder receives protection for the invention, for a limited period of time. For the life of the patent, the patent holder can exclusively control how the invention is made, used, and sold.

3.2.1   Patent rights

In the United States, a patent is a property right granted by the government to an inventor "to exclude others from making, using, offering for sale, or selling the invention throughout the United States or importing the invention into the United States" for a limited time in exchange for public disclosure of the invention when the patent is granted. Issuance of patent rights is, in effect, the granting of a limited monopoly on the market by the government in exchange for full disclosure of the detailed invention and subsequent innovation (reduction to practice of the invention and its application). The advantage to society is the dissemination to the public of the detailed methods by which the invention works and this stimulates the further development of new technology based on this invention. Thus, societies that protect inventors with patents have an opportunity to advance rapidly in science and technology applications.

3.3 Types of patent

3.3.1 Utility patents

This is the most common type of patent; it is filed to protect the way something is made, how a tool or device operates, or how a process can accomplish some useful purpose. Improvements, or any combination of these, are also filed as utility patents. In the broadest sense, a discovery or invention is patentable when it is new, useful, and non-obvious. Among other things, a patent includes a specification, which describes the invention, and a set of claims, which defines the legal boundaries of what the patent protects.

For example, pharmaceutical product patents could include a composition of matter, describing the possible combinations of new chemical compounds that could be used to make the invented drug for the purpose of treating a disease; device patents could include construction of a device, composition of matter of new materials and specific applications of the device; biological drug patents would typically include the process of manufacture of a protein, the engineered protein-producing organism, and any final delivery modifications to the protein as the functional aspect of the protein (its 3-D shape) is not easy to characterize.

Biomedical utility patents can be classified in popular terms (this terminology is not recognized by the USPTO) into the following three types:

(1) *Composition of matter* – where a new composition of a gene or protein that has been isolated and sequenced, or a newly synthesized pharmaceutical drug molecule composition, is claimed for use as a drug, a drug target, a diagnostic, a screening assay; or other application. A composition of matter is patented for all of its uses, whether now known or developed later – so long as the composition has a practical use when the patent is applied for.

(2) *Application or method of treatment* – methods of treating patients with a given disease through the use of a particular gene or protein, or through targeting a gene or protein with a drug. Even if a patent on the gene or protein is already granted, if a new use is discovered, a new patent can be filed on that later invention.

(3) *Device or machine* – where a new machine or medical device is developed to treat a disease, including how the device is engineered and how it is used.

3.3.2   Design patents

This is a patent for a new, original, and ornamental design for an article of manufacture.

3.3.3   Plant patents

Patents can be granted for asexually reproduced plant varieties by design and plant patents.

3.4   What can and cannot be patented?

3.4.1   What cannot be patented (from the US PTO website)

Laws of nature, physical phenomena, abstract ideas, literary, dramatic, musical, and artistic works (these can be copyright protected) cannot be patented. Neither can inventions which are:

- Not useful (such as perpetual motion machines); or
- Offensive to public morality.

3.4.2   Can living things be patented?

The following subsection is reproduced by permission from the Biotechnology Industry Organization website, www.bio.org/ip/primer.

Some living things can be patented, but not all. Like any invention, a living thing must be "new" in order to be patented. More importantly, living organisms under consideration for patenting cannot be those that occur or exist in nature. Thus, one cannot obtain a patent on just any living creature, such as a mouse, because mice have been around for a long time. If someone makes a kind of mouse that never existed before, however, then that kind of mouse might be patented.

> *Microbes* As long ago as 1873, Louis Pasteur received a US patent for yeast "free from organic germs or disease." With the growth of genetic engineering in the late 1970s, the patentability of living organisms was re-examined, and confirmed. A landmark case involved Ananda Chakrabarty's invention of a new bacterium genetically engineered to degrade crude oil. In 1980, the Supreme Court clearly stated that new micro-organisms not found in nature, such as Chakrabarty's bacterium, were patentable. Chakrabarty received a patent in 1981 (US Pat. No. 4 259 444). In the Chakrabarty decision, the Supreme Court stated that "anything under the sun that is made by the

hand of man" is patentable subject matter. Therefore, if a product of nature is new, useful and non-obvious, it can be patented if it has been fashioned by human beings.

Plants In 1930, the US Congress passed the Plant Patent Act, which specifically provides patent protection for newly invented plants that are asexually reproduced. In 1970, Congress provided similar protection for newly invented sexually reproduced plants.

Animals In the 1980s, the question of whether multicellular animals could be patented was examined. The key case involved a new kind of "polyploid" oyster that had an extra set of chromosomes. This new, sterile, oyster was edible all year round because it did not devote body weight to reproduction during the breeding season. The PTO found that such organisms were in fact new and, therefore, eligible for patenting. It found this particular type of oyster to be obvious, however, and thus did not allow a patent for it. Nonetheless, the polyploid oyster paved the way for the patenting of other non-naturally occurring animals. In 1988, Philip Leder and Timothy Stewart were granted a patent on transgenic non-human mammals (US Pat. No. 4 736 866) that covered the so-called Harvard mouse, which was genetically engineered to be a model for the study of cancer.

Natural compounds Natural compounds, such as a human protein or the chemical that gives strawberries their distinctive flavor, are not themselves living, but occur in nature. Thus, they are new and can be patented only if they are somehow removed from nature. Therefore, a compound that is purified away from a strawberry, or a protein that is purified away from the human body can be patented in its purified state. Such a patent would not cover the strawberry or the person.

The human body at the various stages of its formation and development, and the simple discovery of one of its elements ... *cannot* constitute patentable inventions. *The US PTO does not allow anyone to patent a human being under any circumstance.* An element *isolated* from the human body or otherwise produced by means of a technical process, including the sequence or partial sequence of a gene, may constitute a patentable invention, even if the structure of that element is identical to that of a natural element. Criteria of novelty, non-obviousness, etc., still need to be satisfied. As techniques to isolate and sequence DNA and deduce function based on similarity to other genes are becoming more and more commonplace, the US PTO looks at whether the invention is novel and includes an inventive step (is non-obvious), plus other criteria to determine patentability. Among these important criteria are that the patent disclosure provides a written description and an enabling disclosure, sufficient for persons of ordinary skill in the relevant field to make and use the invention. The disclosure must also include the "best mode" for practising the invention that is known to the inventors, at the time they apply for the patent.

3.4.3   What type of invention or discovery is patentable?

Patents are filed with government agencies and their patent examiners evaluate, issue, and register patent rights. These agencies evaluate the validity of an application based on the following criteria (from the US Patent and Trademark Office criteria; similar criteria are used by other governments). Any invention or discovery that is the subject of the patent application, therefore, must have the following characteristics covered in the application:

- Novel (not previously known, used, sold, on sale, marketed, or publicized),
- Utility (useful task, some use for invention),
- Unobvious to person with knowledge in the field,
- Adequately described to public at time of filing,
- Enable a person with knowledge in the field to make and use it,
- Best mode or effective mode must be disclosed,
- Described in clear, unambiguous, and definite terms.

3.5   Protecting intellectual property by filing a patent

3.5.1   How long do issued patents last in the USA?

- Utility and plant patents;
  - Twenty years from the application date,
  - The term of the patent (the right to enforce) begins with the date of the grant and usually ends 20 years from the date you first applied for the patent,
  - This is subject to the payment of appropriate maintenance fees.
- Design patents;
  - Fourteen years from the application date,
  - The term begins from the date you are granted the patent,
  - No maintenance fees are required for design patents.

Note: Pharmaceutical and some device patents have mechanisms by which the patent term can be extended beyond the standard 20 year term. This is a complex issue, depending on specific regulations and circumstances that vary with context and over time, and thus is not discussed further in this book. For further information refer to the Hatch–Waxman Act and a legal counsel versed in regulatory affairs.

3.5.2   How much does it cost to get a patent?

Total government filing fees (in 2006) for issued patents are approximately $2370 (depending on the number of claims and other factors); and $1250 for small business entities (fees are discounted for a qualified "small entity.")

Maintenance fees (in 2006) over the life of patent are about $6500 and $3200 for small business entities.

Typical legal fees to write the first patent application are $5000 to $15 000.

Foreign filing fees – Asia, Europe, S. America, etc., depending on the countries chosen, can range from $30 000 to $50 000 plus lawyer's and translation fees ranging from $40 000 to $80 000.

3.5.3 Considerations before filing a patent

What are the steps involved in capturing an idea and defining it as new intellectual property? Table 3.1 summarizes the process for three different entities, including individual inventors.

Table 3.1 Steps to consider before filing a patent for academics, corporate scientists, or independent inventors

Process steps	Independent inventor	Academic investigator (PI)	Corporate scientist or inventor
Confirm novelty of idea	Search USPTO and EPO websites and conference proceedings, papers, etc.	Search USPTO and EPO websites and conference proceedings, papers, etc.	Search USPTO and EPO websites and conference proceedings, papers, etc.
File disclosure before publishing anywhere	Find a good lawyer and discuss process with them – read other similar patents	With technology transfer office (OTT) of university	Through supervisor, to chief scientist, technology officer or other designated person
Confirm business case – decision to file patent (section below has more details)	Market research activities	PI should write up commercial significance in disclosure to guide OTT personnel in their market research	Depends on company process but often the scientist has to write up preliminary business potential (impact) in disclosure. Commercial, scientific executive committee will make decision to invest in patent
Patent filing	Typically a provisional patent is filed to allow time for further investigation of commercial potential or feasibility	Typically a provisional patent is filed to allow time for further investigation of commercial potential or feasibility	Typically a provisional patent is filed to allow time for further investigation of commercial potential or feasibility
Patent prosecution	Monitor and pay fees	May be asked to comment on technical issues as patent is prosecuted by law firm	May be asked to comment on technical issues as patent is prosecuted by law firm

Considerations before filing patents

- Cost;
  - A decision to file a patent is an investment decision.
- Ability to obtain and enforce;
  - How clear is the patent space for your invention and are you likely to be able to find a way to enforce the patent in the future?
- Business need for exclusivity;
  - This is a key point in filing decisions: will your business be helped with this patent, do you really need the market exclusivity that a patent provides? Is there likely to be much competition and can your product be easily copied or re-engineered?
- Return on investment;
  - Finally, when can you gain a return that justifies the cost and time to file? A business decision must be made and evaluated at each stage in the prosecution (as described below in detail).

3.5.4   Steps to prepare a patent filing

(1) Search for keywords describing your idea among existing patents and published patent applications at the US PTO or the European Patent Office websites (www.uspto.gov or www.epo.org) or in your local public library. Once you have determined that your idea has not been covered by other patents, you can move onto the next search for prior art. The comparison of your invention to prior patents or to the literature can be complex, and includes factual and legal considerations. For example, the legal meaning of terms in the claims of a patent has to be determined before a proper comparison can be made. Typically this is an exercise to be done in consultation with a patent attorney.

(2) Find out if any prior art exists – make at least a preliminary search on conference abstracts, or scientific or technical publications where your idea might have been published by someone else. If you do not find any, you can move ahead to prepare and file a provisional application.

(3) Choose an attorney (unless you are doing it yourself) and file a provisional patent or a non-provisional application (see later sections for more details on patent prosecution) after consultation.

(4) Post-grant, actively monitor for infringement by others and enforce your patent rights.

The next few sections discuss, in more detail, some specific considerations before applying for a patent and details on the prosecution of patents world-wide.

3.5.5   What is in a patent? How to read an issued patent

The best way to prepare a patent is to read a few patents thoroughly, particularly patents in the same or a related field. (You will also have to disclose to the US PTO the closest prior art that is known to you, including patents by others that are background for your work). Also, to determine whether one has freedom to operate or to evaluate the extent of other patents, it is important to know the significance of the various parts of a published patent and this will be instructive in learning how to read a patent.

Patents are composed of four main sections:

Face page this normally contains the patent number, dates of issue and application, inventors, assignees (owners of the patent rights at time of issuance), abstract and title of the patent, and other miscellaneous information. This important information includes the application date and the issue date (from which one can determine the remaining term of the patent), the inventors, and, most importantly, the assignee (the owner of the patent rights).

Claims This section tells you specifically and pointedly what invention is made and claimed for protection under the patent laws. The claims consist of independent claims (these have no reference to any other claim in that patent and can stand alone) and dependent claims. Even if the independent claim may be found to be invalid, the dependent claims may still be allowed, as they may include additional features that allow the prior art. A dependent claim adds one or more features to the independent claim to which it refers. For example, if a chair per se were patentable, an independent claim might be: "(1) A chair comprising at least three legs." A dependent claim might be: "(2) A chair as in claim 1, having four legs and further comprising a cushion and a seat back." Thus, if an independent claim is patentable (new and non-obvious), its dependent claims will also be patentable (because adding features cannot take away the novelty or make the invention obvious). The language in the patent claims is critical to legal definition and defense of the patent holders' rights. The use and interpretation of even a single word can change the legal rights of the patent holder as seen in the example in Box 3.1. This is one important reason to have a lawyer experienced in patent prosecution construct the final patent and claims.

Description This section adds further detail to the claims by virtue of examples and background. This section is very important as it is often used by the examiner to determine patentability and the meaning and scope of the claims. Also, the claims may be modified after the patent applied for, if supported by content in the description, but the description cannot be modified once it is filed. (In special circumstances, the claims may be amended after the patent is granted, in what is called a "reissue" proceeding.) The *description and specifications* must be carefully drafted and reviewed to support the claims and scope of the invention (see Box 3.1).

Drawings these could be images, photos of gels, schematics, process flow diagrams, or graphs of data. They help to convey more specifics of the invention and help to substantiate the application of the invention.

Box 3.1 Why you need legal counsel in writing a patent

An inadvertent choice of words that may seem innocuous in regular spoken or written language can have different meanings and significance in a legal context and may end up reducing the scope of the claimed invention and its uses and, thus, also reduce the subsequent commercial value of a patent. This example serves to highlight the reason why a well written patent is key to commercialization.

An inventor in a university isolated and discovered a novel protein that seemed to have significant application in curing a major cardiovascular disease. Patents to the invention of isolating and preparing the specific protein were filed by the university, claiming the specific sequence, subsets of the protein (active sites), and DNA, antibodies, etc., resulting in a patent family of over five patents. Company A licensed in the patents that were filed by the university, gaining exclusive rights to the patented technologies, thus ensuring that no one else could use that isolated protein to develop drugs (synthetic small molecules or antibodies) against that target. Drugs targeting that protein were then developed in the Company A over many years, requiring significant investment (millions of dollars), on the presumed strength of the patent around the target and on subsequent patents on the composition of matter of new small molecules developed by the company. The market was predicted to be greater than $800 million per year for a successful drug against that target. Six years later, Company A discovered that Company B was also developing drugs against that same target, obviously making and using the target protein to identify the drug and potentially infringing the exclusively licensed patent on the target protein. Company A wrote a letter alerting Company B of its patents and asking them for an explanation. Company B wrote back stating that they were not infringing the patent, because they were making and using a fragment or a subset of the protein (an active site peptide). A closer review by Company A's attorney (a different attorney from the one who filed the patent) revealed the surprising news that in fact, Company B might be right. The patent claims used the wording "consisting of" when claiming and identifying specific subset sequences of the protein. For example, one of the key claims read: "The protein claimed in claim 1, which *consists of* sequence 1 or sequence 2, etc., ..." Company B was making a peptide of the active site of the protein (relevant for analyzing drug targeting activity) that had a few more amino acids than those listed in the subset sequence 1 of the claimed protein.

Anyone who made a peptide that had one or more amino acids than the specified sequence 1 would literally not be infringing the patent (see section 3.3.10 for more details on infringement). Company A would then have to argue in court, if possible, that Company B's peptide is a legal "equivalent" to what was claimed – an exercise with an uncertain outcome. It would have been better to have sought broader patent claims in the first place. In this example, Company

> **Box 3.1** (cont.)
>
> A learned that it would have been far better to use the phrase "comprising" rather than the restrictive phrase "consisting of." The broader language could have included peptides that were longer than the reported Company A sequence 1, such as Company B's peptides. In other words, the patent claims in this simple example turned out to be too easy to design around. This subtle difference in claim-drafting language, that was not a significant difference in normal conversational usage or to an untrained person, had significant implications for Company A. Company A potentially lost the opportunity (at least the inexpensive negotiated option, rather than the expensive and uncertain option of going to court) to block, clearly and unambiguously, a competitor drug developer who was using the patented technology (in spirit, if not in the letter).
>
> In general, the term "consisting of" is more restrictive on the scope of the patent claims than the term "consisting essentially of," which, in turn, is more restrictive than the term "comprising." The goal of the inventor is to claim the broadest possible scope of their invention and it is the job of the patent office in turn to try to use the most precise language to describe the invention. This example highlights the need to use trained patent counsel in the writing and prosecution of a patent.

3.5.6 Provisional patent application

Typically, one would file a provisional patent (filing fee $200 ($100 for small entities) as of 1st January 2006), which can contain just the description of the invention, without any specific format or any claims specified. One year from this submission, if you decide not to file a full patent application (non-provisional application) based on the provisional patent, then the provisional patent lapses and is discarded. You have lost this priority date (see below) for the application. Most people use the one-year period to find a licensee and justify the costs of filing a full patent application, and better evaluate commercialization prospects of the invention. The provisional patent also equalizes the international playing field, as foreign inventors have one year after filing of the patents in their countries to file applications in the USA. To benefit from the priority date, the content of the provisional patent application has to support the claims of the final application, so it is important to review the wording of the invention results or scientific experiment results discussed in this provisional application prior to submission.

3.5.7 Priority date and publicizing inventions

The priority date sets the date from which patent validity can be contested. That is, the patent cannot be invalidated by any publications dated after the priority date;

however, this rule is different in the USA, it allows a one-year grace period for certain prior art. If the priority date for a patent is set at 28 July 2005, then, for the USA, only publications dated before 28 July 2004 will be considered as prior art. In the rest of the world, publications dated before 28 July 2005 are considered prior art that would invalidate the patent. So, in the USA, inventors have one year from the date of publication of a reference to file a patent, but international rights are lost at the time of publication if a US or other patent is not filed. Prior art in the USA means that the patented invention was not original because it was disclosed publicly more than one year before the application was filed.

The USA also follows a first-to-invent rule (current practice as of December 2007). In the USA, the *first to invent* has priority to the patent rights, whereas in the rest of the world, the *first to file* decides the priority rights to patent the invention. This means that competing inventors with close patent application dates will have an "interference" proceeding in the USA, to determine who actually was first. In the rest of the world, the first to file a patent application will get the patent, even if he or she was the second to invent.

How is the priority date set?

A priority date is set by the date a patent application is filed with the US PTO (provisional or non-provisional). For example, if a provisional application is filed on 2 June 2004, and then subsequently a full patent application is filed before 2 June 2005, the issued patent will then acquire the priority date of the provisional filing – 2 June 2004. This assumes that the full patent application claims are covered by the content of the provisional patent. If a non-provisional full application is filed directly, then that date of filing becomes the priority date. An application can also be filed in a foreign country that has a reciprocal treaty with the USA, so that a US application may have the benefit of an earlier foreign filing (if the US application is filed within one year of the foreign application). Most countries are members of the Patent Cooperation Treaty (PCT), which provides rules for a filing on one country to have effect in all member countries (see section 3.3.8 for details on the PCT).

Why is the date of invention important?

If during prosecution (review and decision making by US PTO), two or more patent applications claim essentially the same patentable invention, a patent can be assigned to only one inventor. The US PTO then initiates proceedings known as "interference" to determine who is the first inventor and entitled to the patent. In the USA, the first to invent gets priority over others. Therefore, good practices in keeping laboratory or invention records are critical to establish the date of invention, which may have occurred many months before the filing of a provisional or non-provisional patent application. Typically, invention records should be corroborated by at least one person who is not an inventor, and is under an obligation to keep the invention secret before the patent application is filed (see details below on recording an invention).

Box 3.2 Importance of recording date of invention – case study

Dr. Wall, a dentist, read about balloon angioplasty in 1981 and figured that the arteries would be prone to reclosure, so he sketched out some drawings for a slotted metal sleeve and sent the drawings to his attorney. The original drawings established a date of invention that could be worth a lot of money today, as Dr. Wall claims that the stents being sold in the $5 billion (and growing) market infringe his patent. The date on the first drawings was October 15, 1984. Companies did not show much interest in his idea then. Then he read about Dr. Palmaz' stent being tested in 1987 by Johnson & Johnson and filed his patent on December 8, 1987. Discussions with one company ended with the company licensing in someone else's (Palmaz's) issued patent instead of Dr. Wall's. Dr. Wall instituted interference proceedings that lasted for years, lengthened partly by personal events. After a rejection by the US PTO in 1995, he filed an appeal in the US Circuit court but failed to make timely filings and the court dismissed the case without a hearing and returned it to the US PTO. The US PTO never sent Dr. Wall an official notice and various efforts to find the application in their records had no results. Then, in 2002, the application appeared on a new computerized US PTO database. Dr. Wall redrafted claims that survived the interference proceedings and his petition to reopen the application was accepted by the US PTO. Patent No. 6 974 475 was granted in December 2005. According to Winslow (2006).

"The heart of their case was a 108-page document called a swearback, in which inventors seek to establish they were first with an invention based not on the original filing date, but on the earlier moment when their idea was fully developed. Dr. Wall amassed phone records, affidavits, and drawings that persuaded the patent office that his invention dated to October 15, 1984, beating the date Dr. Wall says the patent office ascribed to the Palmaz stent – November 25, 1984 – by about six weeks."

This interesting story highlights the intricate workings of the patent office and the importance of properly recording the date of an invention.

An example of a patent infringement lawsuit that was based on the establishment of an earlier date of invention is discussed in Box 3.2

What can you do to record the date of invention?

Record your ideas, experiments, thoughts, and any evidence such as photos in a bound laboratory notebook with numbered pages. Invention is a conception or an idea, not just data from experiments, so ideas must be entered in the laboratory notebook. Record contributions made in group discussions to help identify claims of inventorship. Cross out errors instead of erasing. Date each page in the book and have a witness (not a co-inventor) initial or sign each page. No pages should be removed from the book and blank pages should be crossed out and dated.

As electronic record keeping increases, methods have been developed to record, date, and authenticate computer files, e.g., electronic lab notebooks. A knowledgeable attorney should be consulted regarding electronic record and document retention procedures.

3.5.8   International patent filings and the Patent Cooperation Treaty (PCT) process

The PCT is an international treaty, administered by the World Intellectual Property Organization (WIPO), and signed by more than 125 Paris Convention countries (see www.wipo.org). The PCT makes it possible to seek patent protection for an invention simultaneously in each of a large number of countries by filing a single "international" patent application instead of several separate national or regional patent applications. The granting of patents remains under the control of the national or regional patent offices in what is called the "national phase."

Briefly, an outline of the PCT procedure includes the following steps:

Filing   You file an international application, complying with the PCT formality requirements, in one language, and you pay one set of fees.

International search   An "International Searching Authority (ISA)" (housed by one of the world's major patent offices) identifies the published documents which may have an influence on whether your invention is patentable and establishes an opinion on your invention's potential patentability.

International publication   As soon as possible after the expiration of 18 months from the earliest filing date, the content of your international application is disclosed to the world.

International preliminary examination   An "International Preliminary Examining Authority (IPEA)" (one of the world's major patent offices), at your request, carries out an additional patentability analysis, usually on an amended version of your application.

National phase   After the end of the PCT procedure, you start to pursue the grant of your patents directly before the national (or regional) patent offices of the countries in which you want to obtain them.

The next section puts this international process in perspective with respect to the timelines and steps in the patent prosecution process in the USA.

3.5.9   Patent prosecution process

Typical patent processing time line (see Figure 3.1):

Step 1   Document your invention – the invention date is important, and is critical in the US, as the person first to invent (date recorded in lab. note book for example) has priority to patent rights. In the rest of the world, the first to file has a claim to the rights.

Step 2   File provisional patent with US PTO. The clock starts ticking on any patent that might issue from this "priority date." For international patents, you

Patent prosecution

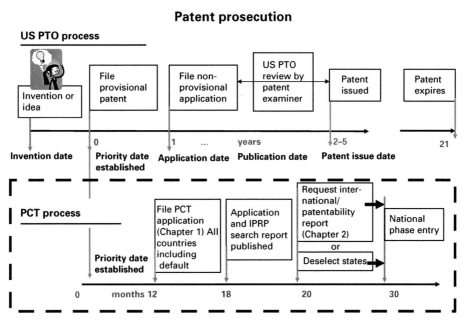

Figure 3.1   Steps for filing and prosecuting patents in the US and through the PCT process.

have one year from this date to submit a full application in other countries through
the PCT process.

Step 3   One year after the provisional filing, submit a full, non-provisional patent
application to the US PTO. Simultaneously, submit a PCT application to a
receiving office (in this case, the US PTO). Since January 2004, all PCT applications
by default include all countries. Selection of specific countries is done later. The
application is now in Chapter I of the PCT process. The PCT application can
usually claim the US-based priority date in most countries.

Step 4   Applications get published and are available for public review typically 18
months after application date. For PCT filing, an International Searching
Authority, typically an examiner in the receiving country patent office, conducts a
search and issues an International Preliminary Report on Patentability (IPRP).
The search results are also published. Chapter I lasts for 30 months with no further
action after unless Chapter II is selected by filing a demand. Meanwhile, at the US
PTO, patents are under review and communications from patent examiners have to
be addressed and claims adjusted.

Step 5   At eight months after PCT submission (20 months from priority date),
the applicant has to select the final countries desired for final filing (national phase
in each country). If demand for Chapter II is filed, a substantive examination
report will be prepared, taking applicants' comments (if any) into consideration.
This step might be helpful in speeding up national prosecution in the receiving
or home country as the examiner is usually the same person in PCT and in the
receiving office.

Step 6   At 30 months from submission into the PCT process (or from the claimed priority date), the patent enters national phase filing in the countries that were finally selected. Fees for individual countries (translations, filing fees, lawyers fees) become due when national phase applications are filed.

Step 7   US patents are issued between two and five years from the initial application, depending on the backlog at the Patent Office and the specific issues in the application. In recent years, the average time for first patentability review by examiner has been about 20 months from filing and the average time for issuance of a patent has been 30 months.

3.5.10   Rough estimate of patent costs for project budgets

Direct costs for IP are composed of legal costs (fees charged by patent lawyer or agent) plus filing fees paid to the government to register and maintain the patents.

Depending on the amount of work put into the project, the legal fees to file a provisional patent can range from $500–$15 000. If a provisional patent filing has high legal fees, there should be a correspondingly lower cost at the time of filing the full non-provisional patent, as most of the work in writing the patent has been done at the provisional stage. However, additional work done by the inventors during the one year between provisional and regular filings can be added to the application. This would of course increase the costs for preparing the application.

Year 1:   ~$500–$15 000 (typically ~$5000): costs for filing a provisional patent depend on the complexity of the technology, the length and depth of the disclosure, the amount of rewriting by lawyer, drafting claims, etc.

Year 2: $10 000–$18 000: non-provisional filing and PCT application filed. The cost depends on the complexity of the patent, the number of claims, etc. Application filing fees have to be paid to the US PTO (check www.uspto.gov for latest fee schedules).

Year 3: $8000–$15 000: continuing fees paid to the US PTO are due for prosecuting the application to obtain the patent.

Year 4 and on: $25 000 (at least 10 countries included) – $175 000: the cost depends on the countries designated for PCT filings. This estimate includes legal fees and government registration or filing fees in about 12 countries.

3.6   Patent infringement and freedom to operate

3.6.1   Patent infringement and protecting your rights

Patents give you the right to block anyone else from selling your invention in the market. Your rights in this regard are limited to the legal boundaries of the country that has granted the patent. Others can infringe your patent if they make, use, or sell the invention specified by the claims of the patent; for example, if they sell a product that has your patented composition of matter in the product. If you have a method-of-use patent that identifies and claims a specific protein as a drug target to treat a disease, anyone who uses that protein target to develop a drug for that disease without your permission can be held in infringement of the patent.

There are two main ways to examine whether someone is infringing your patent or you are infringing someone's patent:

(1) Literal infringement – someone's activities can be seen specifically to infringe on the claims of the patent, literally, i.e., according to the terms of the claims (as properly interpreted according to the patent laws for claim construction). For example, if the drug sold has exactly the formula described in one of the claims in an issued patent, then it is a literal infringement. If the protein being sold by someone has exactly the same amino acid sequence as listed in one of the claims, then it is an infringement.

(2) Doctrine of equivalents – a patent claim that is not literally infringed may be infringed if the accused product or method is legally "equivalent" to what is literally claimed. This is in the grey area, where you believe someone is infringing on the spirit of the patent. If the difference between what is being claimed and what is accused of infringement is not substantial (i.e., it uses substantially the same way to achieve substantially the same result), then there may still be infringement (provided the slightly different methods or materials have not otherwise been disclaimed). In the above example, if the infringer is selling a drug with a subtle twist on the composition to skirt the formula laid out in the claim and still attains the same results, you could argue in the courts that it is equivalent to your composition and the person is infringing. This is a complex argument that relies on prior cases and should be reviewed by an experienced patent infringement lawyer. In general, the literal infringement case is much stronger, and the outcome of arguing equivalents in infringement is largely dependent on the context of the case and the perspective of the judge.

Probably the most contentious area in patent infringement lawsuits is the ability to establish intent to infringe on your patent rights, or "willful infringement," which can result in enhanced damages, up to treble the amount of the actual damage from the infringement. (Intent is not required to prove infringement; only to recover enhanced damages.)

Infringement lawsuits are also very expensive to fight, owing to the legal and technical expertise involved. However, the awards in infringement lawsuits can be very high with one of the highest being the suit between Polaroid and Eastman Kodak in which Polaroid secured a $925 million judgement against Eastman Kodak in 1990. The drug and device industries value patents and have had their share of patent disputes in the past and continuing to the present date.

Owing to the high cost, complexity, and level of technical expertise (both in technology and legal process) involved, taking on a patent infringement issue needs careful planning. It is a good idea to check the validity of the patents (held by the plaintiff) before embarking further into the process. An issued patent can still be ruled invalid and the patent that is being infringed will be tested in court by the defendant, so it is a good idea to run a validity check. If the particular action or product is in direct literal infringement, the case can be put together with more confidence. The main issues remaining then relate to the extent of damages (see Section 3.8.2 and Box 3.8 for more details on determining damages) claimed by the plaintiff and the possibility of establishing willful infringement.

On the other hand, if the infringement is not literal (making, using, or selling a product that is not exactly the same as that claimed or described in the patent), the next step is to put together a complete enforcement plan. In most cases (even in the case of literal infringement), this is probably a good step to take, in order to clarify and get agreement on approaches towards other potential infringers. A good legal team from one or more firms that have no conflicts with the potential infringing parties must be put together so that there is a consistency in the approach through the process.

3.6.2 "Freedom to practice" or "freedom to operate"

A patent allows the holder of the patent to stop others from commercializing products based on the patented invention. However, a single patent may not be sufficient to allow one to develop and sell a product based on the single patent (see example in Box 3.3). For example, a patent holder may have a claim to a drug compound with a known mechanism of action in the body to treat immunology diseases. If someone else discovers a new mechanism by which that drug can treat cardiovascular diseases, they can patent that invention as a novel finding. The primary patent holder now does not have freedom to operate in the cardiovascular area, but can continue to sell the drug for immunology diseases. The holders of the patent for cardiovascular application of the drug also do not have freedom to operate, as they cannot sell the drug until they obtain a license for the drug compound from the primary patent holder.

This means that the holders of a key patent have to make sure that they have the freedom to practice the patented technology in all commercial applications claimed. To make sure that the path to market is clear and protected for the final product, the manufacturer may need to license or own additional patents, in addition to the original invention patent on which basis the product was developed. Typically, when licensing in or buying or selling patents, a "freedom to operate" statement should be sought from a lawyer, establishing the ability to commercialize and capture the value of the patent. Note that this is not risk free, because no freedom to operate search can be guaranteed to uncover every unexpired patent that may be relevant. As a matter of prudence, a pragmatic and reasonable search and analysis should be made, to support a business case for going forward.

If you know about a patent that may "block" your commercialization plans, US law requires a diligent inquiry to investigate whether that patent is infringed or is invalid. Typically, this involves obtaining the opinion of an attorney that the patent is not infringed or is not valid before going forward. Although an attorney opinion

---

Box 3.3 Freedom to operate (case examples)

An example in drug development: if a drug targets the active site of protein X and thus treats a disease or its symptoms, the inventors of the drug can file a patent for composition of matter of the drug, protecting its chemical structure and claiming it as a likely treatment for the disease. That patent may be issued on the merit that the novel composition of matter showed the inventive step and the data in the patent showed the useful step of disease treatment.

However, if some other inventors had found earlier that specifically targeting a ligand to the active site of protein X can successfully treat the disease or its symptoms, they too can potentially be issued a patent claiming that *any* specific ligand for protein X can treat that disease, with some example drugs used to validate and reinforce the claim (not including the novel drug mentioned above). Therefore, the developers of the newly patented drug compound cannot sell their drug in the market to treat this disease unless they have licensed or otherwise obtained rights to the method of use patent described above. Another option would be for either party (typically the holders of the composition of matter patent) to challenge the validity of the other patent in court. Thus, someone buying the company would be well advised to review existing patents or patent applications and check whether the value of the drug compound patent may be compromised by any other patents.

A famous example of the issues that emerge in evaluating freedom to operate can be seen in the Amgen erythropoietin (EPO) patent battle. Erythropoietin is a natural hormone that prevents anemia. Amgen was able to clone and isolate EPO and then transform Chinese hamster ovary (CHO) cells to produce biologically active EPO. Amgen filed for a patent on the vector (the vehicle for inserting the EPO gene into the CHO cell) and the transformed cell (which could be patented, as it was viewed as an engineered production 'machine' for the EPO protein). Amgen also filed for a patent on the EPO protein itself and the process of producing it commercially. The vector and cell patent was allowed but the process patent was denied as it was judged to be "obvious" and, therefore, non-patentable, and the EPO product patent was rejected as a prior patent on EPO had been issued to the Genetics Institute, who had isolated and purified EPO before Amgen. The Genetics Institute had received a patent for human EPO and for pharmaceutical compositions containing EPO but their method of production was to isolate it from urine, making it commercially unviable to produce the quantities needed for therapy. Amgen's patent for the mode of production of EPO made it commercially viable to produce and sell but the Genetics Institute's patent on EPO made it illegal for Amgen to utilize the starting materials to actually produce EPO. Thus neither company (patents) had freedom to operate in the commercialization of EPO. This is a situation that called for a cross-license, allowing both firms to access the market. However,

---

Box 3.3 (cont.)

Amgen and the Genetics Institute fought it out in court in a very expensive and long patent battle, with Amgen eventually winning the case and the Genetic Institute patent being found invalid as it had failed to demonstrate just how it made the purified form of EPO from human urine. During the course of this legal infringement battle, both firms brought their products to market through FDA approval and continued to ramp up revenues. The courts refused to put an injunction on the life-saving medicine.

---

is not strictly required, it is recommended as a traditional way to address potentially complex and difficult patent issues. Going forward without a good faith inquiry, or ignoring the results, could cause serious problems of liability and exposure for patent infringement later on.

3.7   Trademarks

Trademarks are usually some combination of words, phrases, symbols, or designs that identifies and distinguishes the source of the goods of one party from those of others. For example, the colors, font, placement, and other features of the Becton–Dickinson logo 🌀 **BD** are owned by the Becton–Dickinson Company. Similarly, the combination of words that make the product name BD Fluorosensor^{TM} is a trademark owned by Becton–Dickinson. Another example is Lipitor$^®$, a drug name that is trademarked by Pfizer for cholesterol-lowering pharmaceutical preparations. Any representation of this specific product must use the trademarked name precisely as specified by the owner (usually in correct colors, combinations, and order of letters, words, or images).

A service mark is a similar combination of words, phrases, symbols, or designs that identifies and distinguishes the services of one party from those of others.

To claim rights in a mark, use the "TM" (trademark) or "SM" (service mark) designation to alert the public to the claim, regardless of whether an application has been filed with the US PTO. You do not have to register a trademark to use one or have legal claims. Essentially, the first person either to use a mark in commerce or file an intent-to-use application with the US PTO has the ultimate right to the use and registration of a mark. While not required, a trademark registration provides important legal benefits. The federal registration symbol "$®$" can be used only after the US PTO actually registers a mark, and not while an application is pending. Also, the registration symbol with the mark can be used only on or in connection with the goods or services listed in the federal trademark registration. A trademark is renewed every 10 years indefinitely, as long as it is still in use. An intent-to-use application can also be filed to safeguard the trademark before putting it in use.

> **Box 3.4** Trademark disputes (case example)
>
> A famous example of litigation on a trademark is described briefly here. Apple Corps, the record company set up by the Beatles in 1968, took Apple Computer (established 1977) to court over a trademark violation of the use of the name Apple. The two settled in 1981, with the Apple Computer company agreeing not to sell music and settling the dispute with Apple Corps for $25 million. The agreement gave the Apple Computer company rights to the Apple trademark in relation to electronic goods, computers, telecommunications equipment, and data processing equipment. It also allowed for trademark use related to "data transmission services" and "broadcasting services," as well as related promotional merchandising. An additional dispute in 1991, when Apple started making music recordings possible on its computers, ended with another settlement payment to Apple Corps. In 2006, since the Apple Computer company started offering music for downloads on its ITunes website, the Apple Corps took the computer company to court insisting that they were now using the Apple logo and trademark for music, in violation of the 1991 agreement. This case was finally decided in favor of Apple Computer in May 2006.

3.7.1 Why register your trademark?

- Establish ownership, usage and, date of original use,
- Enhanced national exclusivity for use in registered categories – easier to expand business,
- Better legal protection for infringement actions,
- Ability to license trademark.

3.7.2 Filing a trademark with the US PTO

It will cost about $375 (in 2006; $275 for electronic filing) to file an application for use of the trademark in one class of goods or services and additional fees for use in each additional class. If a lawyer is used to file an application, fees can range from $300–$500 for initial application and more if the initial application is challenged by the US PTO.

There is good reason to look for legal assistance on registering trademarks and service marks, because the prosecution process can be quite complex. A trademark is always given for a specific category of goods or services. A trademark holder can use the trademark for several categories but each category of goods would typically require a separate trademark filing. Box 3.4 contains a famous example of a trademark dispute.

3.7.3   International filing of trademarks

The Madrid Agreement and Protocol (effective in the USA from 2003 onwards) allows the US trademark registration to serve as the basis for international coverage in countries party to the Madrid Agreement. A pan-European registration with the European Union is also advisable, as the EU did not sign the Madrid Agreement (although individual countries in the EU did).

3.8   Copyrights

A copyright is a form of protection provided to the authors of "original works of authorship" including literary, dramatic, musical, artistic, and certain other intellectual works, both published and unpublished (www.uspto.gov). The 1976 Copyright Act generally gives the owner of a copyright the exclusive right to reproduce the copyrighted work, to prepare derivative works, to distribute copies or recordings of the copyrighted work, to perform the copyrighted work publicly, or to display the copyrighted work publicly. The copyright protects the form of expression rather than the subject matter of the writing. For example, a description of a machine could be copyrighted, but this would only prevent others from copying the description; it would not prevent others from writing a description of their own or from making and using the machine. Copyrights are registered by the Library of Congress' Copyright Office.

Copyright protection exists from the time the work is created in fixed form. The copyright in the work of authorship immediately becomes the property of the author who created the work and lasts for 70 years after the death of the author.

This topic will not be discussed further here, as copyright protection has limited application in biotechnology. For further details on copyrights and registering copyrights, see www.copyright.gov.

3.9   Trade secrets

Trade secrets are also commonly termed as know-how. Even in a patent or scientific paper where details of a process have to be laid out for anyone to repeat, experienced scientists know that there is an art, a know-how, that is not described in the details. This know-how, if it can be kept a secret, can then build value for a company as its trade secret. However, there are few commercial products where you can sustain a competitive advantage for long by keeping the process or composition of the product a trade secret. The most famous example of a trade secret is the Coca-Cola formula, which has never been patented: workers at the production factories are bound by elaborate agreements and arrangements to keep them from disclosing even the single part of the process they know about.

> **Box 3.5** Trade secrets in drug development
>
> As an example, it is well known that when companies develop crystal structures of drug-targeted proteins, they may publish or patent the crystal structure, but the multiple structures of different proprietary compounds that help them understand how to structure a more potent compound are never published. If the project is to be licensed to a partner for commercialization, the data and tacit knowledge remain a trade secret within the company and have great value as a form of intellectual property – as know-how or a trade secret (data that can help quickly design a potent compound that binds the target protein correctly, eliminating months to years of experimentation).

However, in rapidly moving technology areas like biotechnology or devices, it is rare to be able to sustain an advantage of greater than a year or so by keeping a trade secret (see more discussion in Box 3.5). While trade secrets are not commonly used as the sole means to protect commercialization rights for discoveries or inventions, their use as know-how is increasingly useful in the detailed processes of biopharmaceutical manufacture. Some biopharma companies develop processes that are not disclosed except in FDA filings, which are kept confidential for a number of years. Note, however, that the "best mode" of practising an invention must be included in any patent filed for that invention; it cannot be held back as a trade secret.

3.10 Intellectual property commercialization and technology transfer

3.10.1 Commercial use of intellectual property

Predominantly in the biotechnology industry, and increasingly so in the information industry, business models have revolved around the management of IP rights and the appropriation of maximum value from acquired or developed intellectual property. The limited monopoly granted by a patent gives some degree of assurance of possible revenue streams for a new product, especially products that cost a lot of money and time to bring to market. This reduction of market risk gives rise to a value for the IP itself, a value that is difficult to calculate accurately, but is nonetheless assigned by outside market forces (see additional reading and Section 3.8.2 for more details).

A patent is used to generate revenues (and profits) by building products or blocking others from selling products based on that invention or, in the shorter term, to raise financing, by:

(1) Creating a limited monopoly for the patented product and thus setting a favorable pricing for the duration of the patent term,

(2) Licensing the patent to others who wish to sell the patented product and collecting royalties and payments from them, retaining ownership of the patent,

(3) Selling the patent to someone else (assigning or giving up ownership and all future rights to the patent) in a one-time transaction,

(4) Using the patent position to drive strategic partnerships,

(5) Attracting investment by reassuring investors of future revenues with a strategic patent position,

(6) Getting debt financing on the strength of the value of future revenues to be gained from the patent portfolio (this is a rarely used strategy).

3.10.2   Technology transfer in academic research institutions

While the role and goals of non-profit institutions in commercializing biomedical patents may be questioned, a significant number of breakthrough inventions that have changed and will change markets and technology trajectories continue to be developed at universities or research institutes. Industry has to work with these institutes to gain access to this know-how and turn it into revenue-generating products. Embodying this knowledge (tacit or explicit) in a patent makes one aspect of technology transfer dominate the process – the licensing of patents. However, although easy to overlook, it is important to understand that, in many cases, there exists a know-how that goes beyond the content of the patent. Particularly in those cases, it becomes clear that technology transfer is a "contact sport," wherein scientists from the industrial licensee must interact closely with the inventor-scientist in non-profit organizations. This is the total aspect of technology transfer; not only the transfer of rights to the patented invention but also transferring the more tacit understanding and implementation of all aspects of the invention and technology.

Non-profit academic institutions and for-profit licensees can have inherent misunderstandings as each has a very different context that must be kept in mind as they work together to build value and commercialize inventions (Figure 3.2). It is, thus, critical for both parties to be accommodating, understanding, and, above all, focused on the common goal to successfully work together. Figure 3.2 highlights the different perspectives between the two organizations that come together – one (non-profits) with public good as the driving motive and the other (for-profit small or large corporations) with shareholder profit as the driving motive.

3.10.3   The Bayh–Dole Act

The 1950s–1970s saw an expansion of government R&D and a growth in R&D procurement from universities with increased competition for government research grants. By the late 1970s, there was a recognition of unrealized potential from Government inventions – of 28 000 government patents, only 5% had been licensed. There was little or no uniformity in government intellectual property policies.

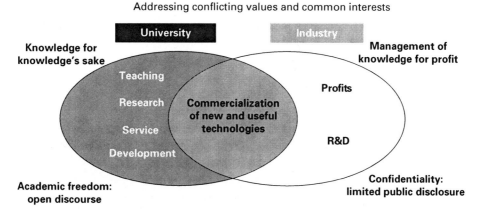

Addressing conflicting values and common interests

Figure 3.2 The difference in perspectives and common interests that intersect in a licensing negotiation between university and industry. Accommodation for each others' perspectives, compromise in terms of engagement, and an understanding of a common goal are required for the two parties to work together successfully. Adapted and reproduced here with permission from Breneman (2003).

In 1980, the Bayh–Dole Act made a fundamental change in this process: title to inventions, made with government funding by small businesses, universities and other non-profit entities, would henceforth belong to those entities, and not to the government. This act also created a uniform intellectual property policy for all government agencies.

However, with these rights to the research institutes came certain duties and obligations:

- Research institutes must file patents on inventions they elect to own,
- There must be a preference for small business licensees,
- Licensed products must be manufactured in the USA,
- Royalties must be;
  – Shared with the inventor, and
  – Used for research and education.
- The government retains non-exclusive right to use the patented technologies for the government's own internal use (this clause may concern some; however, the government seldom manufactures its own products and the government can be a large customer for the manufacturer of the patented technology as they will pay for the products to be made),
- The university has some detailed reporting obligations (e.g., iEdison) on all intellectual property generated with government funding.

Since 1980, many universities and non-profit research institutes have set up offices of technology transfer. Inventions from these institutes have been the source of many successful products that have improved life and health and also contributed to local economic development through the growth of start-up ventures that were built to commercialize specific inventions. Thus, the Bayh–Dole Act has become a landmark act that many other nations are now emulating in the hopes of reaping the same benefits internally.

3.11   Licensing

Patents are assets. Just as land ownership can be converted to cash by leasing rights for development, habitation, or mining, patent rights can be given out. A license is a commercial and legal transaction to transfer patent rights from licensor to licensee. This grant of patent rights is described by a licensing arrangement. The various terms in the license agreement are discussed in detail here.

A commonly asked question: is a contract manufacturer a licensee of my patent?

Since a patent right covers the rights to block someone from making, using, or selling technology based on your patented technology, giving a contract to a manufacturer to make your patented product does imply a limited grant of a license to "make" or "use" your patented technology. However, the terms of this type of license are usually governed by a manufacturing or R&D contract. This type of contract agreement usually explicitly states that all rights to the patent are retained by the contractor.

However, if you wish to ask another party to sell your product in the marketplace and share proceeds with you, it is particularly important to have a written agreement, setting forth the rights of all parties. Such a formal legal agreement would typically grant them a license of your patent rights as appropriate to the joint goals of the parties. For example, the license might be an exclusive grant to a distributor, who would then share in the ability to block commercialization of the patented technology by others. Otherwise, they could technically be in infringement of your patent. Thus, a license to a patent is a way to control the sale of your invention in the market.

Note: when building commercialization strategies around patent rights, you must keep in mind that holding an initial innovation patent may not be sufficient to protect the product in the marketplace and may also not be enough to get the product to market in the face of other existing patents. Investors and business partners should make sure that the due diligence process includes (a) a "freedom to operate" legal opinion on the patent holdings of a new venture as a matter of routine; and (b) an assessment of the scope of your own patent portfolio vis-à-vis potential competitors.

3.11.1   Key non-financial terms of license agreements

The terms of license (commercialization) agreements are influenced significantly by the type of invention or technology and by the needs of the owner of the patent.

Table 3.2 The *grant of rights*

Exclusivity of rights

Exclusive license	Non-exclusive license	Sole license	Partially exclusive license
Only licensee and no one else (including licensor) can commercialize patent	Licensee can commercialize but so can any other licensee or the licensor	Licensor and licensee can both commercialize but licensor will not grant rights to anyone else	Partially exclusive license (Usually limited by territory or field of use) Licensee may have rights to commercialize only in certain applications (e.g., for cancer and not any other disease) or certain countries

Territory and geographic distribution of rights

All-inclusive (world-wide)	Conditional or geographically limited
Licensee has rights in any geographic region (country) in which the patent was issued. This is typically the case for exclusive licenses	Licensee has rights to commercialize or practice the patent in a defined, limited set of countries. Partially exclusive or non-exclusive licenses can use this as one criterion to better control and distribute their patent rights

Field of use

All applications and disease areas	Limited applications and disease areas
All applications included in the patent are typically covered in an exclusive, world-wide license, but the licensor can be creative where appropriate	Licensor can be creative and use segmentation of the license terms in specific therapeutic areas based on licensee expertise or other interests to gain maximum value out of the patent

In general, a license agreement gives the licensee one or more of the following: the rights to make, to use, to have made, or to sell the products based on the patented invention. In consideration of this *grant of rights*, the patent owner is paid by the licensee. The payment terms are the subject of much discussion and debate, as discussed here, but the most important terms in the license agreement are the terms involved in the grant of rights. These include a carefully-worded description of exactly *what rights* are being licensed (patents, trademarks, know-how, etc.), the *field of use* for which the rights are being granted, the *territory* in which the rights are being granted and whether or not the license is to be *exclusive, non-exclusive, or sole*. These types of license are outlined in Table 3.2 and compared in Table 3.3.

It can also be important for a license to specify how the patent rights that are granted can be policed and enforced, for example who can bring a lawsuit for infringement, who pays for litigation, etc.

Table 3.3 Pros and cons of various types of license

Type of license	Pros	Cons
Exclusive license	Greater commitment from licensee Higher fees Higher royalties Closer monitoring of development	Higher risk of failure of product commercialization May be wrong partner or strategy Licensee will typically have single focused market approach, thus not reaching maximum potential of technology before patent runs out Licensee can use exclusivity to block other potentially "good-for-humanity" type development work – the typical goal of the inventor
Non-exclusive or partially exclusive licenses	Several paths to market Several markets addressed simultaneously Increased chances of final commercialization	Multiple market carve-out may raise problems down the road Managing licensees and multiple partnerships may be a challenge Usage is difficult if encumbered by other licensees' efforts, data, or liabilities Lower fees and royalties

Typically, the subject and scope of the license also includes terms that specify rights to any improvements in technology made by the licensee or licensor.

Other terms in the body of the license agreement are important, but these terms are the main defining terms of the license agreement and are also strategically the most important terms for the licensor to decide on a priori. Licenses can be simple or very complex, depending on the circumstances; the examples in Boxes 3.6 and 3.7 are just the tip of the iceberg. Box 3.6 is an example of some terms from a licensing agreement between a university and a company and Box 3.7 contains an example of some terms of a licensing agreement between two commercial organizations.

3.11.2   Financial terms in a license

The various payments by licensees need to be worked through and coming to agreement on these figures can be a rather difficult negotiation in the licensing process. Underlying these discussions of financial terms is the perception of value

---

Box 3.6 Example grant of rights in an exclusive license from university to company

(Note that all capitalized words are defined in specific terms at the beginning of the license agreement document.) A short excerpt from a typical exclusive license given by a University (referred to as "UNIV") to Small Biotech, Inc. ("LICENSEE") for all discoveries related to cancer research from a particular sponsored research agreement, has the following *grant of rights*:

UNIV hereby grants to LICENSEE a royalty-bearing, world-wide, exclusive license under LICENSED SUBJECT MATTER to discover, research, develop, make, have made, use, offer for SALE, SELL, and import LICENSED PRODUCTS for use within LICENSED FIELD. This grant is subject to the payment by LICENSEE to UNIV of all consideration as provided herein (*Note: this consideration usually consists of upfront, milestone, and royalty payments*), and is further subject to rights retained by UNIV to:

(a) publish the general scientific findings from research related to LICENSED SUBJECT MATTER subject to the terms of Article X-X, Confidential Information, provided, however, INVENTOR shall disclose pending publications to LICENSEE in accordance with Section X.X of the SPONSORED RESEARCH AGREEMENT; and

(b) use LICENSED SUBJECT MATTER for research that has not been sponsored by a commercial entity, teaching, and other educationally related purposes. Any transfer of material embodiments of LICENSED SUBJECT MATTER pursuant to this Section X.Xb shall be governed by a material transfer agreement substantially in the form attached hereto as Exhibit X.

Here, the LICENSED SUBJECT MATTER (covering any intellectual findings that may arise in the research area of interest) is defined as:

Inventions, discoveries, assays, and processes covered by PATENT RIGHTS or TECHNOLOGY RIGHTS within LICENSED FIELD.

LICENSED FIELD (defined to restrict the rights of the licensee) is defined as:

... (i) treatment, prevention, diagnosis, or prognosis of solid tumor, sarcoma, skin or blood cancers; and (ii) determination of predisposition to cancer....

and PATENT RIGHTS (specifically written to cover multiple definitions of intellectual property) are defined as:

... UNIV'S rights in information or discoveries covered by a VALID CLAIM ... in patents, or patent applications, whether domestic or foreign, and all divisionals, continuations, continuations-in-part, reissues, re-examinations, or extensions thereof, and any letters patent that issue thereon ...

Additionally, Licensee has rights to sublicense:

X.X LICENSEE may grant sublicenses consistent with this AGREEMENT if LICENSEE is responsible for the operations of its sublicensees relevant to this AGREEMENT as if the operations were carried out by LICENSEE.

Box 3.7 Example grant of rights in co-exclusive license between three companies

In 1997, Angiotech Pharmaceuticals executed a co-exclusive license to Cook Inc. and Boston Scientific (BSC) for its drug, paclitaxel, for use on vascular stents. It retained certain rights for itself. This agreement has since become one of the most famous examples of the convergence of drugs and devices into combination products. The following *grant of rights* illustrates a *co-exclusive license* with all the three parties tied together for successful commercialization.

(Note: words with capitalization of first letters have been formally defined in the beginning of the agreement.)

Grants. Subject to the terms and conditions hereof, the following licenses are granted hereby, each effective as of the date of this Agreement:

(a) BSC Technology License ... Angiotech hereby grants to BSC an exclusive (subject only to the rights granted to Cook and reserved to Angiotech in paragraphs (b) and (c) below ...) world-wide right and license to use, manufacture, have manufactured, distribute, and sell, and to grant sublicenses to its Affiliates to use, manufacture, have manufactured, distribute, and sell, the Angiotech Technology in the Licensed Field of Use solely for use in the Licensed Applications (the "BSC License").

(b) Cook Technology License ... Angiotech hereby grants to Cook an exclusive (subject only to the rights granted to BSC and reserved to Angiotech pursuant to paragraphs (a) above and (c) below ...) world-wide right and license to use, manufacture, have manufactured, distribute, and sell, and to grant sublicenses to its Affiliates to use, manufacture, have manufactured, distribute, and sell, the Angiotech Technology in the Licensed Field of Use solely for use in the Licensed Applications (the "Cook License").

(c) Reservation of Rights. Angiotech reserves all rights to the Angiotech Technology for (i) any use or purpose outside the Licensed Field of Use and Licenced Applications and (ii) non-commercial research purposes in all fields and applications, including the Licensed Field of Use and Licensed Applications.

The following terms were defined in the contract:

"Angiotech Technology" shall mean (a) the patent rights, license rights and existing technology set forth in Exhibit A hereto, (b) any new Angiotech Technology which Cook or BSC, as the case may be, elects to have included in the Angiotech Technology pursuant to Section 2.3, (c) any and all improvements to the foregoing developed by Angiotech, or, subject to limitations and restrictions on Angiotech's rights to technology licensed from third parties, for Angiotech, during the term of this Agreement (including those arising under the CRADA to the extent solely owned by Angiotech), and (d) technical information that is useful or necessary to practice the foregoing.

"Licensed Field of Use" means endoluminal vascular and GI applications.

"Licensed Application" means the use of Angiotech Technology in the Licensed Field of Use on or incorporated in stent products and endoluminal products, but specifically excluding systemic treatments and pastes, microspheres, films, sprays, and similar formulations, in circumstances where such are not applied to or incorporated in either a stent product or an endoluminal product, as the case may be.

Reference

From a Boston Scientific Corporation 10-K SEC Filing (SEC accession number 0000950135-03-002096), period ended December 31, 2002, available at www.sec.gov.

of the technology or patent. However, this has to be tempered with current market trends for the technology or application.

What is the value of the patent?

The value of the patent and invention is a perception and the subjective view of the beholder will change this perceived value. In the end, both parties have to come to a common subjective context within which they agree the value. A calculation on value varies by the defined scope of the application area, resources, and time required to develop the invention, current needs of each party, and other such subjective and objective factors, thus making it hard to fix an accurate value outside of a context. Even quantitative tools, such as discounted cash flow and option pricing models, are subjective in the assumptions that have to be made to run these models. Finally, a close look at comparables in the licensing marketplace is used to give a lower and upper range for the financial terms and is useful in setting expectations on both sides. Thus, valuation of intangible assets such as intellectual property is a context-dependent exercise, where output from any analytical or empirical model must always be tempered by the market forces relevant to the business context for valuation.

A general *list of financial terms* typically included in a license agreement might be:

- *Technology transfer, access fees, or up-front payments*: This lump sum payment, due at signing, recognizes the investment made to date by the licensor both in developing know-how and the technology itself, and also includes consideration that some licensor preparation and effort may be necessary to allow access to the technology.
- *Patent prosecution and maintenance fees*: The licensee can be asked to pay legal and US PTO fees for maintaining the patent.
- *Milestone payments*: If the technology or invention succeeds in further stages of development, the licensee is asked to acknowledge the increased value (lowered risk) of the patented technology by making payments to the licensor.
- *Royalties*: Royalty rates, paid on commercial sales of the products, will vary by the state of the patented technology at execution of the license agreement and will typically be based on industry or market rates prevailing at that time. A rule of thumb sometimes used by many licensors is the 25% rule – it is often accepted that a royalty that is equal to 25% of the expected pre-tax net profits is a fair rate. The royalty rate in the license agreement will then depend on the market forces of each particular product. For example, if the licensee has profit margins of 60%, the royalty paid to the licensor should be 15% (¼ of 60%) of sales revenues. If profits of 4% are expected, the royalty rate should be around 1% of net revenues. Many licensing agreements include adaptive royalty rates that change as the annual revenues reach certain thresholds. Also, see Box 3.8 for a legal viewpoint on what might constitute "reasonable royalty rates" and the Georgia–Pacific factors.

Box 3.8 Determining a reasonable royalty rate: A legal perspective on claiming infringement damages and valuation for licensing

Contributed by Robert Schaffer, Attorney at Darby and Darby PC, NY

If your patent is successfully enforced against an infringer, the infringer may be enjoined from further infringement, e.g., by withdrawing the infringing product from the market. An injunction is not automatic, and recent cases have made it harder for the patent owner to get an injunction. The other remedy for infringement is that the patent owner can recover money damages. This can be all of the profits reasonably lost by the patentee to the infringer, if the patentee has a directly competing product. By statute, the damages cannot be less than a "reasonable royalty" for the invention. In making a "reasonable royalty" determination, courts typically look to a hypothetical negotiation between a willing buyer and seller of the invention rights, and they consider the factors that typically go into such a negotiation.

These factors are laid out in a landmark court case called Georgia–Pacific, and the royalty factors are called the Georgia–Pacific factors. These same factors can be used as a guide during actual licensing negotiations. The calculation of damages in a patent infringement case can be complex and highly contentious. As may be expected, the patentee tends to claim as high a lost profit or royalty as the facts arguably support, while the infringer argues for the lowest possible amount. Both parties are in the hands of the court, and there is often no reason for either party to think that it will get a better deal from the judge than they could have gotten from each other in a good-faith business negotiation. Valuing a patented invention, including the reasonable royalty it can command, is something of an art form and, for a court case, typically includes help from business and economics experts. Because of the high stakes involved, it may be a good idea to undertake a "reasonable royalty" evaluation before seeking to license an invention, and before bringing a lawsuit. This can particularly help to provide a ballpark "low ball" or "worst case" value for the invention, when planning to commercialize an invention or enforce a patent.

- *Sublicensee and sublicense fees*: If the patent is sublicensed to another party by the licensee (if they have been given that right in the license agreement), then a portion of the payments to the licensee are typically passed through to the licensor – this arrangement can be a flat fee or also a staged royalty, as appropriate.
- *Minimum annual royalties*: A minimum annual royalty payment starting with first commercial sales can be used to ensure that the licensor exercises a good effort in generating maximal revenues for the product.

- *Equity considerations (also warrants and options)*: A small licensor may find it beneficial to have a well established licensee purchase equity as part of the payments, for validation of the company as a whole and to increase long-term investors. On the other hand, a university as licensor may accept equity in lieu of cash payments from a start-up licensee that has limited resources to move the patented technology forward. Warrants and options are other methods of acquiring or selling equity in a license agreement.
- *Royalty anti-stacking provisions*: If a licensee also has to license other patents to get the product to market, then royalties payable to all licensed-in patents may stack up to make it economically unfeasible for the licensee to retain any profit from the sale of the product. An example would be a licensed-in drug compound which also requires the licensing-in of a delivery system technology in order to enable the product to be made and sold. In this case, the licensee will want to reduce the burden of the stacked royalties by requesting a subsequent reduction in each royalty while the licensors will want to minimize this reduction. There are several mechanisms and formulas that have been used to calculate the amount of royalty reduction. These terms would be placed under an anti-stacking royalty reduction provision.

3.11.3 "Boilerplate" clauses in the license agreement

There are several standard (boilerplate) parts of almost any business or legal contract that are also part of the licensing agreement contract and these are mentioned here to give an overview of the entirety of the licensing agreement. These clauses will not be discussed further here as there are many available resources that describe these terms in detail.

- Termination provisions,
- Best efforts,
- Warranty and indemnification,
- Arbitration and applicable law,
- General provisions,
- Assignment,
- Severability,
- Entire agreement (contents represent the agreement in entirety),
- Force majeure, contingencies,
- Notices.

3.12 Biotech business models and IP management strategies

Once a patent is licensed, depending on the agreement, the activities of the licensor can range from "collect payments and royalty checks" to active participation in the

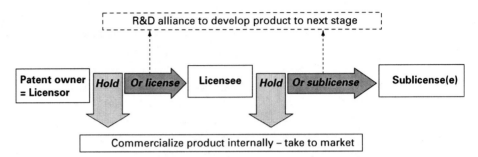

Figure 3.3   Schematic of various choices for a patent owner and licensor and subsequent licensees. A licensor can either (1) license and wait for money to come in, (2) license (singly or non-exclusively) and still develop product to market internally (or not license out), or (3) partner with licensee for co-development towards product.

development (Figure 3.3). Typical biotech-pharma licensing arrangements (especially at a stage before phase III trials) tend towards the latter, with the licensor (biotech company) contributing resources, patents and specialized know-how in a co-development agreement, and the experience-base of the pharma company people and processes helps to build further commercial, regulatory, or operational expertise in the biotech company. Start-ups based on medical device technology and patents most often license the technology or sell the company before entering clinic but after pre-clinical studies that prove the concept (to avoid the high costs of clinical trials). Some device companies form alliances with larger, established device companies for market access. Start-up diagnostic companies usually license out their technology to a commercial partner in order to gain access to an established technology platform, sales channels, and markets. Thus, several considerations guide the structure and terms of the licensing agreement, depending on the strategic needs of the licensor.

In general, the licensor can wait for royalties, or co-develop technology in a partnership all the way to market, or choose to co-develop only in strategic functional areas. The license agreement, as seen above, has a wide variety of terms that reflect the multiple combinations of arrangements possible. The licensee also has similar choices, either to develop the IP to the next step, and then sublicense to a third party to complete commercialization and similarly wait for royalties, or to co-develop or develop the patents through to market (Figure 3.3). The licensee can also bundle various in-licensed patents together to make a more attractive and comprehensive portfolio package for the next sublicensee. There are many companies that operate on a business model that works this way: license patents from one party; take the patent or technology to the next value creation step; and then license it out to someone else, collecting the incremental value created as its revenue or profits. Two examples of companies with this business model that were active from the early 1980s, licensing in from universities and licensing out to corporations, RCT (Research Center Technologies) and BTG (British Technology Group).

	R&D	FDA process and clinical trials	Manufacturing	Marketing and Sales	
				US	International
Do it yourself					
Strategic partners or licenses					

Figure 3.4 Functional look at a business model. This schematic can be filled in to give a good idea of where the company is currently and where it should invest functionally over time.

There are other licensors who follow a business model of a high level of legal activity, controlling and enforcing rights to patents without actually carrying out value-adding development beyond the invention and patent prosecution step. Thus, it is clear that intellectual property management strategies (and subsequent licensing agreements) are closely linked with the specific business model chosen by the company.

3.12.1 What is a business model?

The business model is at the heart of an innovation. A business model describes the means by which an organization generates revenues and profits from an innovation and resultant products. A business model also defines the product (to some extent), positions the company in the value chain (product commercialization process) and describes the mechanisms of getting revenues from the product over time.

A functional approach to defining your company's business model is presented in the value chain schematic in Figure 3.4, where the current status of a company can be clearly depicted in terms of key value creation functions. This same chart can be used to define future activities and engage in business strategic planning. Some questions that frequently arise are:

- Are we focusing the company on R&D – services or products?
- Are we going to manufacture or partner or outsource?
- Are we going to build sales and marketing or go to resellers or commercial partners?

However, within each segment of the functional elements above lie deeper questions (Are we developing services or products, are we making components, or do we want to make systems, and should we build sales and marketing?) that further define the business and operations. Above all, the dynamic nature of the context of business model must be recognized. Continuous changes in the markets, technology, and state of maturity of the sector require adaptability in the business model to sustain success. Although general operational business models based on intellectual property strategies are discussed here, financial models for these companies are better covered in other publications.

3.12.2   Practical note on business models for drug, device, and diagnostic innovator companies

Innovator companies are those that focus on the first step in the value chain – the discovery of new inventions and the development of innovative product ideas from those inventions. Typically, these companies are focused on developing product ideas for large markets, as economic investors in these companies drive the focus towards large valuations (based on achieving large revenues).

In the case of *drug innovators*, early drug discovery is an expensive and challenging area, full of early failures. It is common for most early-stage drug discovery companies to aspire to forward integrate along the value chain, but increasing levels of investments and continued high risk make it a reality that they will have to license their innovative product idea to the large pharma companies that have the marketing and investment power to build portfolios that mitigate risk.

Device innovator companies might find it easier to go to market as each device can find a niche market, but again, the economics of venture-capital-type investors typically focus a company towards large markets, which are probably best addressed by licensing to one of the top device companies that dominate the markets. Some companies have also started as specialty distributors while simultaneously pursuing development of novel products; a model that is largely possible because of the sometimes fragmented nature of the distribution business in medical devices.

Innovator diagnostic companies have a particular challenge in getting their tests to market. The test platform is usually based on a technology that is accepted in the market and has an established base of labs that are familiar with that platform. This is an established market base that is captured by the technology platform manufacturer or larger diagnostic company. If the new test is not accepted rapidly and launched across established platforms, the innovator diagnostic company runs the risk of being beaten by a fast follower who copies their test on another established technical platform. Thus, the innovator diagnostic company has to build an acceptance base and reach a threshold market share to have its test carried by the major centralized diagnostic labs (high volume). To capture various technology platforms and rapidly gain market acceptance and usage, innovator diagnostic companies can non-exclusively license their technology to several large diagnostic companies. They can continue to develop and sell the test themselves, while establishing the test as a "standard of care" through the increased market share gained by allowing larger partners to market the test. An additional and significant consideration is the opportunity to gain reimbursement from payers (Chapter 7) with the acceptance of the new test by many physicians.

3.12.3 Emergent dominant business models among biotechnology (drug) companies

This section refers predominantly to the evolution of business models in the drugs and research tools segment of the biomedical technology companies discussed in this book but also applies to device or diagnostic ventures. The phrase "biotechnology companies" is used in this section to refer to drug companies that are making either small-molecule chemical drugs or biological drugs. Within each type of business model are notes on licensing or on intellectual property management and financial management strategy. These should serve as broad guidelines. The list of business models is ordered by the appearance of these dominant strategies in the industry, but is not meant to imply that the vertical or horizontal strategies, or other strategies, are not relevant today.

The dominant business models that emerged in the biotechnology industry are:

(1) Vertical (product),
(2) Horizontal (tools and services),
(3) Hybrid I – discovery tools forward integrating to product development,
(4) Hybrid II – services back-integrating to products or discovery.

(1) Vertical model

A company with a vertical business model has a product focus with vertical integration over the whole value chain to discover, develop, and market a single technology or set of technologies (usually therapeutic drugs) that are end products for consumers. The first wave of "vertical model" biotechnology companies was founded in the late 1970s and early 1980s, based on breakthrough innovations that enabled increased efficiency and scale of biopharmaceutical manufacturing, making protein therapeutics a reality. Traditional large pharmaceutical companies have a vertical business model. Many smaller biotechnology and device companies focus on research, and work in a "short vertical" model, where the product prototype (having achieved proof of concept in human models) is sold or partnered out to a commercial partner.

Intellectual property strategies in this vertical model would typically include building and owning patents and in-licensing patents to maintain or gain market access. Patents typically focus around novel compounds or blocking patents on processes. Process trade secrets would be important strategic advantage for certain companies. Forming brand recognition for technology platforms can also build advantage.

The financial strategy is for large up-front investments with a long-term wait for returns. This is a high risk model, as resources are focused around a few products that take a long time to get to market, but it is balanced by a high return on investment. This business model captures the maximal value of investment.

The successful companies have emerged as the giants of the small but fast-growing biotechnology industry. Examples of companies with varying degrees of success with the vertical business model are: Biogen-Idec, Immunex, Amgen, Genetech, Medtronic, and Boston Scientific.

(2)   ## Horizontal platform model

Companies following a horizontal model operate at a specific location in the value chain and sell their product or service across products, companies, or industries. Radical innovations that industrialized biological research and created technology platforms and companies promised to be gold mines of information and insight, as they would enable improved success in the drug development process. Companies rapidly emerged around these innovative technologies by capturing intellectual property, proprietary information, or enabling processes (high throughput gene sequencing, expression arrays, etc.) and re-selling them as services, products (e.g., array chips), and intellectual assets (e.g., licensing use of platforms, partnerships to sell output of platforms).

Intellectual property management strategies would typically include owning patents around a core technology area, and would include a strategy to out-license them to gain licensing fees. The intellectual patent portfolio of companies following this model need not be as complete or tightly integrated as those following the vertical model.

In this financial strategy, companies need lower up-front investment, with technology platforms generating revenues through services or licensing or through sales of non-regulated research tools relatively early. Companies may start with venture financing or governmental financing but have the potential to be profitable with a positive cash flow within a few years.

This business model is representative of the second wave of new company formation in the biotechnology industry in the 1990s. Of these companies, a few successful ones built up rapidly on partnership revenues or produced products that are widely licensed and used in all fields of biological research – both academic and industrial. Examples of this business model are: Affymetrix, Lion Biosciences, and Tripos. Also existing within this type of business model are service companies that obtain a comprehensive fee for their service and have no plans to develop an FDA-regulated product on their own. Examples of this type of service are custom manufacturing houses and clinical research organizations (CROs), such as Parexel, Lonza, and Quintiles.

(3)   ## Hybrid model I – tools to product development

This business model occupies a horizontal and vertical position over the value chain. The company usually starts with a horizontal strategy and leverages resources for vertical integration. The evolution of business models after the genomics stock market bubble (September 2000) reflects a diminished value placed on the horizontal model along with shareholder pressures for maintaining the pace of expected returns.

Intellectual property management strategies for these companies would tend to have a mix of internally generated patents and a strong drive towards in-licensing IP to fill a product portfolio as vertical integration strategies emerge.

The financial strategy is for early revenues; derived from platform tools and services sold across the value chain, these are then invested in integrating forward into drug development over a therapeutic product development value chain, merging the two business models described above.

Examples of hybrid I companies are: Curagen, Millenium, Incyte, and Celera.

(4)   **Hybrid model II – services backward integrating to discovery**
This business model, like hybrid model I, predominantly occupies a horizontal position over the value chain. Shared risk models, where the services company takes on a performance risk and gets incentives based on success, have been increasing in recent years. Some companies have also leveraged their existing R&D service functions and revenues to carry out internal R&D on drug discovery, adopting a model similar to the early-stage biotech companies. These hybrid business models have been used with caution in the past, as there is a real risk of alienating existing customers who may feel that the service business is now becoming a competitor. Some examples of service companies that are developing their own internal R&D and product lines are Albany Molecular Research, Structural Genomix, and Accelrys.

3.13   Summary

In this chapter, intellectual property concepts have been introduced, with a clear understanding of their worth in capturing value while commercializing biomedical technologies. Product development is influenced greatly by these strategies and by the nature of intellectual property protection chosen to gain exclusivity in the market. Choices of projects and investment decisions, such as investing in innovation on a new technology platform, are governed by the ability to capture value in the commercialization process through the subsequently created intellectual property. This chapter has covered the main tool (licensing) and business models used to capture and use intellectual property to further product development.

Exercises

3.1. Describe types of intellectual property needed for commercialization of your chosen product for the specific indication chosen.
3.2. Describe how specific patent claims in filed patent applications will provide market protection for the chosen products.

3.3. If you have an initial idea, search the US patent databases to determine if a patent application or issued patent covers your idea. Search scientific and general publications for keywords representing your invention or idea to determine the patentability of the invention.

3.4. Identify future IP that will or might be needed in a commercialization path to access your chosen market. Describe a strategy for IP acquisition (assumptions are fine, just state them clearly up-front). State the necessary key licensing terms for an in-licensing agreement.

3.5. What might be a business strategy or model based around managing your starting IP assets?

3.6. State key licensing strategies in the context of value chain positioning and give a brief rationale. Identify your key assumptions.

3.7. Based on your IP strategy, plan the costs and timeline of patent prosecution, licensing, or acquisition for your chosen product.

References and additional reading

Breneman, L. University–industry collaborations: partners in research promoting productivity and economic growth, *Research Management Review*, **13**(2), 2003.

Goldscheider, R. *Licensing Law Handbook: The New Companion to Licensing Negotiations*. St. Paul, MN: West Group, 2003.

Lerner, P. J. and Poltorak, A. I. *Essentials of Intellectual Property*, John Wiley & Sons, 2002.

Mowery, D. C., Nelson, R. R., Sampat, B. N., and Ziedonis, A. A. *Ivory Tower and Industrial Innovation: University–Industry Technology Transfer Before and After the Bayh-Dole Act in the United States*, Stanford Business Books, 2004.

Smith, G. V. and Parr, R. L. *Intellectual Property: Valuation, Exploitation, and Infringement Damages*, John Wiley & Sons, 2005.

US Department of Commerce. *Patents and How to Get One: A Practical Handbook*, Dover Publications, 2003.

Winslow, R. Will stent makers fight dentist's patent tooth and nail? *Wall Street Journal*, January 26, p. B1, 2006.

Useful websites

www.uspto.gov – *US patent and trademark office*

www.wipo.org – *WIPO*

www.epo.org – *European patent office*

www.uspto.gov/main/trademarks.htm and www.ladas.com/Trademarks/tmprot.html – *Trademark link*

www.uspto.gov/web/offices/com/annual/2005/040201_patentperform.html – *US PTO: patent processing times*

www.patentbaristas.com

www.patentdocs.us

www.orangebook.blog.com
http://patentdocs.typepad.com/patent_docs/ – *Patent blogs*
www.bustpatents.com/biotech.htm
www.dnapatent.com
http://biotech.about.com – *General reading for biotech patents*

4   New product development (NPD)

Plan	Position	Patent	Product	Pass!	Production	Profits
Industry context	Market research	Intellectual property rights	New product development (NPD)	Regulatory plan	Manufacture	Reimbursement

Roadmap of a product commercialization plan. Stage 4

Learning points:

- Define product characteristics at the beginning of a biomedical product development plan using clinical study endpoints and indications,
- How do drug, device, and diagnostic development processes differ?
- Why do many drugs, devices, and diagnostics fail in development stages?
- How to build a product development plan for drugs, diagnostics, or devices,
- When to kill a project,
- How to prepare for clinical trials – what are the specific issues for diagnostics and devices?
- Successfully make a pitch for a project to senior management for funding,
- What ethical issues must be recognized during product development activities?
- When should you outsource?
- Compliance to specific certifications and laboratory regulations when setting up a new laboratory.

Read this chapter going through the book sequentially, and then revisit the exercises in this chapter after reading Chapters 5, 6, and 7. The approach to new product development has to be an integrated, multi-disciplinary approach, taking input from Chapters 1, 2, 3, 5, 6, and 7 into account (see the roadmap in the preface).

This chapter deals with the development of a product that is being developed with some "new-to-the-world" features, requiring a full review by the FDA before reaching market. Drug or diagnostic products that go through abbreviated product development paths (generic drugs, and diagnostics or devices that are largely equivalent to marketed products) are addressed in greater detail in Chapter 5. However, the principles discussed in this chapter apply generally to biomedical product development.

4.1   Why have a new product development (NPD) process – just get it done!

Developing new products requires input from and interaction with almost all functions in a company (Figure 4.1), as new products build revenues on which the entire company depends for growth and sustenance. Most large companies will have an integrated product development team or a review board that has people from different functional areas in the company. Each functional component of the company has a useful and significant role to play in getting new products to market.

Multidisciplinary reviews are as essential as multidisciplinary teams. Product development must constantly and iteratively take input from multiple departments or corporate functions during the planning and development stages, as described in Table 4.1. If you are in a small company and don't have all these functions, you still need to consider the product from the viewpoint of all these disciplines.

Therefore, a structured process of development is needed to help organize different agencies and functions within an organization. The goals of investing in creating and maintaining a process for new product development (NPD) are:

- At some stage, a defined process is required and reviewed by the FDA in order to approve the product (see Chapter 5),
- A standardized process is also critical to get quality certifications like ISO (International Organization for Standardization, Geneva, www.iso.org),
- To bring products from concept to market in an organized, efficient manner,
- Progress through stages of development can be communicated easily,
- To improve management of the process and coordination with other resources,
- To minimize time, effort, and cost,
- To ensure quality and safety in the process and final product,
- A new product development process is itself a valuable asset of a company, where learning can be captured and efficiencies transferred among all new product development projects.

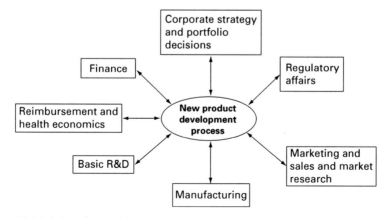

Figure 4.1   Multiple interfaces of the new product development (NPD) process.

Table 4.1 Input and interactions with various departments in the NPD process

Functional input	Purpose
Basic R&D	To work on the project
Reimbursement	To provide input into the economics of the disease state treated (and any associated procedure); to provide input into clinical trial design so that insurers will be willing to pay for the product
Marketing and market researchers	To develop product specifications and possibly test early concepts or prototypes; to work with product cycle planning and to differentiate product from competition
Finance division	To get agreement on budgets and adjustments
Sales division	To discover customer needs
Senior management	To review at level of portfolio; to set strategy, and funding
Manufacturing	To make sure development is scalable and designed with manufacturing in mind
Regulatory affairs division	To guide the results through the regulatory gate keeper and give critical feedback on product development planning

4.2 Planning and preparing an NPD process for biomedical technologies (drugs, devices, and diagnostics)

The development of new biomedical products typically involves three functionally different stages, as shown in Figure 4.2. These functional stages vary in execution and time span between drugs, devices, and diagnostics, as examined further below.

The first few steps in developing a new biomedical product are shown schematically in Figure 4.3. These preliminary planning steps are typically undertaken by engineers, scientists, and project managers for presentation to higher level managers or committees in large companies.

Another level of strategic planning and thinking takes place at the corporate level, where data on the technology roadmap of the industry, the 5–10 year project portfolio planning, finance, marketing, etc., are all considered in the context of an industry and organizational development plan. Development scientists or engineers can be more successful in designing a better product if they understand the target market and its needs (see Chapter 2), the needs of the company, the company strategy, and an overview of the process of final delivery into the market (Chapters 5–7). As described above, keeping these points in mind during the design and development process also helps in planning the product life cycle and subsequent versions of the product. These perspectives will also build a greater appreciation of the significance of the role of a product development engineer or scientist in the entire NPD process.

4.2.1 The project proposal document

The project proposal contains at least the items listed in Figure 4.4 and should give a convincing case for the project, show, specifically, the risks involved, and describe how

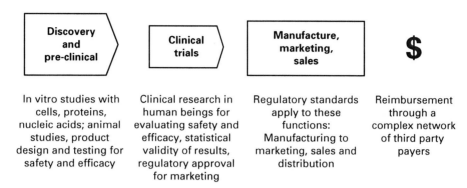

Figure 4.2   A generalized functional and value chain in biomedical product development.

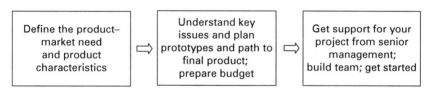

Figure 4.3   Preparatory steps to be made by project manager and team.

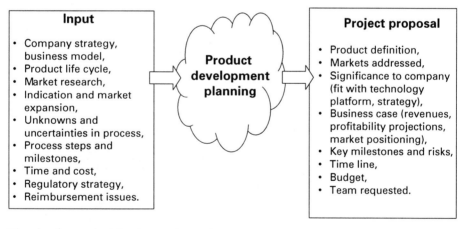

Figure 4.4   Planning for product development overview.

early testing will reduce the risks before the product enters clinical testing on human subjects. Some aspects of the planning process and the inputs are given in Figure 4.4.

4.2.2   Strategy and competency of the company and goal of the project

Most companies have short-term and long-term business plans to grow or sustain themselves. While planning a new product, the context of the business's strategic plan and the available internal competency in technology and functional areas must be kept in mind. It also helps to understand the company's business model and current position in the value chain of the specific industry (refer to Section 1.4 for more details).

4.2.3   Product life cycle planning

Each product has a reasonably well defined life cycle from concept to development, to market, to peak sales, and, finally, to declining sales and obsolescence. The product life cycle from market introduction to peak annual sales for specific industries is well known as a general rule (innovative devices; $\sim$2 years, drugs; $\sim$3–5 years, assuming that patent status is valid, and diagnostics; $\sim$5 years. Note: these lengths will vary for specific products). The new product must fit into the current product line and market-based development cycles to help address internal and external issues and interests, particularly with respect to the long product development cycles for most biomedical products. For example, if a drug is going to go off patent after four years of market launch, then a parallel track development of slow release or inhaled formulation could be part of an NPD plan, so that the new (patented) form of the drug product is ready for release by the time of entry of generic competition into the market. A life cycle planning strategy for a device might be to develop a broader, technically complex, fully configured platform at the first run, and then introduce various parts or features of the device onto the market in a sequential measured fashion, pre-empting competitors who will not be able to match the pace, as redesigning their products will take too long.

4.2.4   Market research

Components of market research are described in Chapter 2. The outcome of the market research should identify the product characteristics and define the product and target market in greater detail. One other specific outcome of market research is the identification of a primary indication and indication expansion strategies. The inputs from market research (the "voice" of the customer (VOC) or customer needs, is one such input) are consciously and quantitatively synthesized into product characteristics by using various design tools, such as a "house of quality" (where design and functional inputs from external and internal sources are weighed against each other by assigning numerical significance, arriving at a better idea of the relative importance of each product characteristic) or some other design matrix that brings a display of market research inputs to design and development teams. This approach is discussed in Section 4.10.1. The product development and design process for drugs (small molecules and biologics) typically involves taking a higher-level view of the market, as NPD design decisions in early drug development typically revolve around mode of administration (oral, intravenous) or specific reduction of side effects. However, business decisions in the drug NPD process involve significant market research and in-depth analysis.

4.2.5 Identify key unknowns and risks

Knowing where the hurdles lie in the NPD process makes it more likely that the choices along the NPD path will be successful. Major risks, such as toxic side effects, must be addressed as early as is feasible. Sometimes, the identification of key unknowns that need to be known can help to clarify the priorities of the studies that need to be done. For example, if the pharmacodynamic behavior of the drug compound is identified and listed as an important parameter that dictates many other product development steps, then specific tests to evaluate and optimize those pharmacodynamic parameters should be prioritized in the product development plan. Or if the long term toxic effect of a material is identified as a key risk for a device then, parallel to other development studies, a long term study with the material in vivo (it may not be the final version of the material, but close enough that the result would be indicative) could be initiated. Having a list of these specifically identified risks or unknowns can be helpful in building an NPD process with greater chances of success. More to the point, *the product development plan should show how the risks will be tested early in the project.*

4.2.6 Build a milestone-based plan for product development

Milestones are results of tests that show key reductions of risk in NPD. For example, a milestone for a device could be the successful mechanical testing of the device functions in repeated cycles to failure for addressing expected device usage lifetime. A milestone for a drug could be the demonstration of efficacy in an animal model. A milestone for diagnostic development could be the satisfactory repetition of a sensitive level of measurement, establishing a level of reliability for the diagnostic test. The more specific the milestones, the easier it will be to build a convincing NPD plan. It is important to plan to do the knock-out tests early. However, *planning to fail can be a conceptual challenge for scientists or engineers in product development, who are focused more on getting the technology to work rather than on figuring out how to get it to fail.*

4.2.7 Specific risks known to occur frequently during the development of biomedical products

Biomedical technology products that fail in development typically fail for one or more of the following reasons.

Drug candidate molecules in development fail to get to market for the following reasons (percent compounds failed, as in Prentis *et al.*, 1988):

- Poor ADME characteristics (absorption, distribution, metabolism, or excretion in the human body; desired product characteristics could not be met) (41%),
- Lack of efficacy – compounds did not show the benefit expected (31%),
- Toxicity (22%),
- Market or business reasons (6%).

Diagnostic products that fail in development typically fail because of one or more of the following (see Box 4.1 for examples):

- Lack of clinical utility: no correlation with clinical outcome.
- The necessary sensitivity or specificity of the assay was not verified in subsequent clinical studies.
- The wrong test principle was chosen (genetic, expression, protein, metabolite).
- The wrong test format was chosen (centralized vs. point of care). Perhaps in the IVD industry more than the others, there is a major issue with setting market standards and testing platforms. This is discussed briefly in Section 3.12.2, and the examples in Box 4.1 illustrate this point.
- The test is too complicated, compared with the existing format. This is a value proposition issue, wherein the new test in development may be more precise and sensitive than needed.
- Reliability: repeatability and precision were not achieved.
- Non-linear response of assay in clinical use.
- Patents are not comprehensive or valid.

Medical devices that fail in development typically fail because of one or more of the following (see Box 4.2 for examples):

- Failure to meet efficacy,
- Safety, toxicity, or instability in device behavior or mechanics,
- Biocompatibility,
- Business or market reasons.

4.3   Kill the project early or try some more?

It is important to understand that, despite good technical progress and data, projects get killed in development. Usually, many considerations enter into that decision, including market and reimbursement issues, competitive pressures, newly discovered patent issues, lack of patentability, regulatory changes, financial constraints, or simply a change of strategy in company due to a management change or merger or acquisition of the company. However, a counter-intuitive point frequently brought up in biomedical product development is discussed here: *Why is early failure sought after (over late failure) in biomedical product development?*

4.3.1   Early failure is better than late failure in biomedical product development

A high cost and rapidly rising rate of expenditure in the later stages of medical product development make it attractive to recognize potential product failure points at the earliest possible stage of development. There are always new product ideas that could be tackled by the resources freed up by failed projects. Also, exhaustive and early tests for potential side effects or toxic effects might help

---

Box 4.1 Failure points in diagnostics development pathway

Examples of failures or problems in diagnostics development and diagnostics products

Sensitivity related failure

An IVD test being developed by a large diagnostics company for sepsis was aimed at locating a surrogate marker so that an intervention decision could be made in a timely fashion. Approximately 100 000 in vitro samples were analyzed and studied with extensive molecular mechanisms of sepsis and cell culture studies. When the designed assay was tested in a clinical setting, the assay was just not sensitive enough on real clinical samples and could not deliver results within the time that a clinical decision had to be made. The exquisitely designed diagnostic test thus failed to show clinical utility owing to lack of clinical sensitivity. According to Dr. Christoph Hergersberg, (Global Biosciences Leader at GE Central R&D): "This is the 'so-what?' factor. You have a great diagnostic test – so what? It has to have clinical utility and be tied to clinical outcomes to be accepted and successful."

Failure due to incorrect choice of test principle

HER2/neu is an epidermal growth factor tyrosine kinase that is known to be over-expressed in breast cancer. This over-expression can be caused by the amplification of the gene, and can be measured by fluorescence in situ hybridization (FISH) or in the circulation of breast cancer patients by immunohistochemistry (IHC). Both tests have been developed commercially but which one is more predictive? Even if you come up with a better principle, is the distinguishing part of the test (which may be scientifically a more rational test principle – e.g., chromosomal level detection of rearrangement) more clinically relevant and will it be competitive in cost and utility with the other? This is again, the "so-what?" question in diagnostic development. . .

Market standard related test format incorrectly chosen

If you are developing a test for use in critical care patients, who are in the intensive care unit, point of care (POC) testing is de rigueur. Therefore, one would start developing and creating a POC test. If, however, a centralized lab could beef up the workflow to run this test with a faster turnaround time, the effort and time to develop a new platform might not be worth it. The competition would be driven by economic value, and the time spent in developing a new POC test might be better served in developing a diagnostic test that could be licensed to a large diagnostic that already has a POC testing system in place. For example, Luminex is a market leader in multiplexing, where several assays are run in one test, making it much more cost-effective.

Box 4.1 (cont.)

Complicated and sophisticated test that may be more accurate but does not add much more value to final clinical outcome

A cascade of activated proteins related to a systemic pathology is discovered and a FISH (fluorescent in situ hybridization) assay on the entire cellular signaling path is developed to get a multi-parameter diagnostic test. This new multi-parameter test is potentially more sensitive or more specific. If the existing clinically used test is a simple blood test to get the same diagnosis, then the more complex (and expensive) test will have to show not only better sensitivity and specificity but also a *much* better predictive value, to replace the current clinical blood test successfully.

Lack of patent protection

A lack of adequate patent protection can result in economic failure for a manufacturer, even though the test works. A strong intellectual property position is sometimes difficult to achieve and protect in the diagnostics industry.

The example of the recent patent dispute between Metabolite and LabCorp highlights a unique patent protection issue for the diagnosis industry. University scientists discovered and patented a way of diagnosing vitamin deficiency by measuring levels of an amino acid called homocysteine in the blood. Metabolite (a small start-up company) licensed the patent from the university and then sublicensed it to LabCorp (a large company). LabCorp paid royalties to Metabolite for a few years while it sold the tests and conducted assays according to the methods described in the patents. When a better assay process was invented by Abbott, LabCorp switched to that and stopped paying royalties to Metabolite. Metabolite took LabCorp to court; LabCorp pleaded that the relationship between homocysteine levels and vitamins was a law of nature and could not be patented, thus the Metabolite patent was invalid. However, Metabolite won an award against LabCorp (LabCorp failed in appeal to the Supreme court on a technical matter), but this case raises some important issues – the diagnosis industry is made up of the kinds of correlation that occur in normal and healthy processes. Will these numerous patents also be challenged? It will become very difficult to develop new diagnostic products and take them to market without some certainty and protection from the patent laws.

References

Pollack, A. High court rethinks what can be patented, *The New York Times*, Monday, March 20, 2006.

> **Box 4.2** Failure points in device development pathway
>
> ## Examples of failures or problems in device development
>
> This is an example of a device that failed to meet its claimed efficacy after market clearance. Curon Medical sold a device called Stretta™ for treatment of gastro-esophageal reflux disease (GERD). Cleared under a 510(k), it had problems with establishing long-term efficacy. The device was rejected by the technology assessment boards of various payers and the company filed for bankruptcy in late 2006 and closed its doors, taking the product off the market (www.gastro.org).
>
> Another example of failure of a marketed product due to inadequate studies in product development: Boston Scientific's Enteryx product for GERD had problems with the mechanics of delivery, causing complications and deaths. Injections of the polymer used to thicken the esophageal wall were frequently wrongly delivered by physicians and caused serious complications, even death in one case of injection into the aorta. This product was taken off the market in 2005 (www.gastro.org).

prevent the liabilities of legal lawsuits (see Section 7.13) in the future when the product is marketed to a broader population. Examples are given in Box 4.3.

Product development in the clinical testing phase can cost tens of millions of dollars. Therefore, there is a significant interest in testing for known safety concerns or for specific problematic aspects of delivery or dosage as early as possible. The goal is to identify the risk correctly as early as possible and then either kill the project or fix the issue and thus reduce the chances of failure later on in the project.

4.3.2   When to kill a project

The decision to stop investing in a project is one of the most challenging issues in biomedical product development for two reasons – (1) people are passionate about their projects, as the projects have a higher goal towards helping better human health and (2) because biology is so complex, it is far easier to kill a project at the first sign of toxic side effects than to allow it to continue to try and reach efficacy. On the other hand, there are many stories where projects that were killed and discarded by one company were developed into very successful products by other companies (see Box 4.4 for case example).

Management is concerned with final outcomes, such as product differentiation (with respect to competitors or existing alternatives), pricing, reimbursement, market acceptance, user convenience, and compliance, and has to show eventually (to the FDA and market payers) that the balance between safety and efficacy tips

---

Box 4.3 Examples of desirable early failure milestones

Device example

A device was known to have a problem with chronic fibrosis forming around it, leading to premature failure of the device functions. In developing a next-generation device, an in vivo test was carried out very early in the material selection and design process to determine the amount of likely fibrotic reaction. The goal was to help learn about the process of fibrosis and was set up as an early go/no-go decision point for the project if the fibrosis could not be reduced. One such material, when tested in this way, had to have its edges reshaped, making them more rounded. This resulted in much lower build-up of the cells involved in the fibrous deposits and thus showed a way to make the final device less prone to failure due to fibrosis in the body.

Drug example

Chronic drugs may fail in late development or regulatory review if they have significant side effects on heart rate. A new class of compounds being developed for a chronic disease should incorporate, in the NPD plan, acute (short-term) ion-channel binding and other cardiovascular studies on molecules in the early design process (lead compounds) so that further investment in certain classes or types of compounds is halted in the NPD process (early failure). The typical process would be to test drug candidate compounds (at a much later stage of development) in expensive long-term cardiac toxicity studies in large animals. Several such efforts, to look for in vitro markers that might help predict specific drug toxicities, are in progress in academia and in industry.

---

towards efficacy and that the product has clinical utility. Therefore, a project will sometimes get killed by management because of changes in regulatory or market environments, frustrating the scientists and engineers, who have achieved the technical milestones. In addition, there are budget allocations and resource constraints that usually factor heavily into a decision to kill a project. For example, if a project has been funded for three years and in the fourth year, the team still has major problems, it is more likely that the project will be killed during the next review. The product development team, focused on showing efficacy, should attempt to gain better appreciation of these external and internal business issues and monitor them as best as possible.

While it may be easier to evaluate and quantify external factors (markets, regulatory, economic factors, competition) as criteria to drop projects, the decision to drop a project for technical reasons alone is the hardest. There are numerous

> **Box 4.4** Old drugs never die – they get revived . . .
>
> A story in *The Wall Street Journal*, dated August 11, 2003, described how a small company, Genesoft, successfully picked up and turned around a drug-development project (brand name "Factive") that a big pharma company (Glaxo SmithKline (GSK)) had killed. SmithKlineBeecham (SKB) had licensed in Factive from a company (LG Group) in Korea. The drug failed FDA review as the FDA was concerned about a rash on the patients. But the product development team had found the rash to be intermittent and carried out more studies to demonstrate this. However, at the time SKB had merged with Glaxo. Glaxo SmithKline dropped the project, never submitting the last findings to the FDA (after having spent five years and $200 million on its development), as they were increasingly focused on billion-dollar drugs and did not feel the last safety hurdle would be overcome. The lead scientist from the Factive project left GSK as a result of the merger and was working for GeneSoft. When he heard over a newswire about the opportunity to license the drug out again, he convinced his CEO to pick it up. They struggled but were successful in raising the funding and obtaining the license from the Korean company. They continued development and in one year filed for FDA approval and successfully put the drug on the market, transforming Genesoft's future and improving patient health.

examples in many industries (typically in larger companies) where a project was officially declared over because of a scientific or technical hurdle but a passionate scientist or engineer with insight kept tinkering with the concept to overcome the hurdle. The scientist or engineer would succeed in overcoming the technical problem after numerous months or years and that would result in renewed funding, development, and launching of the new product. Examples of such products exist in various industries and include GE's digital X-ray, DuPont's BioMax biodegradable polymer and IBM's silicon germanium devices and many others, as described in Leifer *et al.* (2000). Examples such as these will continue to emerge as one-off cases but can also result in significant angst amongst management as the product might have reached market faster if the right investment had been continued. There is no simple answer to this quandary. However, several approaches and concepts from management theory, which relate to better management of product development in high uncertainty and emerging technology domains, are discussed in the next section.

4.4   Uncertainty-based view of product development processes

There are four main uncertainties in all product development – two that management can control are *resource uncertainty* and *organizational uncertainty*, and two that management has to adapt and adjust to are *technical uncertainty* and *market uncertainty* (Leifer *et al.*, 2000).

Technical uncertainties are addressed by engineers and scientists in product development while market uncertainty – in terms of competition and market segmentation, pricing, etc. – can be factored into the product development processes and product definition or characteristics. Resource and organizational uncertainty may occur because the project may not have the right amount of funding assigned to it at the right times, the team in charge of the project may get disbanded, a senior manager supporting the project may leave, expertise in that technical area may not exist in the organization, or market channels may be new or unknown to the organization. However, these types of high internal uncertainty projects are also means for the company to renew itself from within as the company growth trajectory is launched into a steeper curve. Examples include the Avastin drug product at Genentech, which made it a world-leading oncology company in a few short years, the digital X-ray project at GE, the first drug-coated stent at Boston Scientific, Viagra at Pfizer, etc.

As the uncertainties in product development rise, so also does the possibility to give the company tremendous advantage and market share or revenues by radically changing the markets or the technology base for competition. These radical innovations are supported through alternate channels of product development within a company with established incremental innovation systems and need long-term views, typically only afforded by large established companies. If they are not funded, they frequently go underground, using resources obtained through informal networks and volunteer efforts (Leifer *et al.*, 2000). At some point the project comes out of the dark, undergoes examination, and competes for resources. With the desire to reduce time to market, why do these potentially breakthrough projects not receive management attention sooner? Because funding and organizational commitment requires a business plan or business case that reflects a level of certainty that simply does not exist throughout much of the life cycle of a breakthrough innovation project. There are several management books on the market that discuss this particular problem of radical or breakthrough innovation management (see additional reading list at the end of this chapter).

Figure 4.5 highlights the shift in product development approaches, from an environment where all four areas of uncertainty rank very highly (top of Figure 4.5; most small companies with novel products inhabit this space), to the low-risk, incremental projects that are preferred by most managers, where the external risk is very low and the internal uncertainties are also very low. In the three approaches that deal with high-uncertainty projects – the milestone, discovery-driven, and learning plan approaches – the most important assumptions are clearly defined, and tests to prove or disprove the assumptions are developed. However, the purpose of these different approaches is typically as described here: milestone-based planning is used to drive a single, high-uncertainty product; discovery-driven planning is used to develop a new business concept; and

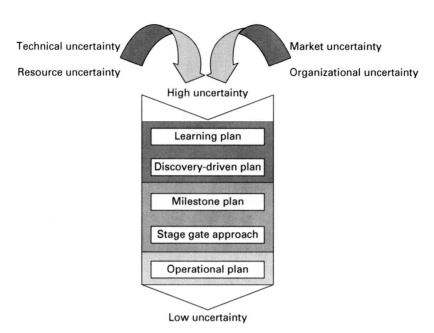

Technical uncertainty

Resource uncertainty

Market uncertainty

Organizational uncertainty

High uncertainty

Learning plan

Discovery-driven plan

Milestone plan

Stage gate approach

Operational plan

Low uncertainty

Figure 4.5   Uncertainty-based view of product development planning (Rice, M. P., O'Connor, G. Colaselli, and Pieratozzi, R. Driving breakthrough innovation: implementing a learning plan to counter project uncertainty. Forthcoming in *Sloan Management Review*.)

innovations to drive that new business concept are explored in the learning-plan approach.

The sequence of milestones is clearly formulated in the milestone and discovery-driven processes as the end goal is quite clear in these approaches, as opposed to the learning plan. The clarity of objectives in discovery-driven planning allows the team to work backwards from the goal, recognizing assumptions and evaluating their validity. Further details on these various approaches can be studied in the management papers and books listed in the additional reading list at the end of this chapter.

This book focuses on the stage-gate process as this process is particularly well suited for biomedical product development. The regulatory gatekeeper (FDA) forces specificity and focus of application (the indication) very early on in the development process making it imperative to develop a defined process. Over the last few decades, most companies (in diverse industries) have adopted some version of the stage-gate process first introduced by Robert Cooper in 1988. The stage-gate process consists of activity stages, between each of which is a decision point or a gate for a go/no-go decision. The content and format of the "gates" are usually based on perceptions of risk at that stage of the project. The actual decision making process (go, no-go, or repeat stage again) depends on the context of the project and also the culture and processes of the company but should usually include the scientific team leader (or members).

4.5 Stage-gate approach

4.5.1 Stages and gates

Stages are key areas of activity that define a functional area or focus. Moving from one stage to the next also generally correlates to major steps along the value chain (see Chapter 1). Gates are the decision-making evaluation points for the results of that stage. Each stage could have several evaluation criteria within a gate. If the outcome from that stage does not meet pre-defined parameters, then the project does not move on to the next stage of activity. For example, if a diagnostic test cannot demonstrate specificity to a certain pre-set level, then it cannot move on to clinical testing (Figure 4.6). An example gate for a drug would be the demonstration of efficacy in an animal model of the disease or the demonstration of adequate stability in formulation; without showing which the drug will not be allowed to move onto formal pre-clinical toxicity testing studies.

Cooper, in his original paper (1988), defined six stages of activity in a product development process and it is conceptually useful to see those original six stages and screening gates as shown in Figure 4.7.

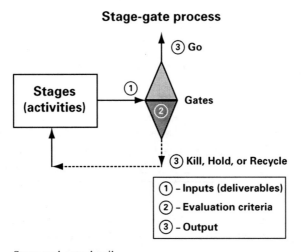

Figure 4.6 Stage and gate detail.

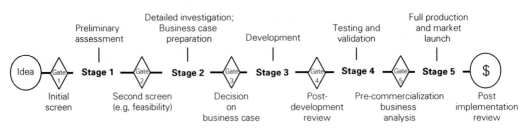

Figure 4.7 Stage-gate process as described by Robert Cooper (adapted from Cooper, 1988). Reproduced by permission of Westburn Publishers, Ltd.

4.5.2   How to configure a stage-gate process plan for my biomedical product

Each stage should be focused on one key functional area with the gates defined by key risk-reducing results of that stage. Within each stage, you can have several sub-stages and gates, representing key areas of evaluation of the project. For example, in a combination product that involves live cells implanted on a bioresorbable material coated with a drug, the first stage of pre-clinical testing could have sub-stages that evaluate each of the individual components with regard to cross-reactivity (e.g., will the implanted cells behave in the right manner when placed on the drug coated resorbable device?).

A brief discussion of the various stages of development for drugs, diagnostics, devices, and combination products is given here, with a conceptual description of the types of evaluation gates. Each company will have different processes and variations of the stage-gate process in place and the reader must apply the general principles described here in the specific relevant context.

While constructing a stage-gate plan, it is important to be as quantitative as possible in defining both the specific parameters in a gate and the interplay among various parameters. With regards to the interplay between parameters, for example, drug solubility may have a set threshold, but a lower value could be acceptable if other pharmacokinetic parameters, such as half-life, are better than expected. Or a device life span may be reduced if the weight threshold is reached. These can be mapped in a matrix with some weights and multipliers in each parameter interaction box. For example, in diagnostic development, the interaction box between specificity and sensitivity gates might have a multiplier of 0.8, so that if the specificity is higher than the expected level, the sensitivity could be 80% of the current threshold and still yield an acceptable product.

The stage-gate plan is the first plan for product development, identifying activities and key milestones, and is useful for generating budgets, financial and resource allocation plans, and time lines (described later in the chapter).

4.5.3   Unique features of biomedical development

The regulatory review of data to obtain market approval is a unique feature of all regulated biomedical products, and affects the new product development process. The FDA reviews data that span most of the development process and it is important to keep detailed records of the development of a drug or device using specific guidelines as suggested by the FDA (Chapter 5). This requirement, to store early product development data for reporting to the government, is unique to this industry. The various multiple iterations in product design and development also need to be well documented and presented with explanations to the FDA. The processes of product testing, the study design, etc., are regulated by the FDA (QSR regulations, see Chapter 5). In particular, once the product is in final preparations to enter human clinical testing, the design is in effect "locked in." Any change in product characteristics during or after that phase of testing requires added notifications to be submitted to the FDA and, in some cases, further progress of the NPD depends on FDA approval. This design lock during early product development (before manufacturing) is another unique feature of biomedical product development.

There are benefits to the public and eventually to the manufacturer, from this onerous regulatory process, as explained in Chapter 5.

4.6   Ethical requirements in biomedical product development

If product development proceeds without regard to general ethical principles and the specific checks and balances described here (and in Box 4.5) and in Section 4.16 the company can face negative consequences, including a complete halt of all product development activities.

Ethics considerations formally enter the NPD process at the time of *pre-clinical testing* of the drug or device and continue through the clinical development and post-approval stages of development. Specific embodiments of these considerations are described in the following sections.

Box 4.5 Regulations for care of animals and human beings during product development

IACUC resources are available online at: http://grants.nih.gov/grants/olaw/references/outline.htm.

The *Animal Welfare Act* has provisions to regulate and ensure that animals used in research, for exhibition, or as pets receive humane care and treatment. Regulatory authority is vested in the secretary of the US Department of Agriculture (USDA) and implemented by USDA's Animal and Plant Health Inspection Service (APHIS). Rules and regulations pertaining to implementation are published in the Code of Federal Regulations, Title 9 (Animals and Animal Products), Chapter 1, Subchapter A (Animal Welfare), available from Regulatory Enforcement and Animal Care, APHIS, USDA, Unit 85, 4700 River Road, Riverdale, MD 20737-1234. File Name 9CFR93.

The Public Health Service (PHS) Policy on Humane Care and Use of Laboratory Animals was updated in 1996 and contains guidelines on what constitutes humane and ethical treatment and care of animals used in research. Information concerning the policy can be obtained from the Office for Protection from Research Risks, National Institutes of Health, 6100 Executive Boulevard, MSC 7507, Rockville, MD 20892-7507

IRB related: FDA regulations that apply to clinical investigations and govern the development of drugs, biologics, and devices are contained in Title 21 of the Code of Federal Regulations (CFR), which can be purchased from the Superintendent of Documents, Attn: New Orders, PO Box 371954, Pittsburgh, PA 15250-7954.

4.6.1 Institutional Animal Care and Use Committee (IACUC)

Any study being done on vertebrate animals, or on tissues or cells taken directly from an animal, requires the establishment of an animal care and use program and policy at the company or institute. This Institutional Animal Care and Use Committee (IACUC; vernacular pronunciation "I-a-cook") will review the specific study protocol. An animal care program must be managed in accordance with applicable federal, state, and local laws and regulations, such as the federal Animal Welfare Regulations and Public Health Service (PHS) Policy on Humane Care and Use of Laboratory Animals (PHS 1996). The IACUC reviews the animal care program and approves any experimental procedure that involves vertebrate animals. The IACUC committee must include a veterinarian. The IACUC reviews facilities and study protocols for the following:

- Minimum standards of care and treatment must be upheld.
- Research facilities must meet required standards of veterinary care and animal husbandry, exercise for dogs, psychological well-being of primates, etc.
- Pain or distress caused by research must be minimized as best as the experiment allows (anesthesia or pain-relieving medication). Note: the Animal Welfare Act also forbids the unnecessary duplication of a specific experiment using regulated animals.

4.6.2 Institutional Review Board (IRB)

An Institutional Review Board (IRB) review and approval of any study protocol that involves interactions with human subjects is required by the FDA. Institutional Review Boards that approve studies of FDA-regulated products must be established and operated in compliance with 21 CFR (Code of Federal Regulations) part 56. An IRB review is mandatory before starting human clinical trials with any biomedical product. The main purpose of an IRB is to ensure the rights and welfare (safety) of the subjects participating in a clinical trial are protected. Thus, the IRB rigorously reviews (in addition to the submitted study protocol) the "informed consent form" that subjects sign to confirm they understand the procedure and risks involved in a clinical trial (see Box 4.6). The IRB also verifies that the sponsor (product developer) has obtained all necessary permissions from the FDA before beginning the trial.

4.7 Define the product and process – indications and endpoints

The goal of all development work in any company is to get a product to market as quickly and as efficiently as possible. For biomedical products to get to market, there is an additional consideration, as the market is defined through very specific language in the approval from the Food and Drug Administration (FDA). The

---

Box 4.6 Informed consent forms

Minimal requirements for protection of clinical trial subjects as per the Code for Federal Regulations (21CFR50)

Title 21 – Food and drugs
Chapter I – Food and Drug Administration, Department of Health and Human Services
Part 50 – Protection of human subjects – Table of contents
Sub-part B – Informed consent of human subjects
Section 50.25 Elements of informed consent

(a) Basic elements of informed consent. In seeking informed consent, the following information shall be provided to each subject:

   (1) A statement that the study involves research, an explanation of the purposes of the research and the expected duration of the subject's participation, a description of the procedures to be followed, and identification of any procedures that are experimental.

   (2) A description of any reasonably foreseeable risks or discomforts to the subject.

   (3) A description of any benefits to the subject or to others that may reasonably be expected from the research.

   (4) A disclosure of appropriate alternative procedures or courses of treatment, if any, that might be advantageous to the subject.

   (5) A statement describing the extent, if any, to which confidentiality of records identifying the subject will be maintained and that notes the possibility that the Food and Drug Administration may inspect the records.

   (6) For research involving more than minimal risk, an explanation as to whether any compensation and an explanation as to whether any medical treatments are available if injury occurs and, if so, what they consist of, or where further information may be obtained.

   (7) An explanation of whom to contact for answers to pertinent questions about the research and research subjects' rights, and whom to contact in the event of a research-related injury to the subject.

   (8) A statement that participation is voluntary, that refusal to participate will involve no penalty or loss of benefits to which the subject is otherwise entitled, and that the subject may discontinue participation at any time without penalty or loss of benefits to which the subject is otherwise entitled.

(b) Additional elements of informed consent. When appropriate, one or more of the following elements of information shall also be provided to each subject:

   (1) A statement that the particular treatment or procedure may involve risks to the subject (or to the embryo or fetus, if the subject is or may become pregnant) that are currently unforeseeable.

Box 4.6 (cont.)

(2) Anticipated circumstances under which the subject's participation may be terminated by the investigator without regard to the subject's consent.

(3) Any additional costs to the subject that may result from participation in the research.

(4) The consequences of a subject's decision to withdraw from the research and procedures for orderly termination of participation by the subject.

(5) A statement that significant new findings developed during the course of the research that may relate to the subject's willingness to continue participation will be provided to the subject.

(6) The approximate number of subjects involved in the study.

(c) The informed consent requirements in these regulations are not intended to pre-empt any applicable Federal, State, or local laws that require additional information to be disclosed for informed consent to be legally effective.

(d) Nothing in these regulations is intended to limit the authority of a physician to provide emergency medical care to the extent the physician is permitted to do so under applicable Federal, State, or local law.

disease for which the product is approved is called the *indication* (the impact on the market is discussed in greater detail in Section 2.5.5). All data collected in carefully designed experiments (clinical studies with human subjects) and submitted to the FDA have to satisfy rigorous evaluation by the FDA and show that the product will perform as stated *for the specific disease condition* that it is being indicated for. Each new indication for the same product needs a separate application to the FDA by the product developer (follow-ons to the primary approval are shorter). On approval, the FDA issues a *label*, which very specifically defines the indication for the product; and the manufacturer cannot market or make any claims outside of treating or diagnosing the disease condition or indication on the label. Therefore, the product development process begins with the selection of the *indication* or the specific state of the disease for which the product is going to be developed (see Section 2.5.5 for more details on how this selection will affect markets and marketing).

The product development studies have to be focused and designed carefully to finally convince the FDA, with statistical analysis, that the product works safely to treat or diagnose that specific indication or disease compared to either placebo or current comparable products. The final outcome of the studies, on which the approval is based, is called the *endpoint* of the study. Clinical endpoints are distinct measurements or analyses of disease characteristics reflecting the effect of a thera-peutic intervention in a clinical trial or study. An endpoint is the hypothesis that a clinical trial is designed to test. An example of a hypothesis is: this putative anti-hypertensive drug, given to patients of a certain type (over the age of 65, with systolic pressures above 200 mmHg) will reduce blood pressure by 10 mmHg. The product development plan and, in particular, the clinical studies are designed and structured to try and reach a statistically significant answer to that hypothesis.

Endpoints can be grouped as single, multiple, or composite and the final claim (marketing, efficacy, etc.) made on the device or drug will depend completely on the evaluation of this set of endpoints. Hence study design must be carried out keeping the endpoints in mind. Examples of simple and composite clinical trial endpoints for drug products are given in Box 4.7. Box 4.8 contains a device example on how to choose a clinical endpoint.

Market research input is used to help identify specific indications but usually the endpoints emerge from the hypothesis defined by the mechanism of action of the biomedical technology and the pathology of the disease (see Chapter 2).

4.8   Typical drug development process

Drug development takes over ten years from the definition of the problem and identification of drug target to market approval from FDA. The process typically costs over $800 million (including the cost of failed prototypes) with the majority of the costs incurred during human clinical testing of the drug. Figure 4.8a shows the average time for each stage of development along with the average cost for each stage of drug development. Figure 4.8b shows, in slightly greater detail, the relative ratio in distribution of costs of drug R&D across various functional stages of development.

The functional segments of the value chain for drug development are outlined schematically in Figure 4.9 (and also discussed in Chapter 1) and the stages for each functional segment of the value chain are discussed in greater detail in the following sections.

4.8.1   Discovery and pre-clinical testing

Target discovery and validation

A drug development project often starts with the identification of a disease problem that is lacking adequate treatment (a "medical need") and the discovery of a pathological mechanism that appears to influence the disease, its symptoms, or its progression. An example would be an initial idea to develop a treatment for Alzheimer's disease, as the drugs currently available are not adequate. A little research on etiology and pathology of the disease will reveal that there are three possible ways to prevent disease progression or possibly reverse the disease – block glutamate neurotoxicity, prevent amyloid plaques, or attenuate neuro-inflammation. Tissue cellular processes that are altered from normal health behavior have some changes in the quantity (decreased or increased levels being made), the form (mutation), or the function (activity) of the proteins that carry out these processes. Either one of the above approaches to developing a new treatment for Alzheimer's would point to a specific enzyme or cell receptor whose activity would have to be

Box 4.7 Primary and composite endpoints for drug studies

Material adapted from an FDA presentation, 2004.

Primary endpoints comprise a set of clinical endpoints based on which clinical benefits are assessed. Clinical studies with the product have to show a statistically significant effect (compared with a control group) to rule that the primary endpoint has been met satisfactorily. Primary endpoints usually provide characterization of various aspects of a disease and are used to describe clinical benefits.

Examples of primary endpoints in clinical trials:

- Anti-hypertension drug trial primary endpoints;
  - Supine diastolic blood pressure.
- Congestive heart failure drug trial primary endpoints;
  - Reduction in incidence of all causes of mortality,
  - Reduction in incidence of stroke,
  - Reduction in incidence of myocardial infarction.
- Alzheimer's drug trial primary endpoints;
  - Alzheimer disease assessment scale – cognitive sub-scale,
  - Clinician's interview-based impression of change.
- Epilepsy device trial primary endpoints;
  - Percent reduction in seizure rate,
  - Percent reduction in drop attack rate,
  - Parental global evaluation of seizure severity.

Secondary endpoints

In a clinical trial, secondary endpoints form a set of clinical endpoints that are intended for possible inclusion in the label, after efficacy has been demonstrated by the primary endpoints.

Composite endpoints

Composite endpoints are a combination of several primary endpoints, used when the disease manifestation is complex.

Example

A study of Losartan (COZAAR) vs. Atenolol in 9193 hypertensive patients had three primary endpoints – reduction in incidence of cardiovascular (CV) death, stroke, or myocardial infarction (MI) – which were summarized in a composite endpoint as below:

Composite endpoint (CV death, stroke, MI) = The time to the first occurrence of either CV death, stroke, or MI.

Box 4.8 Challenges in designing clinical endpoints for device trials

This example is an extract from an FDA guidance document for percutaneous tissue ablation in atrial fibrillation on clinical trial design and endpoints (www.fda.gov/cdrh/ode/guidance/1229.html). This minimally invasive procedure involves the ablation or selective removal of a segment of the tissue that gives the heart muscle its synchronizing pulsation signals.

Clinical study designs for percutaneous catheter ablation for treatment of atrial fibrillation

Introduction and scope

Atrial fibrillation (AF) is a complex arrhythmia; its precise mechanisms remain unclear, and the clinical presentation, arrhythmia characteristics, and underlying pathophysiology are variable. This guidance document addresses study design issues associated with catheter ablation devices intended for treatment of atrial fibrillation. These devices (product code: LPB; electrode, percutaneous, conduction tissue ablation) are class III, requiring pre-market approval applications before marketing (section 513(a) of the Federal Food, Drug, and Cosmetic Act (21 USC 360c(a))).

Study endpoints: primary effectiveness endpoint

In the future, it may be feasible to demonstrate that ablation therapies for AF positively affect disease outcomes. Currently, it is probably most appropriate to evaluate ablation therapy for AF as a palliative therapy and to select endpoints that have the potential to demonstrate clearly a reduction in symptoms caused by AF. The FDA believes that evaluation of the reduction of AF burden (or the reduction in the incidence of AF) is problematic as the primary endpoint for a study designed to evaluate therapy for paroxysmal AF. Measurement of this endpoint post-ablation could be strongly influenced by various, non-therapy-related factors ... *For a primary effectiveness endpoint, the FDA recommends the relatively unambiguous endpoint of freedom from symptomatic atrial fibrillation at one year* [emphasis added]. This outcome should be in the absence of anti-arrhythmic drug therapy ... A one-year follow-up period both minimizes the confounding effects of the clustered, non-random AF recurrence pattern that was previously discussed and provides sufficient time to evaluate adverse events, e.g., pulmonary vein stenosis, that may be manifest or progressive only at late time points in some patients.

Primary safety endpoints

In considering primary safety endpoints, the FDA acknowledges that an ablation intervention arm and a drug intervention arm may have different safety criteria.

Box 4.8 (cont.)

Ablation procedure safety endpoint

For an ablation procedure safety endpoint, the FDA recommends, for the devices addressed in this guidance document, a composite serious adverse event endpoint that includes, but need not be limited to, the following:

- Transient ischemic attack,
- Cerebrovascular accident,
- Major bleeding,
- Pulmonary vein stenosis,
- Pericarditis,
- Myocardial infarction,
- Diaphragmatic paralysis,
- Death.

Composite serious adverse event endpoint

For a drug intervention arm, the FDA recommends a composite serious adverse event endpoint, which includes, but need not be limited to, the following:

- Life-threatening arrhythmia,
- Transient ischemic attack,
- Cerebrovascular accident,
- Anaphylactic reaction,
- Pulmonary hypertension (if amiodarone therapy),
- Death.

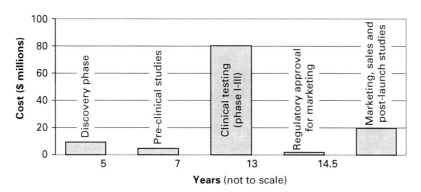

Figure 4.8 Typical time and costs for development of a new drug; Pie chart illustrating, in percentages, the allocation of development costs. Data from Parexel's *Pharmaceutical Statistical Sourcebook*, 2005.

Functionality costs for drug development

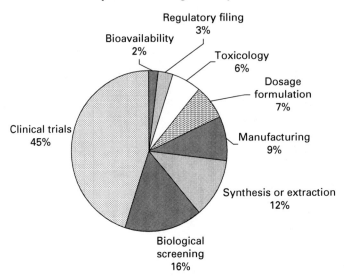

Figure 4.8   (cont.)

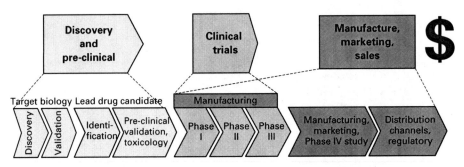

Figure 4.9   Activities in drug development.

blocked, enhanced, or modulated with a drug. These enzyme or receptor proteins then become known as *drug targets*. Target discovery usually takes place in academic settings, where such basic and fundamental phenomena are usually studied but with the advent of industrial scale genomics and proteomics, it is likely to happen in corporate research settings as well.

Target validation: Once discovered, the target has to be validated – experiments must be carried out to show that changing the activity of the target protein will affect the disease outcome positively. In this pre-clinical stage, studies are done using knockout models (where expression of the target protein is completely knocked out by genetic manipulation at the formative stage) or other disease models and interventions. These experiments involve fundamental biological principles and practices, are expensive and time consuming, and can last a number of years.

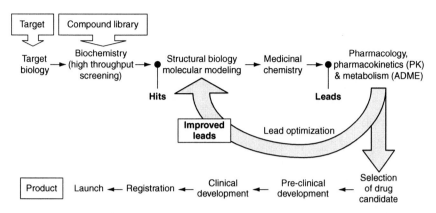

Figure 4.10   Pre-clinical stages of developing a drug product.

Hit to lead to drug product candidate optimization

Once a valid target is selected as the thesis for the treatment, a project proposal can be written up to launch preliminary investigations into developing a product that would either develop a new chemical or biological molecule as a drug treatment for this disease. In these stages, chemical compounds are screened, from libraries to which the company has access. Screening the chemical molecules against the isolated target protein, or against a relevant cell type, (using techniques known as high throughput screening, HTS) will yield a set of molecules that are designated as *hits* (the output of preliminary screening). The project typically moves to its next level of funding, as medicinal chemistry is now involved in refining and optimizing the hit compounds into *lead compounds*. This *hit to lead* optimization and refinement process can take from months to years to yield an acceptable *drug product candidate*.

There are many tools available today to help speed this process up, including computational screens and high throughput crystallography, which can lead to a very detailed understanding of the optimal molecular structure. More discovery tools will continue to be developed as it is necessary to make this part of the process more efficient and productive. As seen in Figure 4.10 and Box 4.9, the lead optimization process from hit to drug candidate involves, in addition to medicinal chemistry, a variety of biological tests (efficacy screening in cells or whole animal models, pharmacokinetics, metabolism, early toxicity) to evaluate the properties of the compounds being synthesized. The process is inherently iterative (Figure 4.10), as are all experimental optimization processes. Boxes 4.9 and 4.10 describe some possible product characteristics for a chemical drug.

At this gate, typically, a full review of the optimized product characteristics is carried out, including a management review of the business case (Figure 4.11), and the design is "frozen" with only minor changes possible after formal toxicity testing (next stage). The lead compounds pass through many tests in this stage, some of which are standard and common to all drugs, while other tests are more specific to the therapeutic area or the specific drug target.

Box 4.9 Sample gate parameters for lead compounds

Lipinski's *rule of five* is a typical set of parameters used as cut-off characteristics to reject or select compounds when good intestinal absorption is important (most oral drugs).

Lipinski's Rule of five states that poor absorption or permeation is more likely when:

- The molecular weight (MW) is over 500,
- $LogP$ is over 5 (or $MlogP$ is over 4.15),
- There are more than five H-bond donors (expressed as the sum of OHs and NHs),
- There are more than ten H-bond acceptors (expressed as the sum of Ns and Os).

The rule of five is called as such since the cutoff for each of four parameters is either five or a multiple of five.

Other parameters used could include characteristics such as solubility (above a certain level) or the potency against the specific drug target, measured in IC_{50} (the concentration at which the compound shows 50% of maximum theoretical activity). For example a cancer compound may be expected to kill all cancer cells in a culture; if it kills 50% of the cells at a concentration of 10 micromolar, the IC_{50} of that compound for that cell line is 10 micromolar.

Reference

Lipinski, C A, Lombardo, F, Dominy, B W, and Feeney, P. Experimental and computational approaches to estimate solubility and permeability in drug discovery and development settings, *Advanced Drug Delivery Reviews*, **23**, 3–25, 1997.

Pre-clinical toxicity

If the drug candidate has passed the screening gates on specific characteristics such as good pharmacokinetic parameters, then it enters a formal toxicity testing program and scale of production under regulatory guidelines. From this stage onwards, *the drug molecule (active pharmaceutical ingredient or API) is usually tested as a formulation (solid, liquid, suspension) with its excipients (other components in the tablet, powder, or solution that do not change biological activity of the API, but may assist in improving solubility or other pharmacokinetic parameters).* Toxicity testing usually requires studies on at least two animal species (typically rodent and canine) to identify the doses at which toxic effects are seen. Additionally, specific effects on various tissues or organs may be indicated, based on the mechanism and characteristics of the drug (e.g., neurotoxicity screening if the compound crosses the blood-brain barrier). The manufacturing method is also established at this point, as the API has to be scaled up. Most of the data at this stage are prepared for submission to

---

> **Box 4.10** Transforming a lead compound into a drug
>
> There are several issues in product development that young companies, and, in particular, inexperienced staff, sometimes fail to consider in pre-clinical tests. In general, the small molecule or biologic must be druggable. Since issues in developing biologics into products are discussed in Section 4.8.2, this box will focus on small molecules. "Druggable" is a term that means "must be capable of becoming a drug product," but this term really covers many characteristics of the small molecule, such as the Lipinski rules mentioned in Box 4.9, manufacturability (if the synthesis has 50 steps or involves toxic reagents, it might not be possible to scale up; or if polymorph crystal forms emerge in the final scaled-up process with different properties from the original compound), stability, protein binding, solubility, and other such parameters. Two examples quoted in an interview by the head of a pre-clinical contract research organization are summarized here. The first example was that of a small molecule that was being tested in experimental animals – the compound was actually degrading into a new compound while stored overnight and the scientists were making their (patent and IND) claims on the wrong molecule. The scientists had not known to conduct a stability check on the small molecule in its final formulation. Another example was that of a group that had developed an anti-cancer agent that was very effective but had to be stored at $-70\,^{\circ}\text{C}$ to be stable. This group wanted to get the drug to market very badly and spent a few million dollars on it, but the drug was destined to fail, as not everyone could store the drug in $-70\,^{\circ}\text{C}$ freezers. There are various parameters that must be satisfied before a drug candidate is anointed. The iterative process shown in Figure 4.10 has several tests that the compound must pass before it can exit the loop.

the FDA and laboratory experiments must be carried out using processes that follow strict FDA guidelines, known as the current good laboratory practices (cGLP), as specified in 21CFR Part 58. These guidelines outline the processes and recording requirements to be followed in data generation, handling, and analysis. These data are submitted to the FDA as part of a petition called an IND (investigational new drug application), requesting initiation of testing in human beings. The compound design is typically locked in prior to these pre-clinical toxicity studies and any change, however minor, must be communicated to the FDA and approved before proceeding further. If the change is deemed *significant*, major sections of the development program might have to be repeated. Compound production is typically scaled up at this point with production information also submitted to the FDA in the IND, and must be carried out under current good manufacturing process (cGMP) guidelines. Only FDA approved and inspected facilities can manufacture the drug compound for human testing. These interactions with the FDA, including the contents of an IND application, are described in more detail in Chapter 5.

4.8.2   Distinctions in pre-clinical development of biotechnology drugs (large molecule biologics)

The large molecule biological drug is usually a protein or a glycoprotein, made by biological processes in a bioreactor full of living cells or in other whole organisms (secreted in the milk of transgenic goats or in a tuber of a transgenic plant, for example), rather than a chemical molecule made by synthetic chemical processes. Subtle changes in the composition of the biotherapeutic molecule can cause significant changes in biological activity and behavior, making it important to work with as close to a final molecule as possible, even in the early stages of drug development. The cell line and the product must be well characterized early on in the process. Although there is always a balancing act with regards to investing in manufacturing-related, well characterized processes early on in the development process (when it is not known if the project will progress to clinical studies) or using prototype drug molecules, biological drugs need more thought and planning in this stage.

A risk factor that is specific to development and testing of biological drugs is the reduction in efficacy that frequently occurs with the development of antibodies in human beings against the protein drug. Strategies to test and reduce the potential for antibody formation in humans must be evaluated and applied early in the development process.

4.8.3   Drug candidate clinical testing to market approval

The FDA suggests that the company arrange its first formal interaction visit before starting human clinical testing. This is not mandatory but highly recommended, as described in Chapter 5. All clinical studies must be carried out using current good clinical practice (cGCP) guidelines. Planning for clinical studies must usually incorporate the following considerations:

- Clinical endpoints must be carefully selected (see Section 5.1 for details). Input from marketing departments and research (Chapter 2) and reimbursement specialists (see Chapter 7 for details) must be incorporated into the study design so that the product is developed with the appropriate data and characteristics.
- Patient inclusion and exclusion criteria must be defined – examples of such criteria are given in Box 4.11.
- Clinical study design and protocol. The measurements made during the study are defined in this document, including details of the dosing schedule. The number of patients to be recruited, group assignment, protocol for drug dosing or delivery, data collection and archival, reporting of adverse events, and many other criteria are defined clearly before the study begins. See Boxes 4.12 and 4.13 for examples and details. The design of the trial and the measurement of the right parameters may become critical in identifying new uses if the drug fails to show efficacy in the trials (see Box 4.12).

Box 4.11 Patient selection criteria for a clinical trial of a new asthma drug

Inclusion criteria

(1) Men and women between the ages of 18–50,
(2) A FEV1 of 80% or greater than the predicted value [Note: FEV1 is the final expiration volume-1 and a measure of pulmonary function that classifies the severity of asthma],
(3) Blood pressure $\geq 110/70$ mmHg,
(4) Pulse rate ≥ 60 beats/min,
(5) No significant health issues,
(6) Non-smoker or ex-smoker < 10 packs/year,
(7) Able to complete diary cards and comply with study procedures,
(8) Women of childbearing age may participate only if they have a negative pregnancy test, are non-lactating, and agree to practice an adequate birth control method (abstinence, combination of barrier and spermicide, or hormonal) for the duration of the study.

Exclusion criteria

(1) History of upper or lower respiratory tract infection within six weeks of first baseline visit,
(2) Currently diagnosed with chronic obstructive pulmonary disease (COPD),
(3) Used short-acting antihistamines within three days of the first baseline visit,
(4) Used cromones (e.g., Intal, Tilade) or long-acting antihistamines within one week of first baseline visit,
(5) Used leukotriene modifiers within 14 days of first baseline visit,
(6) History of any cardiovascular, neurological, hepatic, renal, or other medical conditions that may interfere with the interpretation of data or the patient's participation in the study, in the investigator's opinion,
(7) Smoked within one year prior to first baseline visit,
(8) Any clinically significant deviation from normal in either the general physical examination or laboratory parameters, as evaluated by the investigator at the screening visit,
(9) History of alcohol or drug abuse,
(10) Participation in another research trial within 30 days of starting this trial,
(11) Known allergy or sensitivity to the study drug,
(12) Inability to give consent or unwillingness or inability to comply with study procedures,
(13) Inability to swallow the study medication tablet.

> **Box 4.12** Reconfiguring drug indications
>
> A clinical study protocol is usually written by a multidisciplinary team, which will typically include a clinically trained physician, a biostatistician, a regulatory affairs person, a marketing person, and researchers from the team that discovered the drug. Increased data collection will lead to increased costs, but taking measurements outside of the expected effects has resurrected many drugs that were failing to achieve efficacy in their main development indication.
>
> A classic example is that of Viagra, which was being developed for angina. In Phase I studies the clinician noticed that a majority of the drug-treated volunteers had an unusual side effect (penile erection) while the majority of the placebo subjects did not have any such side effects. Since this was a drug with vasodilatory effects, it made researchers wonder if the vasodilation was predominantly in the penile area. The rest is history. A new blockbuster class of drugs for sexual dysfunction emerged from this finding.
>
> Other studies that have specifically tried to include additional endpoints to see if rescue indications emerged (in case the drug failed the primary endpoint) have not always been successful. Examples include the phase III anti-obesity studies conducted by Eli Lilly, Pfizer, and Regeneron for antidepressive drugs (Regeneron's drug was actually developed for Lou Gehrig's disease) that showed weight loss effects in Phase II and III studies. All of these three drugs with reconfigured indications failed to show sustained and significant effect in obesity.

- The size and length of the clinical study must be determined by a robust statistical analysis, as the final data must show a statistically significant effect for the drug to be valid. This analysis must be done as early as possible in the planning process, as this will give an estimate of the time and cost involved. For example, a 500-patient study that measures the effect of a drug therapy on overall survival of the patient groups will take 1.5 years to recruit patients, 3 years for drug dosing and patient data recording, and half a year for analysis of collected data, at the cost of approximately $12 000 per patient included in the study. This hypothetical study will cost $60M and take 5 years to complete.
- Data analysis techniques have to be laid out a priori as the FDA will want to review the prospective trial and the specific hypothesis the clinical studies will be testing.

Human clinical testing for drugs typically proceeds in four phases:

Phase I clinical studies

The drug (active pharmaceutical ingredient (API) and its formulated carrier compounds) is first tested in a set of normal healthy patients aged between 18 and 45 to determine the toxic thresholds and thus define the therapeutic window for dosage. One of the most difficult product characteristics to determine (owing to the limited

> **Box 4.13** Drug clinical study designs
>
> *Extract from FDA guidance* – www.fda.gov/oc/ohrt/irbs/drugsbiologics.html#
> study (also see Section 7.5.1 for a discussion of the rigor and quality of different trial
> designs)
>
> Before a new drug or biologic can be marketed, its sponsor must show, through
> adequate and well controlled clinical studies, that it is effective. A well controlled
> study permits a comparison of subjects treated with the new agent with a suitable
> control population, so that the effect of the new agent can be determined and
> distinguished from other influences, such as spontaneous change, placebo effects,
> concomitant therapy, or observer expectations. FDA regulations [21 CFR 314.126]
> cite five different kinds of control that can be useful in particular circumstances:
>
> (1) Placebo concurrent control,
> (2) Dose-comparison concurrent control,
> (3) No-treatment concurrent control,
> (4) Active-treatment concurrent control, and
> (5) Historical control.
>
> No general preference is expressed for any one type, but the study design
> chosen must be adequate to the task. It is relatively difficult to be sure that
> historical control groups are comparable to the treated subjects with respect to
> variables that could affect outcome and, therefore, use of historical control
> studies has been reserved for special circumstances, notably cases where the
> disease treated has high and predictable mortality (a large difference from this
> usual course would be easy to detect) and those in which the effect is self-evident
> (e.g., a general anesthetic).
>
> Placebo control, no-treatment control (suitable where objective measurements
> are felt to make blinding unnecessary), and dose-comparison control studies are
> all study designs in which a difference is intended to be shown between the test
> article and some control. The alternative study design generally proposed for
> these kinds of study is an active-treatment concurrent control in which a finding
> of no difference between the test article and the recognized effective agent (active
> control) would be considered evidence of effectiveness of the new agent. There are
> circumstances in which this is a fully valid design. Active controls are usually used
> in antibiotic trials, for example, because it is easy to tell the difference between
> antibiotics that have the expected effect on specific infections and those that do
> not. In many cases, however, the active-control design may be simply incapable of
> allowing any conclusion as to whether or not the test article is having an effect.
>
> For certain drug classes, such as analgesics, antidepressants, or antianxiety
> drugs, failure to show superiority to placebo in a given study is common. This is
> also often seen with anti-hypertensives, anti-angina drugs, anti-heart failure
> treatments, antihistamines, and drugs for asthma prophylaxis. In these situa-
> tions, active-control trials showing no difference between the new drug and

Box 4.13 (cont.)

control are of little value as primary evidence of effectiveness and the active-control design (the study design most often proposed as an alternative to use of a placebo) is not credible.

It is often possible to design a successful placebo-controlled trial that neither causes investigator discomfort nor raises ethical issues. Treatment periods can be kept short; early "escape" mechanisms can be built into the study so that subjects will not undergo prolonged placebo treatment if they are not doing well. In some cases, randomized placebo-controlled therapy withdrawal studies have been used to minimize exposure to placebo or unsuccessful therapy; in such studies, apparent responders to a treatment in an open study are randomly assigned to continued treatment or to placebo. Subjects who fail (e.g., blood pressure rises, angina worsens) can be removed promptly, with such failure representing a study endpoint.

Institutional review boards (IRBs) may face difficult issues in deciding on the acceptability of placebo-controlled and active-control trials. Placebo-controlled trials, regardless of any advantages in interpretation of results, are obviously not ethically acceptable where existing treatment is life prolonging. A placebo-controlled study that exposes subjects to a documented serious risk is not acceptable, but it is critical to review the evidence that harm would result from denial of active treatment, because alternative study designs, especially active-control studies, may not be informative, exposing subjects to risk but without being able to collect useful information.

sets of tests that are possible and the high cost of testing in human beings), but also the most important, is the dosage or therapeutic window definition – how much drug to give or how frequently. Usually, lower bounds of the therapeutic window are set by the early cellular or in vivo animal experiments and upper bounds are set by these phase I studies.

Each participant is given a single dose of the drug and is closely monitored for adverse drug reactions. If none occur, the dose of the drug is progressively increased until a predetermined dose or serum level is achieved or until some event marking toxicity occurs.

Note: phase I studies in cancer therapeutics, which are typically drugs that have high toxicity and are designed to kill cells, are usually carried out in terminally ill cancer patients who have failed other therapies.

Phase II clinical studies

The purpose of the phase II studies is to determine the correct dose–response range (optimizing dosage characteristics) for the new drug and to verify its efficacy for the intended disorder. These studies are carried out in 20–400 patients with the disorder, with patients randomly placed in placebo or drug-receiving groups – called a randomized study. For scientifically more rigorous experimental design, neither the patient, the physician, nor the drug company should know which randomized group is receiving a placebo or the drug until the completion of the study or upon emergence of a (predetermined) significant difference between groups. This type of experiment is called a *randomized, double-blinded study*, where there is little chance of even unconscious bias or manipulation of data or patients. Box 4.12 contains a brief discussion and suggestions from the FDA on clinical study design. The data from this phase are crucial in determining whether to proceed with more extensive studies in large populations (phase III).

Note: sometimes phase I and II trials may be combined into one set of studies, but typically, each phase I and phase II trial has subcomponent studies, titled phase Ia, Ib IIa, IIb, etc. It is advisable to have the FDA review the data at the end of phase II to get their agreement in writing on the design of the phase III clinical trial.

Phase III clinical studies

The purpose of the phase III studies is to verify the efficacy of the drug in much larger populations that better reflect the overall population outside the selected test population, and to detect effects that may not have occurred during phases I and II, so that the sponsor and the FDA can determine that the drug is safe and effective for its intended use. When sufficient data are collected, a rigorous statistical analysis is carried out to prove the efficacy and toxicity; those data and completed analysis are submitted to the FDA with a request for approval to market the drug (NDA: new drug approval). Contents of the NDA are discussed in Chapter 5.

Phase IV clinical studies

This title is given to clinical studies that are conducted after the drug is approved; typically clinical studies in large or select populations. Often, special subpopulations, such as pregnant women, children, or the elderly, are included. The goal of the phase IV studies is primarily to allow the FDA to continue to monitor safety of the drug as the population using it increases. New therapeutic or toxic effects of the drugs can be picked up with greater sensitivity in these larger studies. Reports from ongoing phase IV studies must be sent to the FDA every three months during the first year, every six months during the second year, and annually thereafter. The sponsor must notify the FDA of any unexpected adverse effects, injury, and toxic or allergic reactions.

4.8.4 Manufacturing, marketing, sales, and reimbursement

The manufacture of the drug (major considerations and processes are discussed in Chapter 6) is carried out under strict regulations in approved facilities that are regularly inspected by the FDA. Often, the API is made at one site and combined with the excipients at another location, where the formulation of the final form of the drug – in pill, liquid, or powder form – is completed and packaged for distribution. The drug company has to send in labels and product brochures to the FDA for review. Reimbursement and marketing are discussed in Chapter 7.

4.8.5   Keeping a record for the FDA

The FDA requires the submission of a *drug master file* (see Chapter 5) with all significant development data and records added to this file in order to consider the drug product for market approval. The details of this record, and its content and use are discussed in Chapter 5.

4.8.6   General stage-gate process for new drug development

The stage-gate criteria shown in Table 4.2 for drug development are generalized and will probably differ in specifics based on either the particular nature of the drug being developed or based on the company's internal processes, see Figure 4.11.

4.9   Typical diagnostics development process

Diagnostics are mostly regulated as devices, but since the clinical usage aspects of diagnostics are more closely related to drug therapies, their development is discussed first in this section and device development (which covers several points relevant to diagnostic development) is discussed in Section 4.10.

Diagnostics are developed in two stages – front-end investigative or exploratory research leads to the discovery of a potential marker or diagnostic protein, followed by extensive validation studies. The discovery is then validated in in vitro studies that include analysis of various stratification markers from tissue or serum samples to examine and optimize the accuracy, specificity, sensitivity, and reproducibility of the assay.

Assay development and optimization continues with a chosen clinical-testing technology platform. Before beginning clinical trials, a diagnostic kit that is user friendly, tested, and validated in a clinical environment is developed. The development of a commercial test method (with any needed change of technology platform) is completed before clinical trials are launched. A strong clinical correlation is validated using the configured clinical assay. The testing platform can be changed at this point, as long as the new technology platform can be shown to produce equivalent results. Larger companies now increasingly choose first to configure the assay on their already commercialized technological platform (e.g., immunodiagnostics), so that later optimization issues are reduced. This is akin to bringing final manufacturing considerations into the pre-clinical setting, as is increasingly being done in device and drug development.

The typical development stages and gates for diagnostic development are highlighted in Table 4.3.

Stage 6 may not be necessary if the test is cleared under a 510(k) (see Chapter 5 for details on 510(k) process), but a prospective clinical trial may be needed by the payers (see Chapter 7).

Table 4.2 Stage-gate criteria for drug development

Stage 1 – Target discovery and validation	Gate 1
Biological studies to identify target and indication of interest. If carried out in a company, this is typically part of a larger discovery effort, without a specific project necessarily assigned at this stage.	Primarily a business case review. Potency of target and druggability (accessibility to drug compound) of target are other criteria. Validation data for target must have broad scientific acceptance. Can the target be put into the company's processes? For example, if the company's technical foundation for drug design is based only on the crystal structures of the target and crystal structure of the target is not available, that target might not pass this gate.
Stage 2 – Hit to lead	Gate 2
Lead identification and optimization, includes biology activities. Formal project management in place.	Specific product physico-chemical characteristics, e.g., Lipinski's rule of five, lack of toxicity in early tests, efficacy in animal models of the disease, other project or disease-specific parameters (e.g., blood–brain barrier penetration; oral bioavailability, etc.) For example, the new drug compound must show potency of at least 50% inhibition of cell proliferation at 10 microMolar concentration against a chosen cell line.
Stage 3 – Lead to drug candidate	Gate 3
Formal cGLP studies, toxicity studies, advanced efficacy studies in animal models if needed; also includes formulation and further medicinal chemistry optimization of drug compound; or if biological drug, could include fine tuning of separation procedures, full characterization of post-translational modifications that are acceptable, etc.	Drug candidate meets or passes preferred pharmacokinetic, physico-chemical, pharmacologic and toxicology parameters. No objection by FDA to IND package; approved by FDA to start clinical studies
Stage 4 – Phase I clinical studies	Gate 4
Determine toxic reactions and toxic dose in small group of healthy normal human subjects.	Lack of significant adverse side effects; identification of therapeutic window that is suitable; adequate pharmacokinetic parameters in human subjects.
Stage 5 – Phase II clinical studies	Gate 5
Dose-finding studies, verification of efficacy in 20–400 (or more) patients with disorder.	Efficacy and lack of toxicity; dose-response determined for phase III approval study.
Stage 6 – Phase III clinical studies	Gate 6
Include large scale studies for efficacy and safety with a final report submitted for market approval to the FDA.	Statistical analysis of results from studies supports the claims of efficacy and safety. Obtain FDA approval of NDA after review.
Stage 7 – Phase IV – post market approval clinical studies	Gate 7
Carried out in larger or selected population groups, the FDA reviews data from this ongoing trial periodically.	No significant adverse event and no added toxicity finding. New indication added with selected patient group.

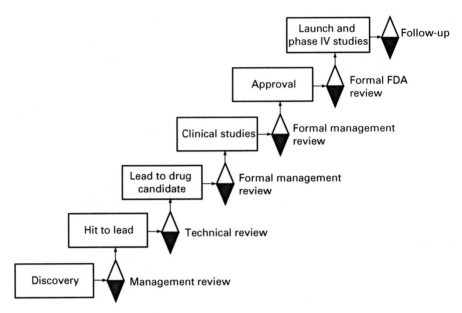

Figure 4.11   Conceptual stage-gate process for developing a drug.

If an instrumentation product is being developed as a technology platform for diagnostic assays, and not a specific diagnostic test, the product development stages are quite different and can be summarized as:

Stage 1   Definition of product specification with input from market needs and product standards.

Stage 2   Manufacturing cost analysis and business case is generated, which become the basis of a go/no-go decision. Cross-functional, multi-disciplinary team is formed.

Stage 3   System and sub-system design. Create a working automated instrumentation process flow for the chemistry and analysis. The generalized assay configuration will flow into the product specifications. Formalized software and hardware specifications are developed.

Stage 4   Validation. Make sure the test system reports the correct results and conforms to customer needs. Protocol testing and beta testing results are used to fine tune or change elements of the instrumentation system.

Typical development of a clinical diagnostic test takes about three to eight years and costs about $30–$75 M, depending mostly on the clinical trial and subsequent investment in commercial activities and market infrastructure. Figure 4.12 points out specific stages in the development of a diagnostic test, with a recognition that the length of the development period depends largely on the type of product and the type of regulatory gateway the product will enter (see Chapter 5 for more details). In essence, some diagnostic products can be sold on the market with minimal clinical development, while others will need a fully fledged prospective clinical trial to be approved for sales and to gain acceptance in the market.

Table 4.3 Stages and gates for diagnostic development

Stage 1 – Biomarker discovery and validation	Gate 1
Biological studies to identify a marker linked to a disease. This discovery research can be carried out inside a company as part of overall basic research activities but is usually discovered in academic medical research centers, which have access to large pools of annotated clinical samples and basic science researchers.	A business case review and a feasibility or proof of concept review. Validation data for biomarker must have strong scientific evidence that links a marker to a disease. The biomarker can be a protein, gene sequence, or specific pattern of genetic changes.
Stage 2 – Clinical test development	**Gate 2**
Development of the assay procedures and the technical method.	A reproducible assay that can be performed on clinical samples. For example, the test should require minimal sample preparation, should be portable across technology platforms with simple operation, show operator independent reproducibility, etc.
Stage 3 – Analytical assessment optimization	**Gate 3**
Assessment and optimization of the analytical methods.	Gates can include good reproducibility, high sensitivity, high specificity, predictability, and a linear response over the relevant range of measures.
Stage 4 – Scale up, manufacturing, and early sales as non-regulated test	**Gate 4**
	Manufacturing cost per test must come under threshold. Reagent sales can proceed for research use only without going through FDA review.
Stage 5 – Retrospective clinical trials, registration, and commercialization	**Gate 5**
Partnerships with access to clinical samples must be set up if needed; registration path is defined and data are collected from analysis of clinical samples from previously completed study (typically for a therapeutic).	Clinical relevance must be clearly shown by good sensitivity and specificity in identifying the clinical outcome. Sales of a diagnostic test can proceed in Europe and US respectively after CE mark and 510(k) FDA clearance (if applicable; see Chapter 5).
Stage 6 – Prospective clinical trials, registration, and commercialization	**Gate 6**
Include prospectively designed studies for efficacy with a final report submitted for pre-market approval (PMA) to the FDA.	Statistical analysis of results from studies supports the claims of efficacy and correlation to clinical outcome. FDA approval of PMA for marketing.

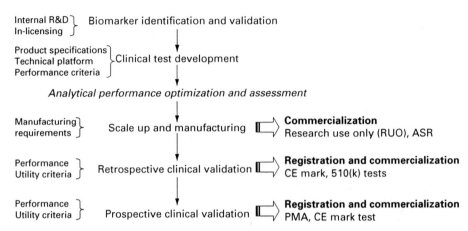

Figure 4.12   Development steps for a new diagnostic. This diagram recognizes that not all diagnostic products will have to go through a prospective trial and that the development pathway is shorter for some types of products, which require minimal regulation.

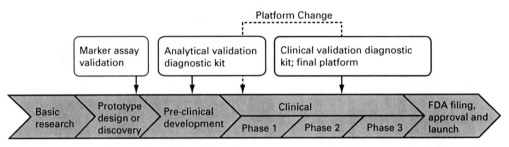

Figure 4.13   This schematic describes the timing of various studies and functions involved in diagnostic development, compared with drug co-development steps. From the FDA white paper on co-development of drugs and diagnostics (see Chapter 5 for more details).

These figures might change significantly in the future if co-development of diagnostics and drugs becomes common (see Section 5.7 for more details), as some of the cost of the clinical trials might be reduced by combining the diagnostic clinical testing with the pharmaceutical clinical trial. The diagnostic could be used to identify a small number of predicted responsive patients for selection in the drug trial, making it likely that the drug will be more effective or less toxic to the treatment. Figure 4.13 lays out the key diagnostic development stages in a time line comparison with the key drug development stages. Biomarker validation is completed in a series of pre-clinical studies that usually includes human samples. The multiple validation studies for the diagnostic test are typically carried out during pre-clinical phases of drug development. A technically validated test with a valid biomarker will then be evaluated for clinical utility, performance, and significance during the clinical testing phases for the drug (Further details on clinical trials for diagnostics are described in Box 4.14).

The process of co-developing drugs and associated diagnostics is also postulated to bring more effective and safer drugs to market much more quickly.

Box 4.14 General considerations for planning and evaluating clinical studies for in vitro diagnostic (IVD) devices

Extract from FDA guidance: www.fda.gov/cdrh/oivd/guidance/1549.html

The following are some general recommendations that may be used when planning and evaluating clinical studies. An additional resource to consider when seeking guidance on reporting clinical or method comparison studies is the STARD (Standards for Reporting of Diagnostic Accuracy) statement (Bossuyt *et al.*, 2003), which is a roadmap for improving the quality of reporting of studies of diagnostic accuracy.

(1) Plan studies to support the intended use claim for the device with data that are representative of the population for whom the device is intended. Include a diversity of ethnic groups if the marker or mutation varies according to ethnicity. Use investigational sites appropriate to the intended use and claims being sought. Clearly outline efforts to define population sampling bias when this issue may affect performance.

(2) Describe all protocols for internal and external evaluation studies. Clearly define the study population and inclusion and exclusion criteria and the chosen clinical endpoint. If literature is to be used to support your intended use, you should clearly explain the study population, inclusion and exclusion criteria, and endpoints in the publication, and reflect how the device will be used in practice. Establish uniform protocols for all external evaluation sites prior to study and follow them consistently throughout the course of data collection.

(3) Determine sample size prior to beginning the clinical study. The sample size should have sufficient statistical power to detect differences of clinical importance for each marker, mutation, or pattern. Consider other approaches in cases with a small available sample size, for example, a disease allele having a low prevalence in the intended use population.

(4) Describe the sampling method used in the selection and exclusion of patients. If it is necessary to use archived specimens or a retrospective design, provide pre-specified inclusion and exclusion criteria for samples, and adequate justification for why the sampled population is relevant to the patient population targeted for the intended use.

(5) For genetic tests, include samples from individuals with diseases or conditions that may cause false positive or false negative results with the device (i.e., within the differential diagnosis), if appropriate.

(6) Analyze data for each individual test site and pooled over sites, if statistically and clinically justified. Justification of data pooling over sites should address variation between sites in prevalence, age, sex, and race or ethnicity.

(7) Describe how the cut-off point (often the distinction between positive and negative, or the medical decision limit) will initially be set, and how it will be verified, if appropriate. If a cut-off point is specified for each of multiple alleles, genotypes or mutations, describe the performance characteristics of

Box 4.14 (cont.)

each cut-off point as it relates to its respective allele, genotype, or mutation. The description of how each cut-off point is determined should include the statistical method used (e.g., receiver operating characteristic (ROC) curve).

(8) Diagnostic devices that assay the presence of a particular pattern (e.g., single nucleotide polymorphism (SNP) set, haplotype pattern), should ideally be validated in a prospective clinical trial. An example of such a device would be a test using a defined SNP set to discriminate between patients who may or may not experience an adverse event associated with a particular drug. Since it is statistically problematic to validate discrimination patterns in the same study in which they were defined, the simplest way to address this is to validate the pattern with an independent data set. Determination of the statistical significance of a retrospectively determined feature pattern may not be possible or minimally would call for careful use of complex statistical procedures, such as bootstrapping, or an explicit cross-validation scheme. Given that it can be easy to obtain a low misclassification rate for a retrospectively determined feature pattern even on random data, a valid procedure for obtaining the statistical significance of such a pattern should be provided. The simplest approach statistically is to evaluate the pattern on an independent data set from a prospective clinical trial, if that is feasible.

(9) Account for all individuals and samples. Perform appropriate data audits and verification before submitting to the FDA. Give specific reasons for excluding any patient or test result after enrolment.

(10) Perform studies using appropriate methods for quality control. Describe the materials and methods used to assess quality control.

Reference

Bossuyt, P M, Reitsma, J B, Bruns, D E, *et al*. The STARD statement for reporting studies of diagnostic accuracy: explanation and elaboration, *Clinical Chemistry*, **49**, 7–18, 2003.

Pharmacogenomics (or personalized medicine) is the term used to describe the identification of such personalized drug therapies, and business and regulatory issues are discussed in more detail in Section 5.7.

4.10   Typical device development process

Owing to the diverse nature of medical devices, development cycles are highly variable across the industry.

Devices can be looked upon as being durable, implantable, or disposable, and perform either therapeutic, diagnostic, or monitoring functions. Examples of each

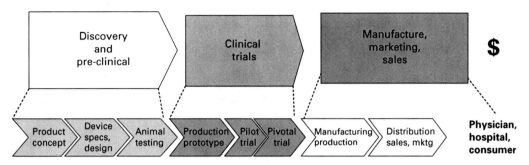

Figure 4.14a   Schematic of device development value chain and process.

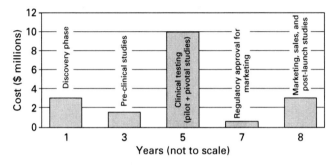

Figure 4.14b   Time and cost for development of an innovative implant device (exemplary data from discussions with industry executives).

type are – durable device: lithotripsy machine used to break kidney stones in vivo; implantable device: pacemaker; disposable device: bandaid. Most in vitro diagnostic products are also looked upon as devices, but will be discussed in a separate section.

The product development process also depends largely on the FDA classification of risk, which will dictate the extent of safety and clinical testing required. Therefore, it is important to understand the classification schema for devices discussed in Chapter 5. Additionally, devices that carry out equivalent functions and are similar to other approved devices will have a shorter development path, and this is discussed later in Chapter 5. Therefore, this section specifically covers new medical devices that have new characteristics or applications and require a full development path with rigorous clinical studies.

Depending on the technology, novelty, application, and other factors, product development may take from a few months to a few years and may cost from a few hundred thousand dollars to millions of dollars (see Figure 4.14b). However, most devices are developed through the key schematic steps shown in Figure 4.14a. These steps are discussed in the following sections.

4.10.1   Discovery, feasibility, and optimization – design and pre-clinical testing

Product concept

The idea for a product usually stems from an invention or discovery, or from examining the needs of caregivers in specific diseases, disorders, or treatment of trauma. Problems in the current method of care give rise to product opportunities but the problems must be carefully analyzed to give product characteristics. Market research is a key activity in this phase (see Chapter 2).

The *indication* for the product and the *specific mechanism of action* are two key factors that will dictate the FDA classification and also the focus of the development efforts, affecting the cost and timeline for development of the device. It is thus important to identify clearly, from market research and technology evaluation, the exact indication and primary mode of action of the device technology.

Usually, a business review is sufficient for a gate decision at this point.

Device design and specifications

Medical device design is controlled and regulated by the FDA, as described in detail in Chapter 5, and the project team must take input and guidance from the regulatory affairs division and also check the FDA Quality System Regulation (QSR, 21CFR 820). At this point, it is imperative to read the requirements for the design process and related documentation in the Quality Systems Regulation Manual (www.fda.gov/cdrh/qsr/contnt.html) and in particular, the Design Controls section of the Quality System Regulation, 21 CFR Part 820, Subpart C, Section 820.30, which outlines the requirements that each manufacturer of any Class II or Class III device, and certain Class I devices, must meet when designing such products or related processes, and when changing existing designs and processes.

The design process for devices also requires input from marketing, sales, manufacturing, and other corporate functions. In particular, the design process must incorporate customer requirements, gained through market research (interviews, surveys, customer input through the sales and marketing organization, third-party market research) and, from those requirements, and customer needs, design and evolve the required product characteristics. Box 4.15 details some aspects of design inputs. In general, design inputs must be formally recorded for regulatory compliance. Typical steps in device design are:

- Identify the need,
- Define the problem,
- Set design objectives and constraints,
- Search for necessary background information,
- Devise alternative solutions (synthesis),
- Analyze solutions,
- Evaluate solutions, make decisions, communicate.

A *product design specifications (PDS) document* is generated after careful evaluation and after striking a balancing act among various criteria and characteristics. In general, customers' needs should be assessed and used to drive product development and design specifications in the PDS. As various choices are made, evaluated, and discarded iteratively in the product development stages at the end of the process, it is important to go back to the starting needs and ensure the adherence of the final output to the initial criteria that were identified as important to the

---

Box 4.15 Design inputs in device development

Design inputs (device requirements) for the selected design project must employ certain procedures, and documents must demonstrate that the design inputs established for the device considered factors such as (this is not a comprehensive list):

- The intended uses of the device,
- The needs of the user and the patient,
- Compatibility with the environment of use and with the safety and performance characteristics of accessories and auxiliary devices,
- Limits and tolerances,
- Risk analysis,
- Toxicity and biocompatibility,
- Environmental issues,
- Electromagnetic compatibility,
- Human factors (see FDA guidance documents on human factors on FDA/CDRH website)
- Labeling and packaging,
- Reliability and stability,
- Voluntary standards,
- Manufacturing processes,
- Sterility.

In addition, the design input sources must be well documented. These design input sources could typically include:

- Customer input through focus groups, surveys, or trade shows,
- Comparison testing of competitor products or benchmarking surveys and activities,
- Internal manufacturing and service department inputs,
- Risk analysis,
- Review of literature, FDA reports, histories of similar products,
- Input from regulatory, quality assurance, R&D, marketing departments.

Finally, these design inputs must be reviewed, approved, and subsequently reviewed again as they evolve. All these processes must be well documented in the DHF.

---

customer (Figure 4.15). This focus on meeting customer needs seems like a simple step but is often forgotten in the process between early development and final stage production.

A popular analytical approach that transforms customer needs (the voice of the customer [VOC]) into engineering characteristics of a product or service is called *quality function deployment* (QFD) or "house of quality." The QFD was originally

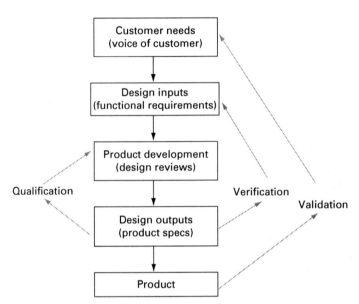

Figure 4.15   Incorporating customer or market-driven design specifications in the design process (figure adapted from talk by Mr. Laurence Roth, Percardia, given at RPI, 2005).

developed in Japan and then imported to the USA by car-manufacturing firms and is now used in virtually all industries. The QFD process prioritizes each product or service characteristic while simultaneously setting development targets for product or service development. A thorough review of customer needs, through observation, interviews, and focus groups, is incorporated into various quantitative measures of product characteristics, as deemed important or demanded by the customer. If a certain characteristic is rated very highly by customers, the product characteristics related to that function or characteristic of the product get higher weightings in the decision matrix. For example, additional weightings may also be added if no competitor product has that characteristic (competitive advantage for the product under development). Various other combinations of considerations can be brought into the matrix to result in a prioritization of design and development activities and product characteristics with the end user in mind.

Recognizing that variability in product quality characteristics is a major cause of customer dissatisfaction and development inefficiencies, a set of statistical, engineering, and design tools called "design for six sigma" have increasingly been adopted by many industries. The successful application of "six sigma" processes in bringing quality into all manufacturing and product development processes in various industries, has created an interest in applying these practices and tools to early stages of product development in the biomedical industry. Further details of the six sigma processes can be accessed on many websites and through the additional readings at the end of this chapter.

Hardware and software design modules must also be specified with similar inputs and formal specifications documents. This is an important area for device manufacturers, with increasing use of computing parts and microprocessors in many

---

Box 4.16 Toxicity testing

Reproduced, with permission, from a 2005 presentation by Lawrence Roth, Vice President, Percardia.

A catheter, which is a limited exposure, blood-contacting device has to be tested for toxicity with the following parameters:

- Cytotoxicity,
- Sensitization,
- Irritation or reactivity,
- Systemic toxicity or pyrogenicity,
- Hemocompatibility.

A permanent blood-contacting device, like a stent or synthetic vascular graft, has to go through the above tests, plus:

- Sub-chronic toxicity,
- Genotoxicity,
- Implantation study (special controls),
- Chronic toxicity,
- Carcinogenicity.

---

devices. Other components in the biomedical device design process include "*human factors engineering*," which looks at user interactions with the device, to design-in ways to prevent human or user error.

Thus, in addition to specifying and designing the characteristics of the device, the design phase includes a significant effort in risk analysis, safety analysis, assessment of human-factor requirements, and formulation of project planning documents.

Animal and toxicity testing

The device prototype is evaluated in animal models before the final production run. These studies are used to optimize product characteristics. Specific biocompatibility and toxicology or safety studies will depend on the type of device (listed under special controls for that device type), the materials used, and the application. For example, a neurological implantable device that contacts cerebrospinal fluid and brain parenchyma may need an animal implant test to determine local effects on brain tissues and fluids, the susceptibility of seizures, and other physiological functions. Another example with more details is given in Box 4.16. In general, biocompatibility and toxicology tests include the following:

- Acute, sub-chronic and chronic toxicity,
- Irritation to eyes, skin, and mucosal surfaces,
- Sensitization,
- Hemocompatibility,

- Genotoxicity,
- Carcinogenicity,
- Effects on reproduction including developmental effects,
- Specific organ toxicity and effects, as needed.

Reliability testing

Medical devices that are not disposable should also undergo a series of reliability tests, typically run in laboratory settings. Reliability is a measure of the potential for failure of a device – mechanical, electrical, or, material failures could be involved in the reliability testing depending on the particular device.

Production prototype

The results of these tests are all factored into the final, optimized design of the device. The development of a production prototype is carried out after senior management meets for another formal design review. At this stage, a design "lock" is implemented. Some aspects of the device design might already be fixed and defined as unchangeable by the biocompatibility tests. The device design must also include consideration for manufacturing scale-up – called "design for manufacturing." The business case is also analyzed and reviewed again, before the commitment to go to production is made. Quality control and engineering divisions should be involved in making production prototypes so that the scale-up can be carried forward seamlessly into manufacturing stage. The design lock-in has to occur before the production prototypes are taken into clinical trials.

4.10.2   Special considerations for device clinical trial design

Clinical trials

The preferred study design in regulated product trials is a double-blind randomized trial, in which patients are randomly assigned to a treatment or control group with neither the care provider or the patient knowing which group is which. However, in device trials it is usually not possible or ethical to mask the device, especially in an implanted or surgical device. Therefore, device clinical trials are typically run as randomized trials with parallel groups in which patients are randomly assigned to only one device or treatment regimen. The control against which the device efficacy or safety is compared is typically an active control, where another currently accepted device or treatment regimen is applied. Since a placebo group cannot usually be included, some trials have no choice but to compare results against historical data. Another design in clinical trials is a crossover study in which a patient sequentially receives more than one device or treatment regimen in the clinical trial and effectively serves as his or her own control.

Most drugs are administered using well established and widely accepted standard modes of administration. However, for devices, the method of use or implantation is a major factor in the success or failure of a device trial and *investigator training and protocol compliance* is a critical aspect of many device trials.

Device trials typically have a short safety or biocompatibility study (comparable to Phase I trials in drugs) and a pilot efficacy or feasibility study (Phase II in drug trials) followed by a larger pivotal clinical study (Phase III in drug trials) that compares the safety and efficacy of the new device with the current standard of care. Box 4.17 describes specific FDA guidance for designing and carrying out acceptable device trials.

Box 4.17 Guidance for clinical trial design for medical devices

Extracts from the FDA guidance document Statistical Guidance for Clinical Trials of Non-Diagnostic Medical Devices *are presented here.* www.fda.gov/cdrh/ode/ot476.html

In the foreword to the document, the FDA states: "It is our hope that this document, along with the additional information and references that have been cited, will help manufacturers save time, money, and human resources in the planning, conduct, and analysis of medical device clinical trials ... The development of this clinical trial guidance resulted from a concern about the quality of clinical trials submitted to the Agency in support of medical device applications. This concern applied to many critical elements of clinical trial design, conduct, and analysis ... While the manufacturer may submit any evidence to convince the Agency of the safety and effectiveness of its device, the Agency may rely only on valid scientific evidence as defined in the PMA regulation section entitled, *Determination of Safety and Effectiveness* (21 CFR 860.7). A thorough reading of that section is strongly recommended."

Design of the clinical trial

The trial objective

An effective and efficient design of a clinical investigation cannot be accomplished without a clear and concise objective. Usually the study objective is posed as a research question, involving the *medical claims* for the device. This research question should be formulated with extreme care and specificity ... to evaluate a particular type of intervention effectively. A question such as, "Is my device safe and effective?" is far too general to be meaningful. What is the proper way to evaluate effectiveness in the target condition and population? What are the unique safety concerns of the device intervention? Is the device as effective or more effective than another intervention? If so, is it as safe or safer? Is the evaluation of safety and effectiveness limited to a particular subgroup of patients? What is the best clinical measure of safety and effectiveness?

The attempt to answer these and similar questions will provide an essential focus to the trial and should provide the basis for *labeling indications*. For example, if a new device has been developed to treat a progressive, degenerative ophthalmic disorder for which there currently exists an alternative therapy using an approved device, how should effectiveness be determined? Does the new device slow or halt degeneration? If so, does it restore functions that had

Box 4.17 (cont.)

previously been lost? Does it reduce pain or discomfort? Is it to be compared with the approved device and is it thought to be as good as or better than the old device for some purpose? Does it have fewer adverse reactions?

Pilot or feasibility studies

The purpose of a limited study (called a pilot or feasibility study) is to identify possible medical claims for the device, monitor potential study variables for a suitable outcome variable, test study procedures, refine the prototype device, and determine the precision of those potential response variables. It may also allow a limited evaluation of factors that may introduce bias. Pilot studies are often used to field test the device.

Identification and selection of variables

The observations in a clinical study involve two types of variable: outcome variables and influencing variables. Outcome variables (also known as end-points) define and answer the research question and should have direct impact on the claims for the device. These ... endpoints ... should be directly observable, objectively determined measures subject to minimal bias and error. Influencing variables ... are any aspect of the study that can affect the outcome variables (increase or decrease), or can affect the relationship between treatment and outcome. Imbalances in comparison or treatment groups in influencing variables at baseline can lead to false conclusions by improperly attributing an effect observed in the outcome variable to an intervention when it was merely due to the imbalance. For example, blood pressure generally increases with age. If a group of individuals in the treatment group is significantly younger, and possesses lower mean pressures than subjects in the control group, and are then compared using blood pressure as the outcome variable, the investigators may falsely conclude that an intervention was responsible for the observed "reduction" in blood pressure. Once the variables or factors to be included in the trial have been identified, the [most informative and least subjective] ... measurement methods ... should be used.

Control groups

Every clinical trial intended to evaluate an intervention is comparative, and a control exists either implicitly or explicitly. The safety and effectiveness of a device is evaluated through the comparison of differences in the outcomes (or diagnosis) between the treated patients (the group on whom the device was used) and the control patients (the group on whom another intervention, including no intervention, was used). A scientifically valid control population should be comparable to the study population in important patient characteristics and prognostic factors, i.e., it should be as alike as possible except for the application of the device.

Box 4.17 (cont.)

There are many types of control groups. For the purposes of this document, four types are described:

(1) Concurrent controls are those who are assigned an alternative intervention, including no intervention or a placebo intervention, and are under the direct care of the clinical study investigator. Any concurrent control can be a treatment control if it is assigned another intervention. If a placebo or sham is assigned, then it becomes a placebo or sham control. If the controls do not receive any intervention, then they are called a "no-treatment" control.

(2) In a passive concurrent control design, patients receive an alternative intervention, including no intervention, but are not under the direct care of the clinical study investigator.

(3) Self-controls or crossover controls are patients who are assigned one intervention (the order of treatment presentation should be specified in advance), for a prescribed period of time and then, following a washout period, receive the alternate intervention. A washout period refers to allowing a period of time to elapse between the end of one experimental condition and the beginning of the next condition . . . [so that] no residual effects of the first treatment remain that may confound the results obtained from the next scheduled treatment.

(4) A historical control is a non-concurrent group of patients with the same disease or condition that has received an intervention, including no intervention, but are separated in time, and usually place, from the population under study.

Concurrent controls and, where applicable, self-controls allow the largest degree of opportunity for comparability. Passive concurrent controls can provide comparability only if the selection criteria are the same, the study variables are measured in precisely the same way as those in the study sample, and assuming there are no hidden biases. The use of historical controls is the most difficult way to assure comparability with the study population, especially if the separation in time or place is large.

4.10.3 Device manufacturing

Device manufacture also has to comply with FDA guidelines and regulations for tracking each and every step of the manufacturing process, including raw material sourcing. These guidelines are known as current good manufacturing practices (cGMP) and each facility that is certified by the FDA is also regularly inspected. Further details on manufacture and regulatory compliance issues are discussed in Chapter 6.

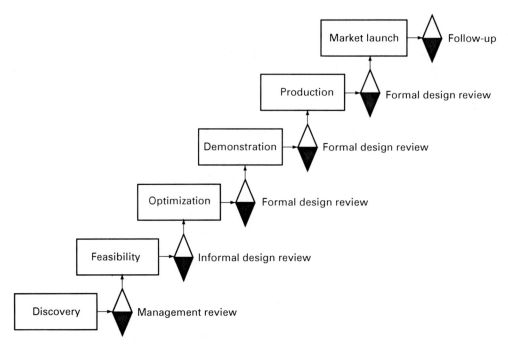

Figure 4.16   Conceptual stage–gate process for device development.

4.10.4   Keeping records for the FDA

The design history file, all pre-clinical studies, and all clinical trial data need to be carefully documented for review by the FDA. These records are maintained in four different formats or records: the Device Master Record (DMR), the Design History File (DHF), the Device History Record (DHR), and the Technical Documentation File (TDF); these are discussed in greater detail in Chapter 5. In particular, the design reviews carried out during product development must be well documented, with all decisions and design changes explained and supported with technical analysis and sound reasoning.

4.10.5   Device development stage-gate process

Figure 4.16 shows the stage-gate process for device development. Table 4.4 explains each step in more detail.

4.11   A few general notes on biomedical product development

Some key dos and don'ts with respect to biomedical product development:

Don't   Carry out extensive studies for alternate diseases or indications once a product has entered formal clinical development for a particular chosen

Table 4.4 Stage-gate process for device development

Stage 1 – Discovery	Gate 1 – Management review
Product concept and preliminary data collection Exploration, brainstorming Sources: R&D, marketing, internal R&D, customers, competitors' literature, academia, conferences	"Gentle" screen; strategic alignment, initial feasibility, magnitude of opportunity Output: "development initiation proposal" Initial resources allocated
Stage 2 – Feasibility and concept testing	**Gate 2: Repeat of previous screen, with more information**
Market size, market potential, market acceptance Technological readiness, proof of principle IP position Product specifications Prototype production Project planning: testing plan, regulatory strategy, budget, timeline preparation	"Must have," "should have" features, market opportunity, Technical feasibility Output: "development continuation proposal" Project contract Spending increases, budget allocated
Stage 3 – Optimization	**Gate 3 – Formal design review**
Design controls implemented Design refined Pre-clinical (animal) testing "Design lock" Materials, equipment, tooling Packaging, sterilization Data for FDA submission gathered – pre-clinical toxicity	Product performance evaluation: customer needs, cost and pricing, safety, efficacy, reliability, target market definition Output: extension of "development continuation proposal"
Stage 4 – Demonstration (if needed)	**Gate 4 – Formal design review**
Validation of manufacturing process FDA submission for clinical trials Pilot-scale production for clinical trials; may also be used for product launch Clinical trials – pilot and pivotal studies	Review of clinical data Review of validation data Output: extension of "development continuation proposal"
Stage 5 – Production	**Gate 5 – Formal design review**

Scale-up of manufacturing process
Validation of GMP compliance
Product QA or QC validation
	Final gate before product reaches public:
	    Review of validation data,
	    Updated financial projections,
	    Operations and marketing plans,
	Output: Approval to launch

Stage 6 – Launch and follow-up	**Gate 6 – Feedback and evaluation**
Marketing launch, sales team Distribution Monitoring of manufacturing (QA, QC) Field support, customer training Educational programs	Adjust programs as needed Feedback to next cycle of development

---

Box 4.18 Failure mode analysis

Adapted from a talk by Mr. Michael Cohen, President of the Institute for Safe Medication Practices

Step 1   Develop a process flow diagram that articulates how the product should be used.
Step 2   Use the diagram and assume the worst possible scenario at each step.
Step 3   Predict the effects of the failure.
Step 4   Rank the likelihood of the occurrence.
Step 5   Rank the estimated severity of the failure.
Step 6   Rank the likelihood of detection.
Step 7   Add steps 4, 5, and 6 and divide by three to develop a criticality index.
Step 8   Develop ranges that are unacceptable.
Step 9   Decide on interventions.
Step 10   Take action and assess the effects of the action.

---

indication. All data involving a product have to be delivered to the FDA. If a vertebrate animal in a study using the same product dies, revealing a new risk, the death has to be reported to the FDA and the main ongoing clinical study may be paused while the FDA re-evaluates the risks involved.

Don't   Fail to obtain appropriate insurance for the human clinical trials.

Don't   Forget to put the adequate ethical controls and regulatory certifications in place in the pre-clinical stage – animal review committees, laboratory certifications for OSHA, biosafety regulations, hazardous materials, department of health certifications, etc. Section 4.16 has a summary of these requirements.

Do   Carry out a failure mode analysis (particularly relevant for device design), as described in Box 4.18.

Do   If the indication changes mid-stream (for example, in human trials, a drug is being developed to treat systemic hypertension, but data from the clinical trial show that it actually seems to work better as a treatment for insomnia) submit an entirely new request to the FDA for renewed human clinical trials, focusing this time on the new indication (in this case, insomnia). If dosage is different for the new indication, check if new toxicity studies need to be done to support new mode of administration or dosage.

4.12   Project management

4.12.1   Project management tools – Gantt charts and critical path

A Gantt chart is a bar chart that shows how project elements (stages), schedules, and other time related systems develop over time. The horizontal black bars in

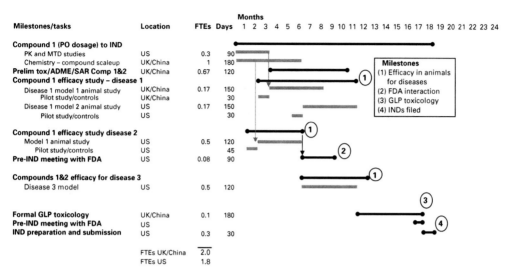

Figure 4:17   Example Gantt chart for pre-clinical development of a drug that has more than one indication.

Figure 4.17 show the summary elements (each summary stage of development), while the shorter horizontal bars indicate sub-stages, activities, or tasks within that summary stage. The vertical bars indicate dependencies, meaning the next task cannot start until the connected previous task has completed. The Gantt chart (or any other related graphical method) is useful as it makes it easy to check visually time lines and job allocations per person (not shown here) so that all team members and management are unequivocal about the tasks and time line responsibilities. Also, progress can be easily tracked against Gantt charts and the software programs available today allow for changes to cascade through the chart, making revisions in time lines and responsibilities easy to communicate. A Gantt chart drawing and planning tool is available in a software package called Microsoft Project (the chart in Figure 4.17 was generated in MS Excel).

Another type of visual representation of the complex set of tasks in a project is the critical path method. The critical path method (CPM) can also be very useful in identifying and allowing specific prioritization of tasks that affect the time line of the project. A brief description of the method is reproduced here (from http://en.wikipedia.org/wiki/Critical_path_method):

The essential technique for using CPM is to construct a model of the project that includes the following:

(1) A list of all activities required to complete the project (also known as a work-breakdown structure),
(2) The time (duration) that each activity will take to complete, and
(3) The dependencies between the activities.

Using these values, CPM calculates the starting and ending times for each activity, determines which activities are critical to the completion of a project (called the critical path), and reveals those activities with "float time" (activities that are less critical). In project

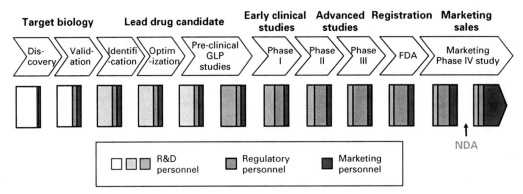

Figure 4.18   Composition of the product development team in a drug development path. Device development teams will have similar configurations and compositions.

management, a critical path is the sequence of project network activities with the longest overall duration, and it determines the shortest time possible to complete the project. Any delay of an activity on the critical path directly affects the planned project completion date (i.e., there is no float time on the critical path). A project can have several, parallel, critical paths. Since project schedules change on a regular basis, CPM allows continuous monitoring of the schedule, allows the project manager to track the critical activities, and ensures that non-critical activities do not interfere with critical ones.

4.12.2   Team composition

Multidisciplinary teams must be formed for a given project, to carry out the varied tasks involved in product development, as seen in the previous sections. In almost all biomedical product development (drugs, devices, and diagnostics), it is necessary to get input from sales and marketing, reimbursement, regulatory affairs, finance, and general management throughout the development process (see Figure 4.18). The level and intensity of engagement with various functions varies over the course of the project. For example, the interactions with marketing, regulatory affairs, and reimbursement would increase steadily as the project went into clinical studies, with each stage seeing more involvement and feedback from marketing, regulatory affairs, and reimbursement as they work on positioning the product in a competitive marketplace. Even within a technical project team, the composition of the team is usually multidisciplinary and the technical backgrounds of team members might change as the project moves along. A new drug project team would typically have a biologist or biochemist, a medicinal chemist (a protein chemist or cell biologist in the case of a biological drug) and a project leader in the team, as the molecule goes through early discovery studies. With progression into advanced pre-clinical stages, a regulatory affairs and manufacturing person might be added to the team to help prepare for the first interactions with the FDA. During clinical stage studies, a physician, regulatory affairs people, biostatisticians, and

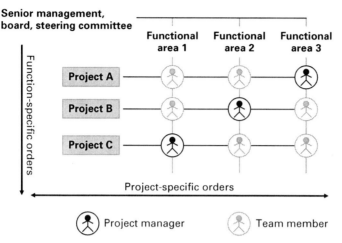

Figure 4.19 Matrix environment in a company, showing the responsibilities of the team leaders and the functional group heads in a typical company. (Reproduced from the BASF corporate website with permission.)

manufacturing staff might be part of the project team, either continuing with the same project manager or with the project, or handed over to a different project manager. In a medical device development project, the engineering (commercial manufacturing) division might get involved as the prototype development stage is reached, and design review and feedback from manufacturing, marketing, and regulatory divisions might become necessary.

4.12.3 Team management in a matrix environment

Sound personnel management practices are important, given the long-term development cycles in the drug and devices industry. Matrix management structures used in most companies today still retain the hierarchical vertical management structure (shown in Figure 4.19 as control of functional areas from top management down). The rigidity of the separation between line management (functional area) and project management depends on the culture and type of matrix organization existing in the company. Matrix management relies on cooperation and communication. In a project environment, the decision-making authority would usually rest with the project manager, but in a matrix environment, all major decisions are reached by consensus between line managers (typically managers of functional areas) and project managers. Project staff have to be committed to both the project and their own departments (functional group).

In larger organizations, there is usually one full-time project manager who leads one project through a process. Often, projects are handed over between project managers specializing in the various pre-clinical, clinical, and marketing functional groupings. In smaller organizations, there may be a doubling up of functional management and project management leadership responsibilities in the same person. There are two organizational extremes in a matrix management environment: (1) all personnel report only to line managers and project managers will have to coordinate through the line managers; (2) all personnel in a project are put in a team and report only to the project manager. In practice, a mix of the two organizational architectures is used. Generally speaking, the matrix environment puts a greater onus on managers to manage personnel, communicate expectations and effectively build consensus for their projects.

4.13   Formulating budgets

It is necessary to estimate a success budget (studies planned have a successful outcome) with some extra padding for slips, error, and repeat studies. One cannot realistically budget for every possibility – for example, you could not have budgeted for the event that the expensive rodent study with a lead candidate drug had to be aborted because the drug compound would precipitate out of solution after three hours and could not be delivered reliably. The best way to put a budget together is to put a success budget together first and then add more resources based on failures of the highest risk events. Try to be realistic and state assumptions. In the end, if there is a technical issue that blows your budgeted amount anyway, there is not much to be done about it but to present the facts. Unless there is a solution in sight for that technical issue, there is a good chance that the project will be dropped, which might be exactly the right choice for a company with stringently limited resources and time lines.

A few key steps that can help in putting a quick annual or total project budget together from a product development plan are described here (see example in Figure 4.20):

(1) *Estimate the personnel resources needed for each stage or sub-stage per year.*
This is typically done by calculating how many people are involved and estimating their time involvement using a full-time equivalent (FTE) measure. This is a way to measure a worker's productivity or involvement in a project. An FTE of 1.0 means that the person is equivalent to a full-time worker. An FTE of 0.5 would signal that the worker is only half-time on the project for one year, or is full time on the project for 6 months. One way to calculate FTEs per stage is to list the total number of people that would be involved, multiply by the number of weeks spent on the project that year and divide that number by the total number of salary weeks in the year. Multiply this result by the FTE cost, estimated per job group by your finance department. The FTE cost rate typically includes overheads, benefits, and other costs. This number will be much higher than the actual salary of the person. For example, medicinal chemists in the USA are typically given a FTE rate of \$200 000–\$250 000 while their salaries may be half that

Stage	Personnel/FTE	Number	Time	Unit	Base Cost (over 1 year)	Cost per year = Base cost × time
4a, and 4b, and 4c	Project manager	1	0.8	FTE	$170 000	$136 000
	Senior chemist	1	0.4	FTE	$250 000	$100 000
	Senior biologist	2	0.75	FTE	$225 000	$337 500
	Biology research assistant	1	0.6	FTE	$115 000	$69 000
	Senior biomedical engineer	1	0.2	FTE	$200 000	$40 000
	Consumables, supplies					
In vivo test in healthy animals, hypertensive animals, toxicity tests	Pressure transducers, assay kits, chemicals, materials costs					$85 000
	Capital expenditures					
	Micro-centrifuge					$18 000
	Contracted, outsourced					
	Outsourced animal study					$92 000
	TOTAL					$877 500

Note: base cost for personnel includes taxes, benefits, overhead costs, some materials

Figure 4.20   Example of a budget worksheet for a stage. Time = no. of weeks on project divided by no. of salary weeks in a year.

    amount or less. The higher number is the actual cost to the company to employ and provide an environment for that person's work.

(2) *Estimate the materials and capital expenditures cost.*

    Direct costs of materials and consumables (expensive antibodies, special probe tips, expensive sensors) that will need to be purchased specifically for the project (even though they may be used later by other projects) must be added up for each stage. Capital expenditures ("cap ex") are usually expense items that have a lifetime longer than a few years and cost more than a company-set threshold amount. Examples are gene sequencing machines, mechanical testing equipment, automated cell-sorting machines, microscopes, etc. Capital expenditure purchases can require submission of a formal justification of the purchase and specific authorization from some chain of command in the company (if the item is significantly expensive).

(3) *Get a quote for any contracted research.*

    For example, animal studies may need to be contracted to a specific animal research contractor who has developed expertise in that model. That quote, and the additional costs of any further analysis of the results or tissues, needs to be specifically included in the budget calculations.

Add these three pieces together for each stage of the project development plan and pretty soon you will have an estimated budget per year and a total for the project. This calculation will at least get you an order of magnitude estimate of the development cost of the project and some idea of the resources that you will need to plan to acquire.

Figure 4.20 shows an example budget preparation worksheet.

4.14   How to get your project funded in a larger organization

First, do not make the mistake of thinking that just because the technology or invention is very exciting, the project will be funded. In a science-driven, pure R&D organization it may be easy to get people excited by a new idea and by the "hot" topical nature of the concept or technology, but a business is also driven by many other considerations, as described in all the chapters in this book.

Communicate, communicate and then communicate some more. That does not mean that one should be redundant and communicate the same message over and over again! Each point of communication must adapt to the audience and to the questions and concerns heard, and the same message may need to be delivered with different perspectives each time. Box 4.19 is an example of how a message was adapted to the audience to help them understand the value and need for a particular project. Communications must cover the elements listed in Section 4.14.1.

4.14.1   The art of persuasion

- Establish credibility,
- Illuminate advantages,
- Provide evidence,
- Connect emotionally;
  - Show commitment,
  - Understand and adjust to audience.

4.14.2   Business case

In general, certain points need to be well researched before taking the project case to senior management:

- Tie to company vision and strategy,
- Tie to current concerns of top management,
- Quantify benefits where possible,
- But do not ignore unquantifiable benefits,
- Demonstrate awareness of risks; show plans to overcome them,
- Use style and format usually preferred,
- Be ready for formal presentations,
- Lobby informally beforehand,
- Options?
- Provide information and counter-arguments to resisters ahead of time,
- Be prepared with other items on project proposal (Figure 4.4).

4.14.3   Valuation decision – net present value (NPV)

Management will frequently carry out an economic analysis (typically a net present value analysis) to determine if the project value fits current financial or economic

---

> **Box 4.19** The art of persuasion – getting your project funded
>
> *Conger, J. A., The necessary art of persuasion,* Harvard Business Review, *May 1998, 76 (3) (reproduced here by permission, all rights reserved by Harvard Business Press)*
>
> Robert Marcell [was] head of Chrysler's small-car design team. In the early 1990s, Chrysler was eager to produce a new subcompact – indeed, the company had not introduced a new model of this type since 1978. But senior managers at Chrysler did not want to go it alone. They thought an alliance with a foreign manufacturer would improve the car's design and protect Chrysler's cash stores.
>
> Marcell was convinced otherwise. He believed that the company should bring the design and production of a new sub-compact in-house. He knew that persuading senior managers would be difficult, but he also had his own team to contend with. Team members had lost confidence that they would ever again have the opportunity to create a good car. They were also angry that the United States had once again given up its position to foreign competitors when it came to small cars.
>
> Marcell decided that his persuasion tactics had to be built around emotional themes that would touch his audience. From innumerable conversations around the company, he learned that many people felt as he did – that to surrender the sub-compact's design to a foreign manufacturer was to surrender the company's soul and, ultimately, its ability to provide jobs. In addition, he felt deeply that his organization was a talented group hungry for a challenge and an opportunity to restore its self-esteem and pride. He would need to demonstrate his faith in the team's abilities.
>
> Marcell prepared a 15-minute talk built around slides of his home town, Iron River, a now defunct mining town in Upper Michigan, devastated, in large part, by foreign mining companies. On the screen flashed recent photographs he had taken of his boarded-up high school, the shuttered homes of his childhood friends, the crumbling ruins of the town's ironworks, closed churches, and an abandoned railroad yard. After a description of each of these places, he said the phrase, "We couldn't compete" – like the refrain of a hymn. Marcell's point was that the same outcome awaited Detroit if the production of small cars was not brought back to the United States. Surrender was the enemy, he said, and devastation would follow if the group did not take immediate action.
>
> Marcell ended his slide show on a hopeful note. He spoke of his pride in his design group and then challenged the team to build a "made-in-America" sub-compact that would prove that the United States could still compete. The speech, which echoed the exact sentiments of the audience, rekindled the group's fighting spirit. Shortly after the speech, group members began drafting their ideas for a new car.
>
> Marcell then took his slide show to the company's senior management and ultimately to Chrysler chairman Lee Iacocca. As Marcell showed his slides, he could see that Iacocca was touched. Iacocca, after all, was a fighter and a strongly

Box 4.19 (cont.)

patriotic man himself. In fact, Marcell's approach was not too different from Iacocca's earlier appeal to the United States Congress to save Chrysler. At the end of the show, Marcell stopped and said, "If we dare to be different, we could be the reason the US auto industry survives. We could be the reason our kids and grandkids don't end up working at fast-food chains." Iacocca stayed on for two hours as Marcell explained in greater detail what his team was planning. Afterward, Iacocca changed his mind and gave Marcell's group approval to develop a car, the Neon.

With both groups, Marcell skillfully matched his emotional tenor to that of the group he was addressing. The ideas he conveyed resonated deeply with his largely Midwestern audience. And rather than leave them in a depressed state, he offered them hope, which was more persuasive than promising doom. Again, this played to the strong patriotic sentiments of his American-heartland audience.

No effort to persuade can succeed without emotion, but showing too much emotion can be as unproductive as showing too little. The important point to remember is that you must match your emotions to your audience's.

value thresholds. The *net present value* is calculated by first projecting all costs and revenues for this project over a certain number of years. The net cash flow for each year is then discounted to the previous year by a certain discount rate (decided by the risk perceived in the project or by a general cost of capital to the company or the expected rate of return for a project – this rate may be set by the company for all projects at that stage of development). The result is sequentially brought down to the present time. The net of the negative discounted cash flows (costs or investments by the company) and positive discounted cash flows (revenues) is typically expected to be a positive number for a project to be approved and sometimes can be compared with other projects to make portfolio decisions among projects. Therefore, if a project has revenues ten years out from the current date, then those revenues will need to be sufficiently large to balance out the closer (less heavily discounted) costs.

Other valuation methods used in the biomedical industry include risk-adjusted net present value, real options, decision tree analysis and Monte Carlo simulations (please see references and general literature for more details on these techniques). In general, every economic decision is built on certain assumptions, and every project manager must pay very close attention to the basis of the assumptions. Additional considerations include health economics (discussed in Chapter 7).

4.14.4 Stakeholders

The next useful step is to carry out a formal or informal stakeholder analysis to prepare to communicate more effectively.

List all stakeholders

- All the people who are affected by your work, who have influence or power over it, or have an interest in its successful or unsuccessful conclusion,
- These include your family, boss, coworkers, future recruits, community, the public, alliance partners, trade associations, etc.

Prioritize stakeholders

- *High power, interested people*: these are the people you must fully engage and make the greatest efforts to satisfy.
- *High power, less interested people*: put enough work in with these people to keep them satisfied, but not so much that they become bored with your message.
- *Low power, interested people*: keep these people adequately informed, and talk to them to ensure that no major issues are arising. These people can often be very helpful with the detail of your project.
- *Low power, less interested people*: again, monitor these people, but do not bore them with excessive communication.

Considerations in preparing to deal with stakeholders

- How can you help the high-power, high-interest stakeholders do *their* jobs better with your project?
- Use the opinions of the most powerful stakeholders to shape your projects at an early stage;
  - To support you,
  - To improve the quality of your project.
- Win more resources – this makes it more likely that your projects will be successful.
- Make sure that people understand the benefits of your project; they are more likely to support you when needed.
- Anticipate what people's reaction to your project might be, and build into your plan the actions that will win people's support.
- What financial or emotional interest do they have in the outcome of your work? Is it positive or negative?
- What motivates them most of all? What information do they want from you? How do they want to receive information from you? What is the best way of communicating your message to them?
- What is their current opinion of your work? Is it based on good information?
- Who influences their opinions generally, and who influences their opinions of you? Do some of these influencers therefore become important stakeholders in their own right?
- If they are not likely to be positive, what will win them around to support your project? If you don't think you will be able to win them around, how will you manage their opposition?

Once this stakeholder analysis is carried out, a clear picture of how communication messages need to be tailored for each particular audience will emerge. In addition, the communication effort can now be focused more effectively.

4.15   Outsourcing product development

Why outsource?

(1) Does it save the company money in the short term? Or in the long term?
(2) Does it bring the product to market faster?
(3) Does it bring in expertise or tools that the company does not have?

Outsourcing work is fraught with problems (many of which are driven by communication issues) and a project manager must not underestimate the time that will be required to manage and complete an outsourced project successfully. In general, outsourcing can add value to a company if it is managed well and integrated into the product development plans and company strategy. Another way to look at the decision of whether to outsource or to build the capability in-house is to evaluate it from a view of the business model of the company. What parts of the value chain will the firm retain or outsource with a long-term view? Figure 4.21 is a useful if simple tool to visualize the company's business strategy and understand internally which component of development is going to be partnered or outsourced.

If the company is never going to build the capability to do cGMP (FDA-regulated process) manufacturing, then the decision to outsource manufacturing is easy to make. If the company does not have animal facilities and only a couple of animal studies need to be done, then, also, the decision to outsource these animal studies is relatively simple. In these cases, outsourcing brings in expertise to the project that is not present in the company.

The debate on whether to outsource (buy) or build capabilities in-house depends on many other considerations, and these considerations will vary with the context of the specific function and project under discussion. For example, if there is a need for speed, it might be faster to outsource a clinical trial to a CRO that has connections in many countries or many sites and can reduce the trial recruitment

	R&D	FDA process and clinical trials	Manufacturing	Marketing and sales	
				US	International
Do it yourself					
Strategic partners, licenses					

Figure 4.21   Strategic business model for planning internal and external development.

times significantly. Alternatively, when working with academic collaborators, it is likely that they are driven by different priorities and might not be able to expand resources rapidly to take on a large job. In this instance, the company might be able to hire people faster to get the job started in-house (build).

Other considerations include the complexity of the task and the concern or sensitivity of intellectual property rights that might be generated or that are embodied in the process. For example, if the process involves the development of new protocols in making a very high-margin, expensive product, the risk of that know-how being disseminated to other players in the industry through the contract house may be too high, as the company might lose its competitive advantage in the market. On the other hand, some jobs that are very complex – like building relevant transgenic disease models for drug testing – may best be outsourced to places where past expertise lies in building these models. If the process requires novel methodology that would require the contractor to reconfigure their infrastructure, it might be cheaper (especially if several products in development go through that facility) to invest in a larger space and build the capability in house.

Figure 4.22 demonstrates the various balances between choosing to buy (outsource) vs. build (internal investment) given certain IP and process complexity issues. When complexity is high but IP concerns are low, outsourcing might be considered, but to a sophisticated provider with whom company personnel will tend to work more as collaborators, to ensure that the process performs as required in a complex environment. If the IP concerns are high, but the project complexity is low, then again an opportunity to contract out only limited parts or specific functional components might be considered – for example, in outsourcing chemistry, one might want the service provider to make compound intermediates, while the final compounds are made in the company. The chart in Figure 4.22 also shows areas where it is probably prudent to build internally, in areas of high complexity and high IP concerns where expertise needs to kept in-house, or in areas where both are low and expertise can easily be built in-house.

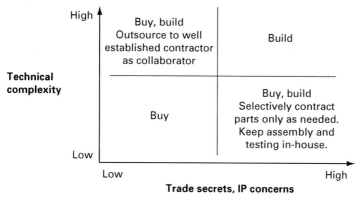

Figure 4.22 Outsourcing decision chart for projects with different levels of complexity and intellectual property concerns.

Here are three practical suggestions to have a successful outsourcing experience, especially when offshoring:

(1) Check references and speak with customers that have contracted similar projects,
(2) Conduct an internal readiness assessment to make sure that existing processes, infrastructure, and assay or testing methods can support an outsourcing development initiative in terms of time commitment, responsiveness, communication tools, etc.,
(3) Try offshore development with small and relatively low risk, internal applications.

4.16   Summary of pre-clinical certifications and laboratory regulations

The summary below is not a comprehensive list, but indicates some key ethical and regulatory compliance issues that must be kept in mind while setting up and running a laboratory. While compliance in some cases is required by federal law or agency (employment law, Drug Enforcement Agency, etc.), in other cases the requirements and procedures vary by state (e.g., Department of Health) (See Box 4.20). It is recommended to peruse their areas of regulation proactively and to determine if company or project activities fall under those regulations.

Pertinent regulatory bodies

- Environmental Protection Agency (EPA),
- Occupational Safety and Health Administration (OSHA): an agency of the US Department of Labor,
- Drug Enforcement Administration (DEA): a US Department of Justice law-enforcement agency, which enforces the Controlled Substances Act of 1970,
- National Institute of Health (NIH; if obtaining federal funds for biomedical research),

---

Box 4.20 A note on understanding US Federal Law and Regulations

Laws are passed by Congress with relatively general language, intended to address a particular issue in a way that can be consistently applied to all instances with the issue. These laws are then passed down to a particular government agency to apply and administer. The government agency then decides how the law must be applied – resulting in regulations, which serve as the practical rules for citizens to adhere to the law.

The regulations by all federal agencies are published and updated in the Code of Federal regulations (CFR). The reference 21CFR 280 = Volume Title 21, section 280 of the CFR. An electronic version of the CFR is at www.gpoaccess.gov/cfr.

- Relevant state's Department of Health,
- Local or institutional committees on environmental health and safety, animal safety, biosafety, radiation safety, and various Institutional Review Boards (IRBs), which review protocols prior to allowing any human testing of new products.

Biosafety

- The NIH requires that organizations conducting recombinant-DNA research have an institutional biosafety committee to ensure that the work meets the safety requirements set forth in the agency's guidelines.
- At many institutions, the biosafety panels, which were first established some 30 years ago, have taken on additional responsibility for overseeing research involving other potentially hazardous biological materials, such as infectious micro-organisms, toxic biological substances, and biological allergens. Fear that those materials could be used by terrorists has intensified the oversight. Federal law spells out strict controls over the use of so-called select agents – that is, organisms and toxins that can pose a severe threat to human health, such as smallpox, botulism, and anthrax. Government involvement with and oversight of local biosafety committees has increased regarding the review of "dual-use" studies – projects with the potential for dangerous as well as beneficial applications.
- An institution must arrange for appropriate hazardous waste disposal, whether of a chemical nature (solvents, toxic volatiles), biological waste (tissues, carcasses from animal studies, etc.) or contaminated materials. Certified contractors must be used. Disposal of radioactive materials must be accompanied by a sound monitoring program of employee exposure.
- Institutions must monitor the use, storage, and disposal of radioactive material. Those regulations emanate from the Nuclear Regulatory Commission. The institutional radiation-safety committee is responsible for the policies and procedures for acquiring and using such materials.

Other certifications and ethical regulatory oversight

- Certifications: in many states, if working with animals, a Certificate of Approval for Working with Live Animals is required by the laboratory. This may require an inspector's visit by the state health department.
- If using controlled substances (e.g., pentobarbital for anesthesia), a Controlled Substances license is required. Registration with the DEA is also required for use of controlled substances.
- Materials Safety Data Sheets (MSDS) must be maintained for all chemicals used in the laboratory and must be made available to all involved employees.
- To follow the NIH guide, a Biosafety Committee and an Institutional Animal Care and Use Committee (IACUC) must be constituted.
- Local labor laws for the state have to be followed – non-discriminatory practices, good safety procedures, and appropriate training for employees all have to be followed in order to avoid problems if an audit is ever carried out.

4.17   Summary

The new product development path listed here for drugs, devices and diagnostics is rather generalized, as each product will have its own nuances and specific gates in the NPD process. In addition, each company will evolve its own NPD process: the general processes discussed here describe key issues that are broadly important to consider during NPD. It is important to realize that Chapter 4 should be read in the context of all the other chapters in this book. It is positioned centrally in the book because the reader is now better informed, while going through the remaining chapters, to develop a sound regulatory path and reimbursement strategy.

Exercises

4.1. Examine carefully the wording of the indication identified in the exercises in Chapter 2. Does it match the target market population? Are the desired product characteristics, identified in Chapter 2, incorporated in addressing the particular indication?

4.2. Identify specific endpoints of a clinical trial that will meet the product characteristics and the needs of the target patient population.

4.3. Identify key risk-reducing milestones. Describe the stages of your product development (use the general templates given in this chapter) and endpoints of each stage or sub-stage.

4.4. Generate a stage–gate development plan or chart with time lines.

4.5. Define gate assessment criteria as quantitatively as possible.

4.6. Summarize the resources needed up to each milestone of development, including final manufacturing: space, personnel, equipment, and consumables. Give high-level approximations of costs (in categories or in blocks of $50 000).

4.7. Generate a Gantt chart using milestones and stages, with all key assumptions annotated.

4.8. Generate a budget with monthly cash flow and large item expenses outlined (make sure that you justify cost assumptions for large ticket items).

4.9. Prepare a presentation with project justification and project plan, budget, and time lines clearly described.

References and additional reading

Block, Z. and MacMillan, I. C. *Corporate Venturing: Creating New Businesses within the Firm*, Harvard Business School Press, 1993.

Christensen, C. *The Innovator's Dilemma: The Revolutionary Book that Will Change the Way You Do Business*, Harvard Business School Press, Reprint 2003.

Cooper, R. G. The new product process: a decision guide for managers. *Journal of Marketing Management*, **3**, (3) 238–255, 1988.

DiMasi, J. A., Hansen, R. W., and Grabowski, H. G. The price of innovation: new estimates of drug development costs, *Journal of Health Economics*, **22**, 151–185, 2003.

Fries, R. (ed.). *Handbook of Medical Device Design*, Marcel Dekker Press, 2001.

Gad, S. C. (ed.). *Drug Discovery Handbook*, Wiley-Interscience, 2005.

Galbraith, J. R., Matrix organization designs – how to combine functional and project forms, *Business Horizons*, **17**, 1, 29–40, 1971.

Gray, C. F. and Larson, E. *Project Management: The Managerial Process*, McGraw-Hill/ Irwin, 3rd edn., 2006.

Justiniano, J. and Gopalaswamy, V. *Six Sigma for Medical Device Design*, CRC Press, 2004.

Krogsgaard-Larsen, P, Liljefors, T, and Madsen, U (eds.). *Textbook of Drug Design and Discovery*, CRC Press, 3rd edn., 2002.

Larson, E. W. and Gobeli, D. H. Organizing for product development projects, *Journal of Product Innovation Management*, **5**, 180–190, 1988.

Leifer, R., McDermott, C. M., O'Connor, G. C., *et al. Radical Innovation: How Mature Companies can Outsmart Upstarts*, Harvard Business School Press, 2000.

Lynn, G. S, Morone, J. G., and Paulson, A. S. Marketing and discontinuous innovation: the probe and learn process, *California Management Review*, **38**(3), 8–37, 1996.

Metzler, R. *Biomedical and Clinical Instrumentation: Fast Tracking from Concept through Production in a Regulated Environment*. Interpharm Press, 1994.

Pisano, G. P. *The Development Factory: Unlocking the Potential of Process Innovation*, Harvard Business School Press, 1996.

Prentis, R. A., Lis, Y., and Walker, S. R. Pharmaceutical innovation by the seven UK-owned pharmaceutical companies (1964–1985), *British Journal of Clinical Pharmacology*, **25**, 387–396, 1988.

Project Management Institute, *A Guide to the Project Management Body of Knowledge (PMBOK®)*, Project Management Institute, 3rd edn., 2004.

Sapienza, A. M. *Creating Technology Strategies: How to Build Competitive Biomedical R&D*, Wiley-Liss, 1997.

Whitmore, E. *Development of FDA-Regulated Medical Products: Prescription Drugs, Biologics, and Medical Devices*, ASQ Quality Press, 2nd edn., 2003.

Useful websites

www.gpoaccess.gov/cfr – *Code of Federal regulations*
http://grants.nih.gov/grants/olaw/references/outline.htm – *Animal care guidelines*
www.fda.gov/cdrh/qsr/contnt.html – *Devices: quality systems regulations*
www.fda.gov/cdrh/ode/ot476.html – *Clinical trials for devices*
www.fda.gov/cdrh/oivd/guidance/1549.html – *Clinical studies for diagnostics*
www.fda.gov/oc/ohrt/irbs/drugsbiologics.html#study – *Clinical studies for drugs (biologics)*
http://en.wikipedia.org/wiki/Critical_path_method – *Product development critical path*
www.iso.ch – *Quality certification standards (ISO)*

5   The regulated market: gateway through the FDA

Plan	Position	Patent	Product	Pass!	Production	Profits
Industry context	Market research	Intellectual property rights	New product development (NPD)	Regulatory plan	Manufacture	Reimbursement

Roadmap of a product commercialization plan. Stage 5

Learning points

- What are the functions of the FDA?
- What is the importance of indications and endpoints in mapping a regulatory route?
- How do FDA regulations affect pre-clinical and clinical product development planning?
- Identify a path through the regulatory process for a drug, device or diagnostic product idea.
- What are the contents of the submissions required by the FDA at various points?
- How does a product with a combination of diverse technologies get approved?
- How are personalized medicines developed through the regulatory process?

5.1   The FDA: its role and significance for biomedical product development

5.1.1   Introduction and history

A brief history of the FDA proves useful to understanding the rationale and role of this organization in the healthcare system of the USA.

Federal oversight for drugs started with the establishment of US customs laboratories to administer the Import Drugs Act of 1848, as the US had become the world's dumping ground for counterfeit drug materials. However, the founding of the modern FDA is in the 1906 Food and Drugs Act. This act, establishing a national agency to put a stop to food adulteration and fake remedies, was passed in the context of trade concerns. Various trades and the public were concerned about the economics of varying state laws and the increasing use of new synthetic chemicals to create cheap and unsafe adulterated food (deodorized rotten eggs, revived rancid butter, substituted glucose for honey). Upton Sinclair's book *The Jungle* highlighted poor health conditions in the Chicago meat-packing plants and precipitated an ongoing discussion in Congress. President Theodore Roosevelt signed the Food Bill in June 1906. This act made it illegal to sell adulterated foods and make false claims on a food or drug and also carried these bans into interstate commerce. An existing Department of Chemistry was designated to carry out tests and enforce the law. The primary concern was to use scientific methods to analyze the risk to human health and safety.

In 1933 the FDA recommended an overhaul of the obsolete 1906 Food and Drugs Act, launching a prolonged legislative battle that came to a conclusion after a crisis in 1937. In that year, the popularity of the S. E. Massengill Company's elixir, sulfanilamide, for the treatment of sore throats in people with streptococcal infections, drove demand for a palatable form for children. The company chemist added diethylene glycol to sweeten the elixir, without any testing of the new additive. Diethylene glycol is known today as antifreeze and ingesting it carries lethal consequences. In 1937, 107 people, mostly children, died before the US Food and Drug Administration was able to gather all of the supply.

The incident led to the Food and Drug Act of 1938, which, among other things, required drug makers to show that their products were safe before they went on the market. This gave rise to the regulatory pathway that drugs in development go through prior to approval, beginning with animal testing prior to human testing. Laws passed by Congress relating to food and drugs safety are written in regulations and interpreted and enforced by the US FDA, as described in Box 5.1.

Box 5.1 Laws and regulations

As described at the end of Chapter 4 (Box 4.20), laws are written by Congress. The United States Code (USC) is the codification by subject matter of the general and permanent laws of the United States. It is divided by broad subjects into 50 titles and published by the Office of the Law Revision Counsel of the US House of Representatives. An electronic version is available at www.gpoaccess. gov/uscode/index.html

Regulations are written by government employees to explain the practical application of the laws. The Code of Federal Regulations or CFR is the book in which all regulations are codified. Title (volume) 21 contains regulations pertaining to food and drugs. These regulations represent how the FDA interprets the Acts or laws that Congress passes. An electronic version of the CFR is accessible at www.gpoaccess.gov/cfr/.

Citation examples: [21CFR302] refers to title 21 of the Code of Federal Regulations, section 302, while [21 USC 321 (g)1] refers to title 21, United States Code, section 321, subsection (g) part 1.

FDA focus on consumer protection

Pre-market	Post-market
Appropriate experimental design	Truthful promotion
Safety studies	Adverse event reporting
Effectiveness	Post-market studies
Pre-approval inspection of manufacturing processes	Manufacturing inspections

Figure 5.1   The FDA focuses on consumer protection (slide courtesy of Dr. Jan Stegemann, RPI, Fall 2004).

5.1.2   Role of the FDA and significance for product development

The FDA is, thus, a federal organization that enacts the laws with the goal of protecting consumer safety in the development and sale of food and medical products (drugs, devices, and diagnostics). The FDA ensures that the claims made by a medical product accurately reflect its risks and benefits so that users and purchasers of the product can make sound judgment on the balance they want to strike between the benefits and risks of taking the product. Figure 5.1 highlights the key issues that the FDA reviews in the pre-clinical and clinical areas.

In effect, from a manufacturer's viewpoint, the FDA is not only the gatekeeper to the market, but the FDA's final marketing approval of a product will also specify the claims that the manufacturer can make. *The specific wording on the approved label strongly influences and defines the patient population to whom the product can be sold.* The label is generated from the data that the manufacturer provides to the FDA. *Thus, it is clear that the product development process has to be designed with the end label (indication) in mind* (see Section 4.1 for details).

5.2   Organization and scope of the FDA

5.2.1   Divisions of the FDA

Key divisions of interest for biomedical product development and review are:

Office of the Commissioner   Policy, planning, administration, ombudsman, *office of combination products, office of orphan products*, financial management and other functions.

Center for Biologics Evaluation and Research (CBER)   Regulates biological products, such as vaccines, blood, devices and tests used to safeguard blood from infectious agents, biologics, cellular, tissue and gene therapies, and xeno-transplantation products. Under this directive, CBER houses the Office of Cellular, Tissue, and Gene Therapies. Categories of therapeutic biological products transferred to CDER from CBER, June 30, 2003 are: monoclonal antibodies for in-vivo use, proteins intended for therapeutic use, including growth factors, cytokines (e.g., interferons), immunomodulators (non-vaccine and non-allergenic products intended to treat disease by inhibiting or modifying a pre-existing immune response), enzymes (e.g., thrombolytics), and other novel proteins, except for those that are specifically assigned to CBER (e.g., vaccines and blood products).

Center for Drug Evaluation and Research (CDER)   Regulates all prescription and over-the-counter drugs (includes biological large molecule drugs since 2003), monitors drug advertising.

Center for Devices and Radiological Health (CDRH)   Regulates all devices including those emitting radiation (ultrasound, electronic). Has under this directive the *Office of In Vitro Diagnostics*, which regulates all aspects of in-home and laboratory diagnostic tests (in vitro diagnostic devices, or IVDs).

Center for Food Safety and Applied Nutrition (CFSAN)   Responsible for the safety of 80% of all food consumed in the USA – the entire food supply, except for meat, poultry, and some egg products.

Center for Veterinary Medicine (CVM)   Assures that animal food products, and drugs used to treat animals, are safe.

National Center for Toxicological Research (NCTR)   Conducts peer-reviewed scientific research that supports and anticipates the FDA's current and future regulatory needs.

5.2.2   What the FDA does not regulate

The products listed in Table 5.1 are regulated by other government agencies:

Table 5.1 Products regulated by different government agencies

Item	Regulated by
Advertising – make sure it is not misleading to consumer	Federal Trade Commission
Alcohol – labeling and quality	Bureau of Alcohol, Tobacco, and Firearms, Treasury Department
Consumer products, e.g., household goods, appliances, toys, paint, packages	Consumer Product Safety Commission
Illegal drugs with no approved medical use	Drug Enforcement Administration, US Department of Justice
Health insurance	Questions about Medicare should be directed to the Center for Medicare and Medicaid Services (CMS)
Meat and poultry	Food Safety and Inspection Service, US Department of Agriculture (USDA)
Pesticides	The FDA, USDA, and Environmental Protection Agency (EPA) share the responsibility for regulating pesticides
Restaurants and grocery stores	Local county health departments
Water	The EPA is responsibile for developing national standards for drinking water from municipal water supplies. The FDA regulates the labeling and safety of bottled water

Table 5.2 Products regulated by the FDA

Blood-related biologics; blood substitutes, etc.	Product and manufacturing establishment licensing; safety of the nation's blood supply; research to establish product standards and develop improved testing methods
Cosmetics	Safety and labeling
Drugs (including biological large molecule drugs)	Product approvals; over the counter (OTC) and prescription drug labeling; drug manufacturing standards
Foods	Labeling; safety of all food products (except meat and poultry); bottled water
Medical devices	Pre-market approval of new devices; manufacturing and performance standards; tracking reports of device malfunctioning and serious adverse reactions
Radiation-emitting electronic products	Radiation safety performance standards for microwave ovens, television receivers, diagnostic X-ray equipment, cabinet X-ray systems (such as baggage X rays at airports), laser products; ultrasonic therapy equipment, mercury vapor lamps, and sunlamps; accrediting and inspecting mammography facilities
Veterinary products	Livestock feeds; pet foods; veterinary drugs and devices

5.2.3   What does the FDA regulate?

The FDA regulates the products listed in Table 5.2.

There are three main divisions (see Section 5.2.1) at the FDA that receive and review human health product applications for market approval:

CDER   Regulates drugs (including large molecule biologic drugs),

CBER   Regulates the collection of blood and blood components used for transfusion or for the manufacture of pharmaceuticals derived from blood and blood components, such as clotting factors,

CDRH   Regulates medical device manufacturers,

OIVD   (Office of In Vitro Diagnostics; part of CDRH) Regulates all aspects of in-home and laboratory diagnostic tests.

5.2.4   Friends not foe

The FDA's goal is to get safe and effective biomedical products to the public. This is conceptually the same goal that the manufacturers have. Conflicts usually arise, owing to the uncertainty of the science and a different view of risk versus benefit between the company or sponsor and the FDA reviewers. In general, while the FDA is obliged to fulfil its duty to get biomedical products to the public as quickly as possible, the FDA is not driven by commercial concerns and will not change its process or make exemptions to reduce costs to the sponsor. However, the PDUFA (Prescription Drug User Fee Act, 1992 and reauthorized several times since) has made the FDA more answerable as a service organization to the public and to industry. This Act increased the application fees paid by industry sponsors to the

FDA to help fund the review of new drugs; in turn, the FDA has made several performance promises (e.g., set a maximum time for review of applications). A similar act, called the Medical Device User Fee and Modernization Act of 2002 (MDUFMA), charges user fees for device pre-market reviews. (Note: other significant provisions of the MDUFMA allow for establishment inspections to take place by accredited third parties and put in place new regulatory requirements for reprocessed single-use devices.)

The FDA has also made great efforts in recent years to work with industry to help sort through complex new product applications (such as combination products; see Section 5.7) and to give them guidance and clarity on internal processes and reviews at the FDA. The FDA website is a great example of this effort and is a handy reference on most policy and process questions. The FDA also presents at industry conferences and delivers talks to convey their current thinking and opinions to industry.

A 2004 initiative called on the FDA to modernize the *Critical Path* – the scientific process through which a potential human drug, biological product, or medical device is transformed from a discovery or "proof of concept" into a medical product; including scientific tests and tools used to predict whether a product candidate will be safe and effective and used to guide sponsors in selecting dosages or device size or placement, etc. The drivers behind the initiative were the following observations:

- A reduction in new biomedical product submissions despite increasing investment by industry,
- Product development is not becoming more efficient over time – a drug entering Phase 1 trials in 2000 was not more likely to reach the market than one entering Phase 1 trials in 1985,
- An increased rate of failure in the later stages of product development – the most expensive way to fail,
- The FDA, at their unique interface of industry, society, and government could help identify and focus efforts by numerous bodies and organizations on efforts to help improve the medical product development process.

The first public meetings and industry feedback for this Critical Path modernization initiative resulted in a *Critical Path Opportunities List* (published March 2006) that describes how scientific discoveries in fields such as genomics and proteomics, imaging, and bioinformatics could be applied to improve the accuracy of the tests used by the FDA to predict the safety and efficacy of investigational medical products. In particular, the purpose of the Opportunities List is to provide a focus for public and private efforts and investments in new tools that could revolutionize medical product development. The FDA hopes that the suggestions and guidelines on usage of new scientific discoveries will reduce the uncertainty for companies to adopt and apply these new methods and data to their product development processes and applications. This is just one more example of how the FDA is trying to work with industry for better public health.

5.2.5   Science rules – most of the time

The FDA is an organization driven by the scientific method and scientific principles of analysis. The product development plan and, in particular, the clinical study, thus have to be designed to collect data using accepted scientific and experimental methods of inquiry. Statistically valid analysis of the results must be used to support the claim for the indication. However, the FDA usually err on the side of caution in the interpretation of the data and evaluation of risk. They are always playing a delicate balancing act in considering the final approval of new drugs, where political pressure (take the case of the application to make the "morning-after pill" available without prescription; see Box 5.2), internal scientific review and public pressure (for example, in creating a process to make AIDS drugs, and now other drugs, available to patients before final approval) play a significant role. In general, despite existing public opinion or controversy, the sponsor organization must interact with the FDA solely on the basis of data and scientific evidence, wherein the dialogue with the FDA is a formal and highly specific interaction.

Box 5.2 Science, religion and society – a debate over approval of Plan B

An emergency contraceptive (called the morning-after pill or Plan B, which needs to be taken within 72 hours after unprotected sex to prevent ovulation or, in some cases, implantation of a fertilized egg) comprising two levonorgestrel pills (a synthetic hormone used for over 35 years in birth control pills) were approved in 1999 for prescription use. An application for converting Plan B to an over-the-counter (OTC) drug (non-prescription purchase) was not approved despite strong internal (CDER) and external (the external scientific advisory board voted 23 to 4 in favor of approval) support for the scientific evidence. There was a tremendous amount of pressure from President George W. Bush's administration, conservative groups (who felt that this would condone sexual activity for pre-teens and teenagers and let them avoid medical care) and anti-abortion-rights groups (who see this as an abortion pill). Despite overwhelming evidence that the drug is safe and effective, the FDA did not approve it. Dr. Susan Wood, who headed the FDA's Office of Women's Health until August 2005, supported approval of the OTC label. She resigned in August 2005, when the then-head of the FDA, Lester Crawford, announced that the agency had postponed decision on Plan B for months or years. The debate continued at the state levels and at many pharmacies, where individual pharmacists refused to fill prescriptions for Plan B. In mid 2006, the FDA finally approved Plan B for over-the-counter sales to women over the age of 18 only.

Should agencies like the FDA be divorced from the debates and current opinions that are prevalent in society?

5.2.6   International harmonization

The FDA also works outside US national borders to protect US consumer health, as over 80% of seafood, 20% of all fresh produce and millions of other FDA-regulated products come from other countries. On another perspective, most US manufacturers that want to sell their FDA-regulated products outside the US need to be aware of international differences in regulation. In recognition of the increasing global trade in medical products and the myriad complex regulations in place in various countries, there is an ongoing effort to harmonize the regulatory regimes in the three largest markets – the European Union, Japan, and the USA, eventually hoping to generate a common filing process and format for these regulatory agencies. The US FDA is an active participant in this International Conference for Harmonization (ICH). The goals of the ICH are to make the international regulatory processes for medical products more efficient and uniform. A clear example of inefficiencies is seen in the fact that despite similar concerns among these three regions about safety, efficacy, and quality, time-consuming and expensive clinical trials need to be repeated in each region. For more details visit www.fda.gov/oia/Harmonization.htm and www.ich.org. Guidelines created in joint discussion at the ICH are then adopted by individual regulatory bodies (the EU, Japan, Canada, and the USA). Guidelines on various topics have been published by the ICH, including safety and toxicology studies and common format for submission of data prior to first-in-human testing (Common Technical Document), and have been integrated and published as FDA guides to industry (refer to websites listed in Table 5.3 for more information).

5.3   Regulatory pathways for drugs (biologicals or synthetic chemicals)

A drug is defined (at www.fda.gov/cder/drugsatfda/Glossary.htm) as:

- A substance recognized by an official pharmacopoeia or formulary,
- A substance intended for use in the diagnosis, cure, mitigation, treatment, or prevention of disease,
- A substance (other than food) intended to affect the structure or any function of the body,
- A substance intended for use as a component of a medicine but not a device or a component, part, or accessory of a device.

Biologic products are included within this definition and are generally covered by the same laws and regulations, but differences exist regarding their manufacturing processes (chemical process vs. biological process.) Note: the definition of a drug is originally found in 21 USC. 321 (g)1.

A biologic product is defined (in www.fda.gov/cder/drugsatfda/Glossary.htm) as "any virus, serum, toxin, antitoxin, vaccine, blood, blood component or derivative, allergenic product, or analogous product applicable to the prevention, treatment,

Table 5.3 Some useful FDA websites for drugs and biologics

Biologics and small molecule drugs (CDER and CBER)	
Starting point – CDER home page	www.fda.gov/cder/
CDER handbook for review process	www.fda.gov/cder/handbook/
All guidance documents for CDER	www.fda.gov/cder/guidance/index.htm
CBER home page	www.fda.gov/cber
CBER guidance and guidelines	www.fda.gov/cber/guidelines.htm
Drug master files	www.fda.gov/cder/guidance/dmf.htm
Institutional Review Boards (IRBs)	www.fda.gov/oc/ohrt/irbs/default.htm
CDER Manual of Policies and Procedures	www.fda.gov/cder/mapp.htm
Access past drug approval letters and reviews – Freedom of Information Act	www.fda.gov/cder/foi/index.htm
Office of Generic Drugs	www.fda.gov/cder/ogd/index.htm
Office of Orphan Products	www.fda.gov/orphan/
Office of Cellular, Tissue, and Gene Therapies, CBER	www.fda.gov/cber/genadmin/octgtprocess.htm
Good laboratory procedures (GLP)	21CFR Part 58 www.access.gpo.gov/nara/cfr/waisidx_03/ 21cfr58_03.html
Drug approval process overview	www.fda.gov/cder/regulatory/applications/ default.htm
IND details and guidance documents	www.fda.gov/cder/regulatory/applications/ ind_page_1.htm
NDA details and guidance documents	www.fda.gov/cder/regulatory/applications/ nda.htm
ANDA details and guidance documents	www.fda.gov/cder/regulatory/applications/ anda.htm
Office of Combination Products	www.fda.gov/oc/combination/
International Conference on Harmonisation of Technical Requirements for Registration of Pharmaceuticals for Human Use (ICH)	www.ich.org
ICH-pre-clinical safety studies guidelines	www.ich.org/LOB/media/MEDIA506.pdf
Food, Drug, and Cosmetic Act	www.fda.gov/opacom/laws/fdcact/fdctoc.htm

or cure of diseases or injuries." Biologic products are a subset of "drug products" distinguished by their manufacturing processes (biological process vs. chemical process). *In general, the term "drugs" also includes therapeutic biological products (the meaning used in this book)*. While many biologics are treated as drugs, others may be treated as devices and have to pass through the CDRH (Section 5.5).

This section gives a general overview of how a new drug passes through the FDA and describes the impact of the regulatory process on the product development plan. Figure 5.2 shows a schematic of the regulatory paths for marketing approval for generics (copies of already approved drug molecules) and new innovative drug molecules. While planning the regulatory path for drugs, some of the following points are useful to keep in mind:

● Define the exact indication and clinical trial endpoints (Section 4.1) to obtain the desired marketing claims for the product.

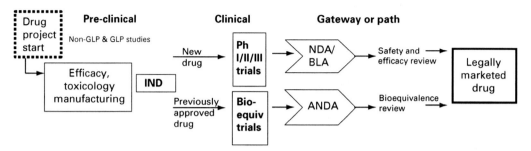

Figure 5.2 Regulatory paths to market for a drug (biological or chemical). IND = investigational new drug; NDA = New Drug Application; BLA = Biologics License Application (equivalent to an NDA for a biologic drug); ANDA = abbreviated NDA. The bioequivalence trials and ANDA path for generic medicines requires much less data and is much shorter compared to the NDA. Note: Over-the-counter (OTC) products do not typically need review and are not shown here.

- Decide if this is an orphan drug product – see Section 5.4.
- Complete required toxicity, manufacturing, and other pre-clinical packages for the IND application.
- Meet with the FDA before filing the IND (see Section 5.3.3) and then at designated times afterwards to keep open discussion on the design of the clinical trials and to gain agreement on the endpoints. Key issues in these meetings are clarification of the size, scope, and characteristics of the clinical trial and the manufacturing process.
- Follow guidance documents and regulatory requirements to file INDs, NDAs, BLAs, etc. Smaller companies may want to work with an outside regulatory affairs consultant or legal counsel who can help make sure that they are fully compliant with the requirements and ensure a smooth path to approval.
- Understand that the review team from the FDA will consist of the following;
  – Project manager,
  – Medical officer,
  – Chemist,
  – Microbiologist,
  – Statistician,
  – Pharmacologist,
  – Establishment or facility reviewer
  – Support personnel.

In brief, there are three main regulatory gateways and paths for a drug product to reach the market: 1) approval of an NDA, 2) approval of an ANDA, and 3) OTC.

Note: the regulatory pathway for a new drug product is discussed first in the sections below, followed by generics and OTC pathways.

5.3.1 Pre-clinical studies regulated by the FDA

Pre-clinical studies that are submitted to the FDA should be well described and summarized and the data should be completely transparent with detailed records.

Formal pre-clinical studies should be carried out following the guidelines in 21CFR58, which are generally described as current good laboratory practices (cGLP). Early efficacy studies and other in vitro studies can be non-GLP as long as the experiments are scientifically well designed with controls and the data are analyzed using statistically valid methods.

Before market approval of a drug, the FDA *will* inspect and audit one or more of the following: development facilities, planned production facilities, clinical trial sites, institutional review boards, and laboratory facilities in which the drug was tested in animals.

Specific pre-clinical studies that are evaluated by the FDA include:

- Efficacy data establishing the utility of the drug in treating the specific indication,
- Pharmacology data on drug behavior,
- Toxicology data on drug safety,
- Full characterization of the drug molecule using current knowledge and technologies,
- Manufacturing process for the drug.

A pre-IND meeting (as described in Section 5.3.3) can be held to discuss the planned GLP (good laboratory practice) toxicology studies and the plans for phase I and II clinical studies.

Toxicology data submitted prior to the start of clinical studies should support the length of exposure to the drug planned in the phase I studies. The primary goals of pre-clinical safety evaluation are: (1) to identify an initial safe dose and subsequent dose escalation schemes in humans; (2) to identify potential target organs for toxicity and for the study of whether such toxicity is reversible; and (3) to identify safety parameters for clinical monitoring. Some chronic toxicity-testing studies may continue in parallel with Phase I clinical testing. Pre-clinical toxicology or safety studies must be carried out under strict GLP guidelines and include the following:

- Safety pharmacology studies,
- Single and repeat dose toxicology studies in two species of mammals (to exceed or equal duration of human trials),
- Genotoxicity studies (in vitro studies evaluating mutations and chromosomal damage),
- Reproduction toxicity studies (animal studies),
- Other supplementary studies if safety concerns are identified (e.g., neurotoxicity studies, cardiotoxicity studies).

Regulatory guidelines for these studies can be accessed at *www.ich.org/cache/compo/276-254-1.html*.

Pharmacology studies are reviewed by the FDA to understand the effect and behavior of the drug molecule in the body. Pharmacokinetic (PK) studies (the half life of a drug, exposure, etc.) and an examination of the absorption, distribution, metabolism, and excretion (ADME) behavior of a drug molecule must also be submitted to the FDA. Additionally, data on the effect of the drug on various key enzymes or on the targeted protein and physiology (pharmacodynamics; PD) are usually collected.

Chemical and manufacturing details (known as the CMC – chemistry, manufacturing, and controls) are also provided, including a detailed description of the drugs' manufacturing process and adherence to established standards and FDA guidelines. Specifically, the drug must be manufactured in facilities that follow general current good manufacturing practices (cGMP) and adhere to specific FDA guidance that pertains to the product at hand. Manufacturing practices are further discussed in Chapter 6.

Specific issues for pre-clinical testing of biological drugs (proteins, glycoproteins, and other biological macromolecules) are addressed in guidance documents published by the FDA. These concerns generally review issues related to local tolerance (most biologics are administered by injection) and immunogenicity studies. Other genetic and reproductive toxicology studies may be requested by the FDA for certain classes of drug. Other tests that may be required for biologics include mutagenicity (e.g., growth hormones or other receptor agonists may induce or stimulate growth of malignant cells expressing the receptor). Gene therapy products may be evaluated for tissue distribution and activation, while monoclonal antibodies may be studied for the formation of neutralizing antibodies, and vaccines may be studied for the formation of non-specific antibodies that may cause immunogenicity or adverse reactions to the vaccine. However, the specific studies required for safety pharmacology endpoints are determined on a case-by-case basis with guidance documents issued for specific classes of therapeutics.

As an example, ICH guidelines on pre-clinical safety testing of biological drugs illustrate one such specific concern: "With some biopharmaceuticals, there is a potential concern about accumulation of spontaneously mutated cells (e.g., via facilitating a selective advantage of proliferation) leading to carcinogenicity. The standard battery of genotoxicity tests is not designed to detect these conditions. Alternative in vitro or in vivo models to address such concerns may have to be developed and evaluated." (*ICH Harmonised Tripartite Guideline*, Pre-clinical safety evaluation of biotechnology-derived pharmaceuticals, S6, 1997).

Other points of detailed review for biologics include an analysis of the ingredients used in the biological manufacturing process, with risks coming from host cell contaminants (cells used to make the biological drug molecule), and the detailed physical characterization of the product and its formulation and stability. In all cases, the product should be sufficiently characterized to allow an appropriate design of pre-clinical safety studies.

5.3.2 Filing an investigational new drug application (IND; or form FDA 1571)

An IND must be filed to conduct a clinical study on an unapproved drug (a full IND is required, as described below) or on an already-approved drug that is being tested for new unapproved indications, at new doses, or in novel combinations with any other drug (a much shorter IND is filed).

An IND is submitted by a sponsor-investigator, defined as one who initiates and conducts a clinical trial (if submitted by a physician to whom the manufacturer will supply the drug, then the physician is the sponsor for that IND submission). Therefore INDs are usually of two types – a commercial IND and a research IND (commercial sponsor vs. physician or researcher driven). An academic researcher who wants to carry out a study using an approved or generic drug must file an IND that describes the new studies as discussed below. In general, there are far more research INDs submitted to the FDA per year than commercial INDs. A new IND application comprises several volumes and hundreds of pages, whereas a research IND may only be tens of pages, as a research IND mainly describes rationale and the clinical protocol for the proposed study and references the content of the original IND.

The IND application can reference a prior IND for the same drug and indication if accompanied by a letter of permission from the sponsor of the original IND. Clinical studies can be initiated 30 days after the date of receipt of the IND by the FDA, unless the sponsor receives requests for more information by the FDA within those 30 days. No specific approval will be sent at the expiry of the 30-day period if no concerns or questions are found by the FDA, and tacit approval to initiate clinical studies is assumed (but a quick confirming phone call or communication with the FDA is advisable).

Exemption for research use for cancer: recent guidelines for clinical testing of cancer drugs exempt them from IND filings, provided the clinical studies (i) will not be filed with the FDA, (ii) will not be used to promote use in any indications other than approved indications, and (iii) will not be used to file for expansion of indications. Then it falls on the Institutional Review Board (IRB) to determine the risk for the study.

An IND submission must include the following (see 21CFR312 and guidelines for more detail):

- *Introductory statement and general investigational plan*: a summary overview of the investigational drug (formulation, dosage, administration) and the sponsor's plan for development.
- *Investigator's brochure*: contains all key non-clinical, clinical, and CMC data that support the clinical trial, providing the investigator and IRB (Institutional Review Board) with scientific rationale for the proposed trial. It should provide enough data to allow them to make an unbiased risk–benefit assessment.
- *Clinical protocol*: (described in detail in 21CFR312.23 and other documents) describes how clinical trials will be carried out, with an estimate of number of subjects, inclusion criteria, dosing plan, etc.; phase II studies should have even more detail, including endpoint measurements and detailed statistical analysis methodology.
- *Chemistry manufacturing and controls (CMC) section*: must provide enough information to demonstrate the identity, quality, purity, potency, and

formulation of the drug product. This includes description of substance and evidence to support its structure, overview of the manufacturing and packaging process, analytical methods used to measure identity, potency, purity, stability, etc. Assurance must be given that the drug product is made under current good manufacturing practices (cGMP).

- *Pharmacology and toxicology information*: Includes characterization of toxic effect with respect to target organs, dose dependent effects, etc. Single and repeat dose toxicity studies in more than one species are usually required.

5.3.3 Working with the FDA in formally arranged meetings

Pre-IND meeting

An IND (investigational new drug) submission is filed before beginning clinical testing. The purpose of a pre-IND meeting is to discuss the design and scope of pre-clinical and animal studies required to initiate clinical trials and also to discuss the design and scope of the clinical trials. This is a formal meeting requested in writing. A record of the minutes will be kept by the FDA and made available to the sponsor after the meeting. A list of objectives, outcomes and specific questions, along with a briefing document, should be sent to the FDA before the meeting. The discussion is focused on data and scientific methodology without any commercial or emotional issues being raised with the FDA. The sponsor would typically propose a study design with explanations based on scientific analysis or statistical methodology and seek agreement from the FDA rather than asking the FDA to suggest protocols. This is also typically a multidisciplinary meeting, including FDA representatives from clinical, chemistry and statistical disciplines.

End-of-Phase II meeting

This is typically the next meeting with the FDA, although an end-of-Phase I meeting can also be requested. In particular, if the program is fast-tracked, then an end-of-Phase I meeting is usually appropriate. The end-of-Phase II meeting is a critical meeting in the development process, as the protocols and endpoints of Phase III studies and other details on dosing and manufacturing expected in a strong NDA (for small molecule or synthetic drugs) or BLA (for large molecule or biological drugs) are agreed on during this meeting. The sponsor is expected to provide proof of efficacy and other data to support the Phase III design and endpoints and to show that the drug is performing a desired function. Figure 5.3 (from the FDA website) shows the various points of interaction with the FDA during the drug development process.

5.3.4 New drug application submission

The submission of the NDA is the key component in the regulatory approval process. The NDA contains clinical and non-clinical test data and analyses, drug chemistry information, and a description of manufacturing procedures. The NDA consists of thousands of pages of information to be reviewed by highly qualified individuals or teams from clinical, pharmacology, toxicology, chemistry, statistics,

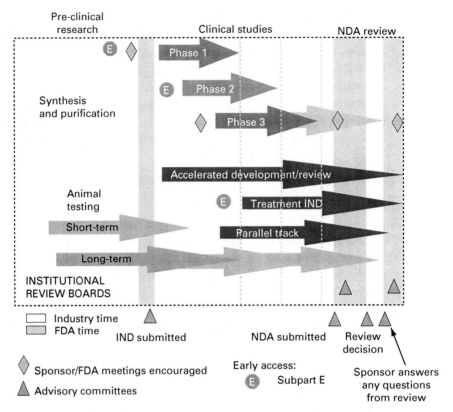

Figure 5.3   Chart showing FDA–sponsor interaction points (from the FDA website). Interaction points are marked in the drug development process chart above as yellow diamonds. An interactive version of this chart is at www.fda.gov/cder/handbook/. Subpart E refers to an expedited evaluation process for life-saving medicines where no alternative exists.

biopharmaceutical, and microbiology disciplines. The FDA has specific and highly detailed guidelines on formatting, assembling, and submitting the NDA. The NDA has over 20 sections which include the following key sections:

- *Application summary*: all review groups read this summary (50–200 pages) of the entire application and it must give a clear idea of the drug and its application. This must include the proposed package insert (label), pharmacologic class, scientific rationale, indication or intended use, potential clinical benefits, any foreign marketing history, CMC summary, non-clinical studies, human pharmacology studies, microbiology summary (for antibiotics only), data and summary of clinical results, statistical analysis, and discussion of risk–benefit relationship.
- *CMC chemistry, manufacturing, and controls section*: describes the physical and chemical characteristics, methods of analysis, stability, etc., and the manufacturing process. It also includes a drug master file (Section 5.3.5), authorization letters, drug product packaging details, etc.
- *Non-clinical pharmacology and toxicology*: Summary or description of all animal and in vitro studies with the drug, including individual study reports.

- *Human pharmacokinetics and bioavailability*: data from Phase I and summary of all pharmacokinetic studies performed with overall conclusions.
- *Clinical data*: includes clinical pharmacology, controlled clinical trials, with an integrated summary of effectiveness data demonstrating substantial evidence of effectiveness for each indication claimed. Clinical trials done in foreign countries can be submitted as long as certain provisions (described in Section 5.3.5) are met. This section also contains a statistical analysis of the data, with clinical trial reports, a summary of effectiveness and safety, and a summary of risks and benefits.
- *Safety update reports*: this section is used to update new safety information that is collected while the application is in review.

5.3.5 Clinical trials done in foreign countries

Data submitted in a 510(k) or PMA can be gathered in foreign countries as long as the studies are conducted:

- In accordance with the Declaration of Helsinki or local laws and protocols, whichever is stricter,
- On a patient population that is representative of the US population,
- Under a standard of care similar to that given in the USA,
- with data being available for audit by the FDA,
- individual patient data are presented to the FDA.

(see *www.fda.gov/cder/guidance/fstud.htm* for more details)

5.3.6 Drug master files

Master files are used by CDER and CBER in a similar manner to the device master files (Section 5.5.7). A drug master file (DMF) is a voluntary submission to the Food and Drug Administration (FDA) that may be used to provide confidential detailed information about facilities, processes, or articles used in the manufacturing, processing, packaging, and storing of one or more human drugs. The information contained in the DMF may be used to support an investigational new drug application (IND), a new drug application (NDA), a supplemental NDA (SNDA) or an abbreviated new drug application (ANDA). Drug master files are generally created to allow a party other than the holder of the DMF to reference material without disclosing to that party the contents of the file. For example, an IND or NDA sponsor can refer to a DMF submitted by a contracted manufacturing facility to support their application. Further details and guidance are available at www.fda.gov/cder/guidance/dmf.htm.

Drug master files are classified by content into five types by the FDA:

- Type I: manufacturing site, facilities, operating procedures, and personnel,
- Type II: drug substance, drug substance intermediate, and material used in its preparation, or drug product,
- Type III: packaging material,

- Type IV: excipient, colorant, flavor, essence, or material used in their preparation,
- Type V: FDA accepted reference information.

5.3.7   Regulatory pathway for copies of already approved drugs (generic or biosimilar drugs)

When a company wishes to market a copy of a drug that has been on the US market after its patent has expired, an abbreviated NDA (ANDA; or ABLA for biologics) is filed. The ANDA must be filed for indications that were already approved for the original drug molecule with no adverse findings since approval. This ANDA filing requires the manufacturer of the copy drug to certify that the original patent is expired and to demonstrate biological and pharmaceutical equivalence to the original drug.

The FDA maintains the key patents and a description of therapeutic equivalence standards for each approved drug in a regularly updated book called the *Orange Book* (for the color of its cover). Therapeutic equivalence is demonstrated by showing bio-equivalence (same rate and extent of absorption, with a 20% difference permissible) and by pharmaceutical equivalence (same dose, dosage form, strength).

The path to market for *biosimilars*, or copies of biological drug molecules (also called *biogenerics*), is not yet clear in the USA (as of early 2007), although biosimilars have made it to market in several countries, including some European countries. These biological drugs are complex molecules that are much more difficult to characterize than small molecule synthetic chemical drugs. Both the FDA and manufacturers of innovative biologicals that are losing patent protection are suggesting a longer process for approval of these copies (compared with small molecule generics) that would require more tests, including clinical efficacy studies.

5.3.8   Regulatory pathway for OTC (over-the-counter) drugs

Over-the-counter (OTC) drug products are those drugs that are available to consumers without a prescription. There are more than 80 classes (therapeutic categories) of OTC drug, ranging from acne drug products to weight-control drug products. As with prescription drugs, CDER oversees OTC drugs to ensure that they are properly labeled and that their benefits outweigh their risks. There are more than 100 000 OTC drug products marketed, encompassing about 800 significant active ingredients. The FDA maintains a list of OTC drug monographs. These monographs are a kind of "recipe book" covering acceptable ingredients, doses, formulations, and labeling. Products conforming to the monograph do not need FDA clearance to be marketed. New ingredients entering the OTC marketplace for the first time, especially those that had previously been approved through NDAs, must apply for the switch to OTC through the NDA process.

5.3.9 Post-market clinical studies (Phase IV) and safety surveillance by FDA

Phase 4 studies are post-marketing studies that may be imposed upon a pharmaceutical firm as a condition for drug approval. Phase IV investigations that are voluntarily conducted by the industry are typically used to support additional indications or to extend the life cycle of the product. Note: supplemental NDAs (SNDA) are filed for each new indication.

The FDA has an active surveillance program that requires sponsors to report any serious side effects not listed on the label within 15 days of learning of such events, and to submit quarterly safety reports for three years post-approval. The FDA has a separate office that specifically tracks adverse events in the post-approval marketplace through various sources, the manufacturer being one of them. The reach of this program and the sources it uses to monitor for safety in the post-approval phase are shown in Figure 5.4.

Drug experience and epidemiologic sources available to FDA
(for post-marketing surveillance and risk assessment)

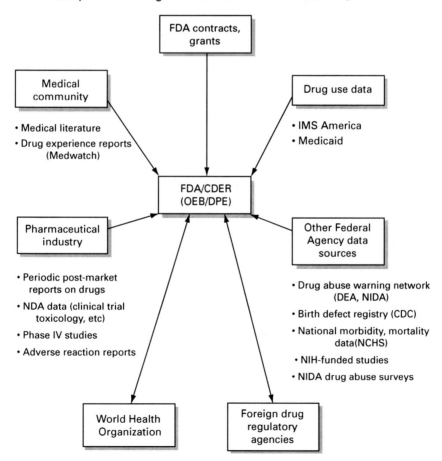

Figure 5.4   Safety surveillance program sources. Chart from the FDA CBER website.

5.3.10   Schematics of IND, NDA, and ANDA review processes

Figures 5.5 to 5.7 are taken from the FDA website and schematically show the CDER review process for IND, NDA and ANDA submissions. The flow charts in Figures 5.5 through 5.7 are largely self-explanatory.

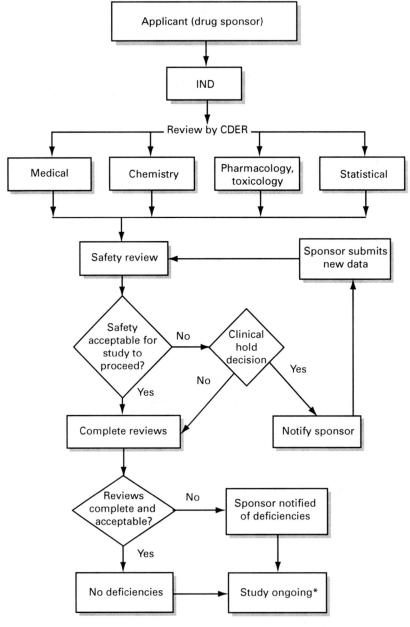

*While sponsor answers any deficiencies

Figure 5.5   IND review process. From www.fda.gov/cder/handbook/ind.htm.

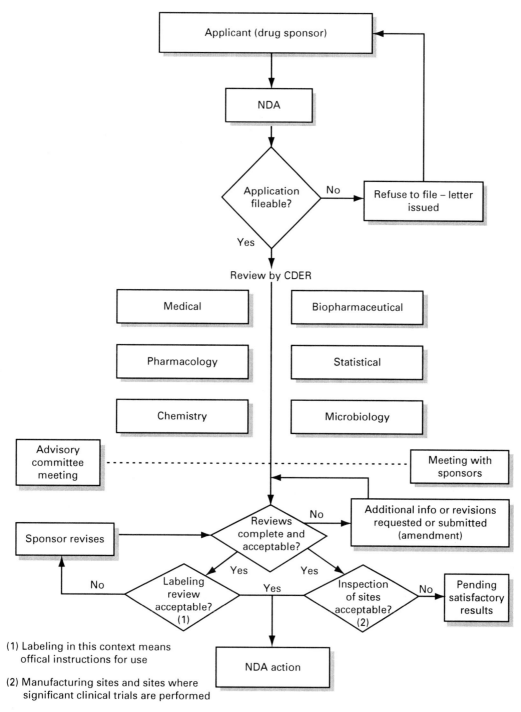

Figure 5.6   NDA review process. Chart from www.fda.gov/cder/handbook/nda.htm.

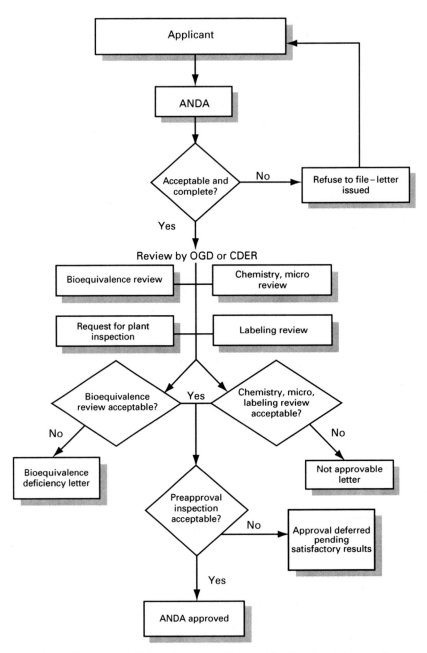

Figure 5.7   Generics review process. Taken from www.fda.gov/cder/handbook/generic.htm.

5.3.11   Speeding up access to drugs

Four separate initiatives are the Fast Track Program, accelerated approval (subpart H), priority review and subpart E.

Fast track process (the following information is from the FDA website www.fda.gov/oashi/fast.html)

The Fast Track Drug Development Program facilitates the development and expedites the review process of drugs intended for the treatment of a serious or life-threatening condition. The fast-track drug program was first initiated in section 112 of the FDA Modernization Act of 1997. Guidance documents are available at www.fda.gov/cder/guidance/5645fnl.htm and on the CBER website for Fast Track; www.fda.gov/cber/gdlns/fsttrk.htm.

A drug can receive fast-track designation if it meets three criteria:

(1) The drug must be targeted for use by a person who has a serious or life-threatening condition,
(2) The drug must be intended to treat a serious condition, and
(3) The drug must have the potential to address unmet medical needs.

A drug that receives fast-track designation is eligible for some or all of the following:

- More frequent meetings with the FDA to discuss the drug's development plan and ensure collection of appropriate data needed to support drug approval.
- More frequent written correspondence from the FDA about issues such as the design of the proposed clinical trials.
- Eligibility for accelerated approval, i.e., approval on an effect on a surrogate, or substitute, endpoint reasonably likely to predict clinical benefit.
- Rolling review, which means that a drug company can submit completed sections of its new drug application (NDA) for review by the FDA, rather than waiting until every section of the application is completed before the entire application can be reviewed. The NDA review usually does not begin until the drug company has submitted the entire application to the FDA.
- Dispute resolution if the drug company is not satisfied with an FDA decision not to grant fast-track status.

Fast-track designation must be requested by the drug company. The request can be initiated at any time during the drug development process. The FDA will review the request and make a decision within 60 days based on whether the drug fills an unmet medical need in a serious disease.

Once a drug is designated for fast-track review, the FDA works closely with the sponsor, with frequent reviews of the data and protocols, often allowing parallel clinical and continuing pre-clinical development. In addition, most drugs that are eligible for fast-track designation are likely to be considered appropriate to receive a priority review (see below).

Example of fast track drug development: in November 2004 a drug called Tarceva was approved by the FDA through the fast-track program. Tarceva is used for the treatment of people with locally advanced or metastatic non-small-cell lung cancer. In early data from clinical trials, Tarceva showed that people taking the drug had two months' additional survival (from five months to seven months). Although this increase in improvement may seem rather small, the potential of the drug to bring additional benefits and improvements was enough for acceptance into the fast-track program.

Accelerated approval or subpart H (information from the FDA website www.
fda.gov/oashi/fast.html and in 21 CFR 314.500 and 601.400)

The accelerated approval process allows earlier approval of drugs that treat serious
diseases, and that fill an unmet medical need, based on a surrogate endpoint. The
FDA bases its decision on whether to accept the proposed surrogate endpoint on
"adequate and well controlled" studies that demonstrate the effect of the drug and
may usually require longer term post-approval confirmatory studies. For example,
instead of having to wait to learn if a drug actually can extend the survival of cancer
patients, the FDA might now approve a drug based on evidence that the drug
shrinks tumors because tumor shrinkage is considered reasonably likely to predict a
real clinical benefit. In this example, an approval based upon tumor shrinkage can
occur far sooner than waiting to learn whether patients actually lived longer. The
drug company will still need to conduct studies to confirm that tumor shrinkage
actually does predict that patients will live longer. These studies are known as Phase
IV confirmatory trials. The fast-track program is most useful in clinical product
development up to the submission of the final NDA application.

Priority review (information from the FDA website www.fda.gov/oashi/fast.html)
Prior to approval, each drug marketed in the United States must go through a
detailed FDA review process. In 1992, under the Prescription Drug User Act
(PDUFA), the FDA agreed to specific goals for improving the drug review time
and created a two-tiered system of review times – standard review and priority review.

A standard review is applied to a drug that offers, at most, only minor improvement over existing marketed therapies. The 2002 amendments to PDUFA set a goal
that a standard review of a new drug application be accomplished within a ten-
month time frame.

A priority review designation is given to drugs that offer major advances in
treatment, or provide a treatment where no adequate therapy exists. Priority review
status can apply both to drugs that are used to treat serious diseases and to drugs
for less serious illnesses. A priority review designation means that the time it takes
FDA to review a new drug application is reduced. The goal for completing a
priority review is *six months*.

The distinction between priority and standard review times is that additional
FDA attention and resources will be directed to drugs that have the potential to
provide significant advances in treatment.

Such advances can be demonstrated by, for example:

- Evidence of increased effectiveness in treatment, prevention, or diagnosis of disease,
- Elimination or substantial reduction of a treatment-limiting drug reaction,
- Documented enhancement of patient willingness or ability to take the drug
  according to the required schedule and dose, or
- Evidence of safety and effectiveness in a new subpopulation, such as children.

A request for a priority review must be made by the drug company. It does not
affect the length of the clinical trial period. The FDA determines within 45 days of
the drug company's request whether a priority or standard review designation will

be assigned. Designation of a drug as "priority" does not alter the scientific or medical standard for approval or the quality of evidence necessary.

Subpart E (21 CFR 312.84) allows for approval after phase II efficacy is shown. The drug must provide treatment where no alternative exists, and the need must be severe. For example, Tysabri was approved for treatment of relapsing multiple sclerosis patients under subpart E, as they had no other options for this severe disease.

5.3.12 Market exclusivity for new drugs and the Hatch Waxman Act 1984

A five year period of exclusivity is provided by the Federal Food, Drug, and Cosmetic Act under sections 505(c)(3)(E) and 505(j)(5)(F). Exclusivity is available for new chemical entities (NCEs), which by definition are innovative, and for significant changes in already approved drug products, such as a new use. A five-year period of exclusivity provides the holder of an approved new drug application limited protection from new competition in the marketplace for the innovation represented by its approved drug product. This exclusivity was specifically provided in the 1984 Hatch Waxman Amendments to the Food, Drug, and Cosmetic Act, to encourage R&D investment and innovation and also *to speed entry of generic drugs* into the market. As a balance against that exclusivity, ANDAs, filed by generic manufacturers, could now reference NDAs containing data that had not been developed by the generic manufacturers. No ANDA may be submitted during the five-year exclusivity period, unless it contains a certification of patent invalidity or non-infringement, in which case it can be submitted after four years. Additionally, the FDA grants a specific six-month exclusivity after expiry of the patent term, if the drug manufacturer carries out studies to test the drug in pediatric populations.

5.3.13 Drugs: helpful FDA websites and the Electronic Orange Book

The list of websites given in Table 5.3 provides a starting point for exploration of specific processes or issues.

The Orange Book: Information on drugs that have been approved is listed in the Orange Book and Supplements or the *Electronic Orange Book* (actual title: *Approved Drug Products with Therapeutic Equivalence Evaluations*). See www.fda.gov/cder/ob/default.htm for the *Electronic Orange Book*.

The Orange Book is composed of four lists: (1) approved prescription drug products with therapeutic equivalence evaluations; (2) approved over-the-counter (OTC) drug products for those drugs that may not be marketed without NDAs or ANDAs because they are not covered under existing OTC monographs; (3) drug products with approval under Section 505 of the Act administered by the Center for Biologics Evaluation and Research; and (4) a cumulative list of approved products that have been discontinued from marketing, have had their approvals withdrawn for other than safety or efficacy reasons subsequent to being discontinued, have never been marketed, are for exportation, or are for military use. This publication includes indices of prescription and OTC drug products by trade or established name (if no trade name exists) and by applicant name (holder of the approved application). The Orange Book also has an addendum with patent and exclusivity information on each drug.

5.4   Orphan drugs

The FDA's Office of Orphan Products only designates orphan drugs (that treat rare diseases affecting US patient populations of less than 200 000) and provides grants and guidance, but does not influence the approval and review process of CDER or CBER. An orphan drug designation is given to a specific drug molecule for a specific indication (disease). The Orphan Drug Act (1983) gives seven years of market exclusivity for the orphan drug that gains approval. This market exclusivity is given to the sponsor as an incentive to develop treatments for rare diseases. Additional incentives include tax credits for clinical research undertaken by a sponsor in support of the application. The success of this Act is seen by the fact that fewer than 10 such products were approved in the period from 1973–1983 while over 200 orphan drugs were approved from 1983 to the present. Additionally, the European Union has since also put in place an Orphan Drug program with a 10 year market exclusivity and other regions and countries are considering such legislation. Other countries, such as Australia and Japan, have similar programs, with slight variations.

5.5   Devices: regulatory pathways and NPD considerations

This section presents a general understanding and overview of the device review processes (Figure 5.8). Diagnostics (most of which are regulated as devices) are also covered in this section where relevant but are discussed separately in more detail in Section 5.6. Also discussed here are specific regulatory controls that the FDA will use to review the data generated during pre-clinical and clinical testing of the devices. In particular, it is extremely important to read the general guidance documents or special controls for devices and to address those issues thoroughly during testing of the devices.

In brief, there are three regulatory pathways for devices and an additional one for diagnostics to get to market: (1) exempt from FDA review, (2) 510(k) clearance process, (3) PMA review, and, for diagnostics, if they are exempt from (2) and (3), they have to go through CLIA categorization. These are explained in greater detail in the sections below.

A 510(k) (described in greater detail in Section 5.5.8) is a pre-marketing submission made to the FDA to demonstrate that the device to be marketed is as safe and effective (i.e., substantially equivalent (SE)), as a legally marketed device that is not subject to pre-market approval (PMA). A PMA (described in Section 5.5.9) is an application submitted to the FDA to request approval to market, or continue marketing, a class III medical device. Pre-market approval is based on scientific evidence, providing a reasonable assurance that the device is safe and effective for its intended use or uses. The differences between these two main pathways through the FDA are highlighted in Table 5.4.

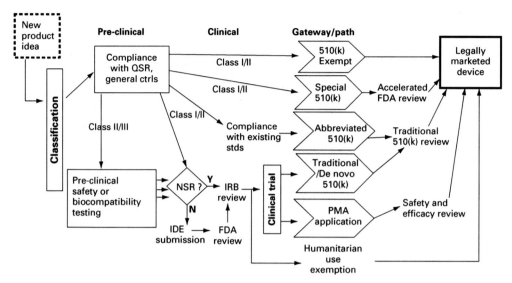

Figure 5.8 Regulatory paths to market for a medical device. QSR = quality system regulation; NSR = non–significant risk study; IRB = institutional review board.

5.5.1 Step 1: determine the jurisdiction of the FDA center – is it a device?

Medical devices range from simple tongue depressors to complex programmable pacemakers with micro-chip technology and, X-ray machines, and include in vitro diagnostic products, such as general purpose laboratory equipment, reagents, and test kits, which may include monoclonal antibody technology. Diagnostics are discussed in a separate section below, but are usually classified as a type of device.

A device is defined by its primary mode of action in the indication specified by the company. For example, a wound dressing containing antibacterials has as its primary mode of action the creation of a physical barrier for the wound and hence is not regulated from the standpoint of the antibacterials, which only enhance the primary mode of action. On the other hand, if the wound dressing is made of a biodegradable matrix whose sole purpose is to deliver the antibacterial compound, the dressing is then reviewed as a drug, with the matrix being an inactive component.

The specific definition of a device is (section 201(h) of the Federal Food and Drug Control Act [21 U.S.C. 321(h)]).

An instrument, apparatus, implement, machine, contrivance, implant, in vitro reagent, or other similar or related article, including a component part, or accessory which is:

● Recognized in the official National Formulary, or the United States Pharmacopoeia, or any supplement to them,
● Intended for use in the diagnosis of disease or other conditions, or in the cure, mitigation, treatment, or prevention of disease, in man or other animals, or
● intended to affect the structure or any function of the body of man or other animals, and which does not achieve any of its primary intended purposes through chemical action within or on the body of man or other animals and which is not dependent upon being metabolized for the achievement of any of its primary intended purposes.

Box 5.3 Drug or device?

Here is an example of why it is important to be very careful in this process of classification: a company (unnamed by request) that was already marketing several catheters designed a new system with which a bolus of CO_2 gas could be injected into a blood vessel. This bubble of gas displaced the blood and gave good images of large vessels and higher resolution images of the small vessel during imaging. The submission for requesting classification of the device under a Class II described the intention of use of the gas as a "contrast medium."

The FDA wrote back that this system would have to be reviewed as a drug as all "contrast media" were automatically reviewed as drugs. Also, CO_2 gas, although used for decades in medical procedures, had no indication and, therefore, could not be the basis for approving a product for its delivery. This reclassification led to a fivefold increase of project costs and a threefold increase in time to market.

If the product fits this definition, it will be regulated as a medical device and is subject to pre-marketing and post-marketing regulatory controls. See Box 5.3 for an example of why defining the device by FDA guidelines is important.

5.5.2   Step 2: classify the medical device – what controls and regulations apply?

To understand the impact of the regulatory process on your product's commercialization path, the next step is to classify the device by its indication and intended use and the risk it poses to the patient or user if it malfunctions or fails. This classification of devices will indicate the type of submission to be made to the FDA to commercialize the device.

Class I   General controls apply (exemptions / without exemptions),
Class II   General controls and special controls apply (exemptions / without exemptions),
Class III   General controls apply and pre-market approval required.

Even the lowest-risk devices (Class I) are subject to certain general controls (see Section 5.5.5). The regulatory controls increase through perceived risk (Class II to Class III). Enter the keyword or device name into the classification database at the FDA website (*www.accessdata.fda.gov/scripts/cdrh/cfdocs/cfpcd/classification.cfm*) to see how other similar devices have been classified. If the device is completely novel, you will still look for descriptions of other devices with similar indications, methods of use or other such comparison within the medical specialty of intended use to gain a better idea of how the FDA will classify the device – both for its regulation number and the risk class. Box 5.4 contains an example of the various records associated with a scalpel blade (a scalpel handle has a separate classification) classified as relatively low risk (Device Class I) in the FDA database.

Box 5.4 Product classification database

Device	Blade, scalpel
Regulation description	Manual surgical instrument for general use.
Regulation medical specialty	General and plastic surgery
Review panel	General and plastic surgery
Product code	GES
Submission type	510(k) exempt
Regulation number	878.4800
Device class	1
GMP exempt?	No

This result of a search of the classification database at the CDRH shows that a scalpel blade has a device regulation number 21 CFR 878.4800, three-letter product code GES, and is a Type I device exempt from reporting to the FDA before marketing, but not exempt from showing that GMP processes for manufacturing are in place.

5.5.3   Step 3: determine marketing application required to be submitted

Class I *exempt* devices do not need to get approval before marketing but still need to adhere to some general controls (guidelines for making, storing, packaging, and selling). Class I and Class II devices that are not exempt can go through a 510(k) submission to get clearance or a PMA process to get approval and will be subject to special controls, such as FDA guidance documents, FDA accepted international standards, and the Quality System Regulation (QSR).

The 510(k) submission is dependent on first locating a substantially equivalent device (predicate device) already on the market and then filing data that demonstrates such equivalence of the new device. Substantial equivalence has to be established both in the technological characteristics and intended use of the new device in comparison to a chosen predicate device.

To locate predicate 510(k) devices, start with a known device currently on the market, and enter the manufacturer's name in the product classification database (see Section 5.5.2). Note the three-letter code (product code) for the classified device. Enter this product code again in the 510(k) products database (www.fda.gov/search/databases.html) search function and you will see a list of all possible predicate devices. On submission of the appropriate data in a 510(k) submission, the FDA will review the data (on average a 90–120 day process) and if they agree, the new device will receive *clearance* (the terminology and process are distinct from the PMA "approval" process) for marketing under regulation 510(k). If the FDA determines that the device is not substantially equivalent to a previous legally marketed device, the sponsor must now go through a de novo 510(k) application (see Section 5.5.7), a PMA (see Section 5.5.8) or a product development protocol (PDP is a contract with the FDA towards faster approval of Class III devices with established technology, see www.fda.gov/cdrh/pdp/pdp.html for more details).

A pre-market application (PMA) process is necessary when the new device is not substantially equivalent to any other device that has been cleared through the 510(k) process. The PMA process is more complex and will usually take two formal submission steps (refer to Figure 5.8) depending on the perception of significant risk (SR) or non-significant risk (NSR) prior to clinical testing of the device. The first step (if SR established) is the submission and approval of an Investigational Device Exemption (IDE) to allow clinical trials to be conducted. These clinical trials will ascertain the safety and efficacy of the device in its intended use. The data will be submitted in a (PMA) to the FDA. On review of the safety and efficacy data, the FDA *approval* will establish market indication and label along with post-approval studies or follow-up. The typical review time is one year.

5.5.4   Working with the FDA in formal meetings

Devices

A pre-IDE (Investigational Device Exemption; similar in concept to the IND) informal meeting is welcomed. This meeting should be used to verify the approach to approval and to evaluate the clinical protocol and any pre-clinical studies that may need to be done. This meeting should not be used to gain an early review of an IDE before submission.

Two formal meetings are encouraged before launching clinical trials for devices, the proceedings of which are binding and recorded.

(1) Only for devices requiring a PMA (pre-market application; requiring submission of detailed clinical tests for approval):

A determination meeting, described in [section] §513(a)(3)(D) [of the Federal Food, Drug, and Cosmetic Act; cite as 21USC 360c(a)(3)(D)], is intended to provide the applicant with the Agency's determination of the type of valid scientific evidence that will be necessary to demonstrate that the device is effective for its intended use. As a result of this meeting, the FDA will determine whether clinical studies are needed to establish effectiveness and, in consultation with the applicant, determine the least burdensome way of evaluating device effectiveness with a reasonable likelihood of success. The applicant can expect that the FDA will determine if concurrent randomized controls, concurrent non-randomized controls, historical controls, or other types of evidence will be acceptable. (quoted from the FDA guidance document).

(2) For devices requiring PMA or 510(k): the agreement meeting, described in §520(g)(7) [of the Federal Food, Drug, and Cosmetic Act], is open to any person planning to investigate the safety or effectiveness of a Class III product or any implant. The agreement meeting is available to submitters of a 510(k) for eligible devices. The purpose of this meeting is to reach a concensus on the key parameters of the investigational plan (see 21 CFR 812.25), including the clinical protocol.

Table 5.4 Comparison of the PMA and 510(k) processes

Characteristic	PMA submission	510(k) submission
Time to collect data	Several years	Several months
Submission size	Several thousand pages	Much less
Manufacturing details	Process, methods, details required	Typically not required
Pre-approval inspection of device manufacturing facility	Required	Not required
Clinical trial site review	Often required	Not required
Review time	1 year	90 days
Post-approval annual reports	Required	Not required
Submission availability through Freedom of Information (FOI) Act	Not available	Available
Scientific advisory panels convened to assist FDA in review	Sometimes	Rarely

Diagnostics

Interactions with the FDA, CLIA, and OIVD offices are similar to those described above, as most diagnostics are classified as devices. The timing of interactions will differ based on the development path and type of diagnostic. See OIVD website (and Table 5.4) for more details.

5.5.5 General controls and exempt devices

Some Class I devices may also be exempt from pre-market notification [510(k)], which means that there is no need to inform the FDA before launching onto market. However, these devices are not exempt from other *general controls*, meaning that they must be:

- Manufactured under a quality assurance program,
- Suitable for the intended use,
- Adequately packaged and properly labeled.

Additionally, as part of the general controls,

- The production and distribution company must be registered with the FDA, and
- Device-listing forms must be on file with the FDA.

5.5.6 Pre-clinical considerations – special controls and QSR for Class II and III devices

Special controls are specific issues that the FDA has identified for a type of device (all scalpel blades, for example) and would like to see addressed by the sponsor when submitting either a 510(k) or a PMA for any product that falls under a similar classification. The FDA issues guidance documents detailing these concerns. These

---

Box 5.5 Example of a special controls guidance document

Guidance for industry and FDA staff
  Class II Special Controls Guidance Document: Dental Bone Grafting Material Devices
  (content below is an extract from the original document)

Table of contents

 (1) Introduction
 (2) Background
 (3) The content and format of an abbreviated 510(k) submission
 (4) Scope
 (5) Device description
 (6) Risks to health
 (7) Material characterization
 (8) Biocompatibility
 (9) Sterilization
(10) Labeling

(6) Risks to health

In the table below, the FDA has identified the risks to health generally associated with the use of the bone grafting material device addressed in this document. The measures recommended to mitigate these identified risks are given in this guidance document, as shown in the table below. You should also conduct a risk analysis, before submitting your 510(k), to identify any other risks specific to your device. The 510(k) should describe the risk analysis method ...

Identified risks	Recommended mitigation measures
Ineffective bone formation	Section 7 – Material characterization
Adverse tissue reaction	Section 8 – Biocompatibility
Infection	Section 9 – Sterilization
Improper use	Section 10 – Labeling

Sections refer to additional parts of the document not reproduced here.

This type of FDA special controls guidance document is a critical tool in designing and carrying out the right experiments and studies with the device in development. Deviation from the guidance document suggested protocols should be done only with good reason and justification provided to the FDA staff, who will use this guidance document as a template when reviewing an application for approval.

special controls guidance documents must be read and thoroughly addressed in pre-clinical design and testing of the product and in clinical trial designs. An example of special controls guidance is given in Box 5.5.

The QSR (Quality Systems Regulation) (21 CFR Part 820) is the device equivalent of the pharmaceutical good manufacturing process (GMP) regulations.

However, unlike the GMP regulations, which primarily affect final manufacturing processes, QSR impacts the pre-clinical stage significantly, as it includes design controls (21CFR 820.30) that apply to pre-clinical studies for all Class II and III (and some Class I) devices as soon as they move beyond initial concept and feasibility testing studies. The design controls section of the Quality System Regulation outlines the requirements that each manufacturer of any Class II or Class III device, and certain Class I devices, must meet when designing such products or related processes, and when changing existing designs and processes. The design control process has multiple components and steps (e.g., a list of design inputs; a design verification process) that require the company to manage and document the entire design and development process formally, with standard operating procedures (SOPs) that comply with, and specifically address, regulatory requirements. All relevant activities must be documented in the design history file (DHF), as further described in Box 5.6. The DHF must be regularly updated during the development process and filed with the FDA. Most importantly for regulatory purposes, *design review activities and results* must be documented and personnel participating in the review must be identified. This NPD plan must be in place (with modifications recorded in the DHF) before development begins. Internal audits must be performed to improve and monitor quality systems continuously.

Box 5.6 Design history file (DHF)

What type of records are maintained in a DHF?

A DHF must be created and maintained for each device made under design controls. The firm should first put into place formal procedures that detail how the DHF will be established and maintained. The DHF should contain the following records (this is not a comprehensive list) or references to specific records and their location:

- The design and development plan along with evidence showing that the device was designed in accordance with this plan and in compliance with Subpart C of the Regulations,
- Design input documents (see Section 4.10.1),
- Engineering notebooks, which contain relevant information recorded after design control began,
- Risk analyses documents,
- A device history file (DHF) index and copies of controlled documents used during the design process, including records of product builds and testing,
- Design output,
- Pre-production design change control records,
- Design review and transfer records,
- The initial device master record (DMR),
- Issues tracking matrix.

The QSR also requires the firms to demonstrate that specific management systems are in place for controlling the device development, production, and marketing processes. These control systems are discussed further in Chapter 6 and in Appendix 6.2. The final stages of development (process and production controls) also require documentation of the production history of a particular batch in the device history record (DHR) and the documentation of the device specifications and manufacturing procedures in the device master record (DMR). The DMR is the term used in the QSR for all of the routine documentation required to manufacture devices that will consistently meet company requirements.

The recording requirements of the QSR (DHF, DHR, and DMR) thus regulate the device from concept to development. The goal of the QSR is to create a set of self-correcting systems that will reliably produce a high quality design, with a controlled and predictable production process.

The QSR manual on the FDA website is recommended reading and can be found at www.fda.gov/cdrh/qsr/contnt.html.

5.5.7   The use of master files (MAF)

Master files are data submitted to the FDA by non-sponsor organizations to allow the FDA to review technical or scientific data from a process or some technical test related to a sponsor's IDE or PMA application. The sponsor can reference the master file in the submission (with the permission of the other party) while still maintaining secrecy between the sponsor and the other party that filed the master file. Thus, master files are typically accepted from those organizations or persons who have not submitted or will not directly submit the information in a PMA, IDE, 510(k), or other device-related application to FDA.

Information in a master file may be incorporated by reference in a client's PMA, 510(k), IDE, or other submission to FDA. The use of information in a master file can only be authorized by the master file holder or by a designated agent.

5.5.8   510(k) submission type and content

There is no specific 510(k) form but instead a format for the submission is described in 21 CFR 807 and in multiple guidance documents by the FDA. The term 510(k) refers to the original section of the CFR that described the process of clearing a device that demonstrates *substantial equivalence* to a device already on the market before 1976 or another 510(k) cleared device on the market currently (a *predicate device*). Since the 510(k) process is much shorter than the PMA route, most companies try to qualify their devices into the 510(k) pathway. *However, as this process may not generate adequate clinical data to satisfy insurance companies or other payers, often manufacturers will benefit by performing more extensive clinical studies to show the specific clinical benefits of the new device or technology* (see Chapter 7 for detailed discussion). To identify a list of 510(k) cleared devices that might be predicate devices, see Section 5.5.3.

To show substantial equivalence, the sponsor has to show:

- That the new device has an intended use that is substantially equivalent to a predicate device, and
- That the technological characteristics of the new device are substantially equivalent to the predicate device.

Typically, a device may be used for multiple indications. Each indication for use must be cleared with its own 510(k). Design inputs, required as part of the design controls, typically contain the information that establishes the technological characteristics in comparison with predicate devices.

The four types of 510(k) submission are:

(1) Traditional 510(k) – if the new device is not a modification of one of the sponsor's own previously cleared devices and does not need to conform to any special control or guidance document from the FDA. The FDA has 90 days to review this submission.

(2) Special 510(k) – if the sponsor has modified its own 510(k) cleared device, but has not added a new indication or altered fundamental scientific technology of the device. The FDA has 30 days to review this submission.

(3) Abbreviated 510(k) – if the new device has to conform to a special control or guidance, a Declaration of Conformance has to be included in this abbreviated 510(k), stating that the device meets the referenced standards. Detailed test reports, like those required in a traditional 510(k), are not required. The FDA has 90 days to review this submission.

(4) De novo 510(k) – this is a 510(k) without a predicate device, where the sponsor can demonstrate that the device has few risks and that the detailed PMA reviews for safety and effectiveness are not required. A de novo 510(k) submission requires more data than the regular 510(k) but fewer than the usual PMA and is usually followed by a request by the manufacturer for classification into Class I or Class II. If classified as Class II, a special controls guidance document is issued by the FDA, allowing subsequent manufacturers to submit traditional or abbreviated 510(k)s. This approach should be confirmed with the FDA.

A 510(k) submission typically contains the following sections:

- *Statement of substantial equivalence* (optional): narrative description or rationale with list of predicate devices,
- *Labeling*: all printed material associated with device and patient information brochures,
- *Advertising and promotional* material (optional),
- *Comparative information*: this is the most important section, containing data with critical choice of comparison parameters and including comparison charts with new device and predicate device data, bench and clinical testing data, and any relevant supporting materials: clinical data may be requested by reviewers,
- *Biocompatibility assessment* (if necessary): the FDA version of the international standard ISO 10993 at www.fda.gov/cdrh/g951.html is used to determine

testing, and discussion with the FDA before conducting any such testing is important,

- *shelf life* (if necessary): stability data,
- *Indication for use* form: list of indications for use; new indications in an abbreviated 510(k),
- *510(k) summary*: publicly released information on the FDA website once the 510(k) is cleared.

5.5.9   PMA submission content

Typically, PMA submission documents take up 1500 pages or more. Many years of effort go into compiling and collecting data necessary for the PMA. A PMA must provide a "reasonable assurance" that the new device is both safe and effective. The evidence is typically a compilation and statistical analysis of data from clinical trials, the majority of which are designed as controlled studies with patients randomly assigned into treatment or control groups. There are administrative elements of a PMA application, but good science and scientific writing is a key to the approval of a PMA application.

A PMA submission includes the following sections:

- *Summary of safety and effectiveness,*
- *Device description, intended use and manufacturing data,*
- *Performance standards referenced,*
- *Technical data (non-clinical)*: non-clinical laboratory studies' section includes information on microbiology, toxicology, immunology, biocompatibility, stress, wear, shelf life, and other laboratory or animal tests. Non-clinical studies for safety evaluation must be conducted in compliance with 21CFR Part 58 (Good Laboratory Practice for Nonclinical Laboratory Studies).
- *Technical data (clinical)*: the clinical investigations section includes study protocols, safety and effectiveness data, adverse reactions and complications, device failures and replacements, patient information, patient complaints, tabulations of data from all individual subjects, results of statistical analyses, and any other information from the clinical investigations. Any investigation conducted under an Investigational Device Exemption (IDE) must be identified as such. Data collected in clinical trials done in foreign countries can be submitted as long as the trials meet certain provisions (described in Section 5.3.5).
- *Labeling*: any printed matter associated with the device, including directions for use, warnings or other labels,
- *Environmental assessment.*

5.5.10   Types of PMA submission

Traditional PMA submission: this is a one-time complete submission, usually made when the device is approved in another country and has already completed clinical testing.

Modular PMA submission: each pre-agreed component of the PMA submission is reviewed and locked in until the final module is received, at which point the entire PMA is complete. The review period is thus shorter, with rolling submissions based on the sponsor's timetable.

Streamlined PMA submissions: in this program, being piloted by the Division of Clinical Laboratory Devices, the clinical trial protocol is discussed and an agreement reached between the sponsor and the FDA, typically addressing a guidance document prepared by the FDA. This up-front agreement and familiarity with the device and protocol allows for a faster review.

5.5.11 Humanitarian use devices (HUDs)

A humanitarian use device (HUD) treats or diagnoses a disease or condition that affects fewer than 4000 individuals in the United States per year and can be approved by the FDA under the Humanitarian Device Exemption (HDE). The HDE is similar in both form and content to a pre-market approval (PMA) application, but is exempt from the effectiveness requirements of a PMA. An HDE application is not required to contain the results of scientifically valid clinical investigations demonstrating that the device is effective for its intended purpose.

The FDA recognizes that sometimes a condition is so unusual that it would be difficult for a company to demonstrate scientifically the effectiveness of their device in the large number of patients that must usually be tested. Additionally, the applicant must demonstrate that no comparable devices are available to treat or diagnose the disease or condition, and that they could not otherwise bring the device to market.

In these special situations, the FDA may grant a HDE to market the device, provided that: (1) the device does not pose an unreasonable or significant risk of illness or injury, and (2) The probable benefit to health outweighs the risk of injury or illness from its use, taking into account currently available devices or alternative forms of treatment.

Table 5.5 gives a list of helpful FDA websites for devices.

5.6 Diagnostics: regulatory pathways and NPD considerations

In vitro devices (IVD) are mostly regulated as medical devices and are subject to all the processes for devices outlined above. The specific office that reviews IVDs is the CDRH's Office of In Vitro Diagnostic Device Evaluation and Safety (OIVD). The FDA defines IVD products as:

Those reagents, instruments, and systems intended for use in diagnosis of disease or other conditions, including a determination of the state of health, in order to cure, mitigate, treat, or prevent disease or its sequelae. Such products are intended for use in the collection, preparation, and examination of specimens taken from the human body. (21 CFR 809.3)

Table 5.5 Some useful FDA websites for devices

All devices (CDRH)	
Starting point	www.fda.gov/cdrh
Device advice (another good starting point)	www.fda.gov/cdrh/devadvice/
Information on exempt devices	www.fda.gov/cdrh/devadvice/3133.html
List of exempt devices	www.accessdata.fda.gov/scripts/cdrh/cfdocs/cfpcd/315.cfm
Classifying a device	www.fda.gov/cdrh/devadvice/313.html
Classification database for devices	www.accessdata.fda.gov/scripts/cdrh/cfdocs/cfpcd/classification.cfm
Registration of an establishment	www.fda.gov/cdrh/devadvice/341.html
Medical device listing requirement	www.fda.gov/cdrh/devadvice/342.html
Labeling requirements	www.fda.gov/cdrh/devadvice/33.html
QSR manual and design controls details[a]	www.fda.gov/cdrh/qsr/03desgn.html and www.fda.gov/cdrh/qsr/contnt.html
Biocompatibility and toxicity tests for devices	www.fda.gov/cdrh/g951.html
GMP manufacturing and quality systems regulation	www.fda.gov/cdrh/devadvice/32.html
510(k) guidelines and details	www.fda.gov/cdrh/devadvice/314.html
PMA guidelines and details	www.fda.gov/cdrh/devadvice/pma/
Guidance on FDA meetings for devices	www.fda.gov/cdrh/ode/guidance/310.html
Early (pre-IDE) meetings with the CDRH	www.fda.gov/cdrh/modact/earlymtg.pdf
Select and search from a list of all databases on the FDA website	www.fda.gov/search/databases.html
Information on master files	www.fda.gov/cdrh/dsma/pmaman/appdxc.html#P7_2
Device recalls	www.accessdata.fda.gov/scripts/cdrh/cfdocs/cfTopic/medicaldevicesafety/recalls.cfm
In vitro diagnostics (OIVD/CDRH)	
Starting point	www.fda.gov/cdrh/oivd/index.html
Devices that are also regulated and reviewed by CBER	www.fda.gov/cber/dap/devlst.htm
List of approved classified IVDs	www.accessdata.fda.gov/scripts/cdrh/cfdocs/cfcfr/showCFR.cfm
Assignment of CLIA categories	www.fda.gov/cdrh/clia/
Regulatory process FAQs	www.fda.gov/cdrh/oivd/regulatory-overview.html
Labeling requirements for IVDs	www.fda.gov/cdrh/devadvice/332.html
Analyte Specific Reagents guidance	www.fda.gov/cdrh/oivd/guidance/1590.html

[a] Excellent advice and guidelines for product development

A few key differences in the review and approval of IVDs, compared with other medical devices are highlighted in this discussion.

In addition to CDRH device reviews and controls, IVDs are subject to the Clinical Laboratory Improvement Amendments (CLIA) of 1988. This law established quality standards for laboratory testing and an accreditation program for clinical laboratories. The requirements that apply vary, according to the technical complexity in the testing process and the risk of harm in reporting erroneous results. The regulations established three categories of testing on the basis of the complexity of the testing methodology: waived tests, tests of moderate complexity, and tests of high complexity. Laboratories performing moderate-complexity or high-complexity tests, or both, must be certified under the CLIA and must meet requirements for proficiency testing, patient test management, quality control, quality assurance, and personnel. The OIVD determines the appropriate complexity categories for clinical laboratory devices as they evaluate pre-market submissions.

In vitro device pre-market submissions (PMA or 510(k)) may also be reviewed by the drug or biologic reviewing divisions (CDER/CBER). Pre-market notification 510(k)s, PMAs, and IDEs for medical devices associated with blood collection and processing procedures as well as those associated with cellular therapies and vaccines will be reviewed by CBER. The medical device laws and regulations still apply.

In vitro devices also have special labeling requirements and distribution restrictions under 21 CFR 809 as discussed next and in Chapter 6.

The regulation of molecular diagnostics (nucleic acid tests or genetic testing) is an emerging area where the FDA is challenged to keep up with emerging technologies. Maintaining a dialogue with the FDA throughout the product development process is a critical part of the regulatory planning for new IVDs. The example of Intergenetics (Box 5.7) shows the impact that regulatory changes can have on new product development in this area.

5.6.1 In vitro devices – regulatory clearance or approval steps to market

In summary, IVD products that are exempt from 510(k) or PMA processes must then go through CLIA categorization, and other IVDs that are not exempt must go through the CLIA categorization in addition to the 510(k) or PMA reviews (see Fugure 5.9).

Step 1: Classify the IVD – Class I, II, or III. [21CFR862/864/866] (see website in Section 5.5.2) provides a list of approved and classified IVDs and is a good starting point to identify possible classification of the planned product and identifying predicates (see Section 5.6.4).

Step 2: Determine path to clearance or approval – 510(k), PMA, or exempt (or analyte specific reagent, see Section 5.5.3 for more detail).

Step 3: After approval, special labeling requirements will apply. The IVD test will be categorized in the CLIA process based on complexity of the test and this will dictate the laboratories to which the test can be sold and where it can be performed.

Historically, there are two regulatory pathways for bringing diagnostic tests to market; one through CLIA regulation of laboratory developed tests and another through FDA review (PMA or 510(k) clearance) of diagnostic kits for sale to third-party labs. The FDA has historically exempted CLIA approved laboratories and laboratory-developed-tests performed under CLIA from FDA controls or review processes (see Section 5.6.4 for further details). Thousands of routine laboratory

---

Box 5.7 Intergenetics and a delayed launch

Adapted from a story reported in The Oklahoman, *October 5, 2006, by Jim Stafford*

Intergenetics, a diagnostics company based in Oklahoma, had shown that its genetic test could assess a woman's risk of getting breast cancer by analyzing DNA signatures from cells obtained in mouthwash samples. It had developed this test over 13 years and had carried out studies on over 8000 women to prove that it worked. A few weeks before the product was scheduled to launch at a large number of breast cancer centers nationwide, a new guidance document for such multivariate tests was issued by the FDA. This document essentially raised the bar for multivariate genetic tests, requiring the test to go through PMA approval process.

The summary of the FDA guidance document released Sept 7, 2006 reads:

The FDA believes that in vitro diagnostic multivariate index assays (IVDMIAs) do not fall within the scope of laboratory-developed tests over which the Agency has generally exercised enforcement discretion. The FDA believes that IVDMIAs must meet pre- and post-market device requirements under the Act and FDA regulations, including pre-market review requirements in the case of Class II and III devices IVDMIAs to assure the public that these tests are safe and effective.

Intergenetics had to postpone the commercial launch, raise more venture capital and put a PMA package together. The company filed an IDE and was able to gain some revenues from launching the test on a limited basis in seven certified labs nationwide that were able to fulfill the CLIA requirements for the (now deemed to be) higher complexity test. This incident highlights the need to keep in touch with the FDA throughout the development process, to make sure that any new regulations or guidances are known to the company in advance.

---

tests that are used in clinical practice are currently exempt from FDA review. See Section 5.6.3 for more details.

Note: Almost all *molecular diagnostic testing* (also referred to as nucleic acid tests (NATs) or genetic testing) today is CLIA-regulated and is currently exempt from FDA review. For example, out of the almost 1000 genetic tests on the market only a handful (five) have gone through FDA approval. Cystic fibrosis testing, HIV genotyping, and phenotyping are examples of commonly performed CLIA laboratory-developed tests. The FDA is now considering regulation of a certain subset of laboratory developed tests called IVDMIAs (in vitro diagnostic multivariate index assays) but has indicated that they have no intention of regulating all laboratory-developed tests.

5.6.2   Pre-clinical and clinical considerations for in vitro devices

The FDA review of a 510(k) of an IVD is based on the evaluation of the analytical performance characteristics of the new device compared with the predicate, including:

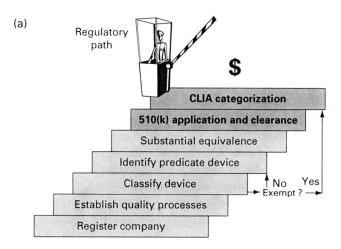

(b) FDA regulatory clearance class I/II diagnostic device
      (6–9 months)

      – Register company as medical device manufacturer with FDA
      – Establish quality process – design, packaging, labeling, and
        manufacturing
      – Classify device-Class I exempt, Class I, or Class II for some
        tests. If exempt, apply directiy for "CLIA categorization only"
      – Identify predicate devices for application
      – Establish substantial equivalence with approved tests
      – Pre-market notification (510(k) submission); CLIA
        categorization request
      – Post-marketing reporting

Figure 5.9   Regulatory path to market for a medical diagnostic device. (a) schematic (b) description of
                 regulatory path steps towards diagnostic approval.

- The bias or inaccuracy (accuracy) of the new device,
- The imprecision (or precision) of the new device, and
- The analytical specificity and sensitivity.

Therefore, pre-clinical studies must offer valid data to satisfy the reviewer in these areas.

The types of studies required to demonstrate *substantial equivalence* include the following:

- In the majority of cases, analytical studies using clinical samples (sometimes supplemented by carefully selected artificial samples) will suffice.
- For some IVDs, the link between analytical performance and clinical performance is not well defined. In these circumstances, clinical information may be required.
- The FDA rarely requires prospective clinical studies for IVDs (see exception with recent guidance in Box 5.7), but regularly requests clinical samples with sufficient laboratory or clinical characterization to allow an assessment of the clinical validity of a new device. This is usually expressed in terms of clinical sensitivity and clinical specificity.

5.6.3   Clinical Laboratory Improvement Amendments program

Congress passed the Clinical Laboratory Improvement Amendments (CLIA) in 1988 establishing quality standards for all laboratory testing after inaccurate results on Pap smear tests led to questions on how labs functioned and what quality control procedures existed. The CLIA program was put in place to ensure the accuracy, reliability, and timeliness of patient test results, regardless of where the test was performed. Some 12 000 labs (of some 200 000 registered labs) were in the program in 1988, and over 170 000 labs were regulated as of 2002 under this program. The CLIA require that clinical laboratories obtain a certificate from the Secretary of Health and Human Services before accepting materials derived from the human body for laboratory tests (under 42 USC § 263a(b)).

The Centers for Medicare and Medicaid Services (CMS) (formerly the Health Care Financing Administration) assume primary responsibility for financial management operations of the CLIA program, which is self-funded by user fees from regulated labs. The CMS thus pays the FDA for CLIA categorization of commercially marketed tests. This task is regulated by the CDRH and CBER divisions at the FDA, and the FDA also has an ongoing partnership with the Centers for Disease Control (CDC) in this program. The CDC was in charge of categorizing tests before 2000. An example of the throughput is that 3642 tests were categorized by the FDA in the 28 month period from Jan 2000 to Apr 2002.

The FDA CLIA program assigns commercially marketed in vitro diagnostic test systems to one of three CLIA regulatory categories based on their potential risk to public health: waived, moderate complexity, or high complexity. Laboratories performing moderate-complexity or high-complexity testing, or both, must meet requirements for proficiency testing, patient test management, quality control, quality assurance, and personnel.

5.6.4   Analyte-specific reagents or "home-brew" tests

In the past, the FDA was not actively involved in regulation of in-house (so-called "home-brew") tests or in regulation of the building blocks sold and used to create these tests. In 1998, FDA classified the building blocks of in-house tests as analyte-specific reagents (ASRs) and began to regulate them, but still puts very few controls on most ASRs.

From the FDA website: "ASRs are defined as 'antibodies, both polyclonal and monoclonal, specific receptor proteins, ligands, nucleic acid sequences, and similar reagents which, through specific binding or chemical reaction with substances in a specimen, are intended for use in a diagnostic application for identification and quantification of an individual chemical substance or ligand in biological specimens.' 21 CFR 864.4020(a). Most molecular diagnostic tests or nucleic acid tests (NATs) or genetic tests fall under the description of ASRs and are restricted devices. Among the restrictions on ASRs is a requirement that advertizing and promotional materials for

---

Box 5.8 Example of a warning letter by FDA on incorrect sale of ASRs
by a company

Excerpt of letter taken from the FDA website; identifying names are omitted here.

August 26, 2005

    Dear Dr. [ ]

The Office of In Vitro Diagnostic Devices (OIVD) has reviewed information on your [ ]^{TM} Brand Internet website ... Diagnostics that are marketed as analyte-specific reagents (ASRs).

    Our review indicates that each of these products is a device under section 201(h) of the Food, Drug, and Cosmetic Act (FDCA or Act), 21 USC 321(h), because it is intended for use in the diagnosis of a disease or other condition, or in the cure, treatment, prevention, or mitigation of disease.

    According to your instructions for use/methods for use, each of the gel-based [ ] genetic assays is intended for "in vitro diagnostic use" to detect various human genetic mutations. In addition, a press release issued by [ ] on March 17, 2005 claimed that, "the [ ]^{TM} family of kits for in vitro diagnostic use provide laboratories simple and cost-effective assays for use in genetic screening programs. Industry-leading [ ]^{TM} kits are available for the genetic analysis of human diseases such as cystic fibrosis and cardiovascular disease..." ...

    ... Based on information on your website, these devices do not adhere to the restrictions on the sale, distribution, and use of ASRs. Your website makes specific analytical and performance claims, such as that your devices can detect multiple mutations per device and screen for particular diseases. Statements on your website describing your devices indicate that they are intended for the detection of mutations related to a clinical diagnosis of, for example, ... In addition, the instructions/methods for use supplied for your assays provide detailed procedures (along with directions and guidelines for the interpretation of results) that are unique for your assays and that constitute analytical and performance claims ...

    A review of our records shows no clearance or approval for your gel-based [ ] genetic assays ... These devices are therefore adulterated under section 501(f)(1)(B) ...

    ... You should take prompt action to correct these violations. Failure to correct these violations promptly may result in regulatory action being initiated by the FDA without further notice. These actions include, but are not limited to, seizure, injunction, and civil money penalties. Also, Federal agencies are informed about the warning letters we issue, such as this one, so that they may consider this information when awarding government contracts ...

    Please notify this office in writing, within fifteen (15) working days of receipt of this letter, of the specific steps you have taken to correct the noted violations, including an explanation of each step being taken to prevent the recurrence of similar violations ...

ASRs may not 'make any statements regarding analytical and clinical performance.' 21 CFR 809.30(d)(4)." See Box 5.8 for an example of this restriction.

In simple terms, an analyte-specific reagent (ASR) is the active ingredient of an in-house test. Most ASRs are classified as Class I devices, exempt from the pre-market notification process. Thus, ASRs represent a lucrative market opportunity as the product development is relatively short and the product can readily be marketed by meeting the low-burden requirements described below. However, these are rapidly developed tests that may not have adequate levels of clinical validation or outcome data that would be required to establish adequate levels of reimbursement (see Chapter 7 for detailed discussion).

Analyte-specific reagents are used in conjunction with other general purpose reagents and general purpose instruments by a laboratory to set up an in-house ("home-brew") test or laboratory testing service. While specimens can travel to the lab setting up this service, the test itself is not marketed outside of the single lab setting up this service. Analyte-specific reagents must have clear activity as the active ingredients of an in-house test but should be provided without instructions for use or performance characteristics. It is the responsibility of the laboratory using the ASR to develop a recipe for the test at hand and to take responsibility for establishing and maintaining performance.

Both the manufacturers of ASRs and the laboratories using them are subject to incremental regulation with controls (based on classification as Class I/II/III ASRs) to:

(1) Assure the quality of the materials being used to create these tests (Quality System Regulation 21CFR820 applies).
(2) Assure that laboratories preparing these tests were able to establish and maintain performance and understood their responsibility for accomplishing this (test results using Class I ASRs must be labeled as not cleared or approved by FDA).
(3) Provide appropriate labeling so that healthcare users would understand how these tests were being validated. (As per 21 CFR 809.10(e)(1)(x): "Analyte specific reagent. Analytical and performance characteristics are not established.")

The manufacturer of an ASR has to register and list their establishment with the FDA and can only sell the ASR to:

(1) In vitro diagnostic manufacturers,
(2) Clinical laboratories qualified to perform high complexity testing, as regulated under the CLIA,
(3) Organizations that use the reagents to make tests for purposes other than providing diagnostic information to patients and practitioners, e.g., forensic, academic, research, and other non-clinical laboratories.

Additional guidance released in 2006, clarifies that the following practices are inconsistent with the marketing of an ASR:

• Combining, or promoting for use, a single ASR with another product such as other ASRs, general purpose reagents, controls, laboratory equipment, software, etc. (see Box 5.8),
• Promoting an ASR with specific analytical or clinical performance claims, instructions for use in a particular test, or instructions for validation of a specific test using the ASR.

Specific ASRs involved in blood screening are classified as Class III, or, in selected cases, Class II devices, and require pre-market approval. Analyte-specific reagents used to diagnose life-threatening contagious diseases with high public health impact are also classified as Class III products. Examples of these include tests for HIV and tuberculosis. Manufacturers and healthcare facilities must report deaths and serious injuries that an ASR has or may have caused or contributed to in accordance with 21 CFR Part 803.

5.7 Emerging regulatory guidelines for co-development of pharmacogenomic diagnostic tests and drugs

The difference between pharmacogenetic (specific DNA sequence comparison studies) testing and standard genetic testing is described in a FDA guidance document released in 2006 (www.fda.gov/cdrh/oivd/guidance/1549.html):

Pharmacogenetic tests for clinical use ... aid in selection of certain therapeutics. When sufficient clinical information is available they may also aid in dosage selection of the therapeutic. Therefore, a pharmacogenetic test target population will typically be composed of candidates for a particular therapeutic. Target populations of genetic tests, on the other hand, will usually be composed of those who are suspected of having, or are at risk of developing, a particular disease or condition.

Additionally, pharmacogenomic (PGx) tests compare inter-individual differences in whole genome patterns (SNPs, mutations, etc.), differentiating this term in practice from the pharmacogenetic tests, which typically test specific DNA sequences.

According to the FDA: "The promise of pharmacogenomics lies in its potential to help identify sources of inter-individual variability in drug response (both effectiveness and toxicity); this information will make it possible to individualize therapy with the intent of maximizing effectiveness and minimizing risk. However, the field of pharmacogenomics is currently in early developmental stages, and such promise has not yet been realized."

The area of pharmacogenomic (PGx) testing of patients to help select more responsive groups for clinical trials or as a screening tool for identifying and selecting patients for prescription of a drug is of great interest in the future area of personalized medicine. A PGx test could be used to identify the population most likely to respond to the drug, while another PGx test can help screen out people that are likely to have toxic reactions to the drug; both tests helping to reduce dramatically the number of subjects required for the clinical studies. An example would be a PGx test that identifies people with a rare mutation of a liver enzyme that can slow down the breakdown and hence the clearance of a drug, causing it to remain in the body much longer at higher concentrations, leading to more toxic effects.

There are several business and regulatory issues that make the development of pharmacogenomics-based "personalized" medicines challenging: if the patient population is limited to those identified by the pharmacogenomics tests, will the current pressure on drug pricing make it possible to develop a profitable business in such personalized medicines that only address a small market? How will the use of pharmacogenomic testing (used to help screen study subjects and improve the rates of success) in clinical trials be regulated by the FDA? Although the use of pharmacogenomics is potentially beneficial to developers who could see reduced costs of development for both drug and diagnostic, due to smaller and faster clinical studies, there is uncertainty on how the data will impact the final indication. Will the FDA use this data to limit the final label and indication and make the market so small that it is economically not viable or attractive for the developer? These uncertainties will need to be addressed through adaptive business models and through extensive dialogue with the regulatory and reimbursement agencies.

To clarify the process of developing a pharmacogenomics based test that is tied to drug therapy, the FDA published a suggested co-development path through the regulatory pathway, as shown in Figure 5.10. This schematic (and the associated Figure 4.13) were intended to stimulate discussion with industry as final guidance and regulatory pathways for this co-development have not been clarified (as of November 2006). Figure 5.10 indicates the various regulatory actions and interactions with the FDA that will take place for a drug–diagnostic combination, referenced against similar actions for drug development. While an IND is filed for the drug development, an IDE must be filed simultaneously for the diagnostic–device development process. A PMA or 510(k) will be filed

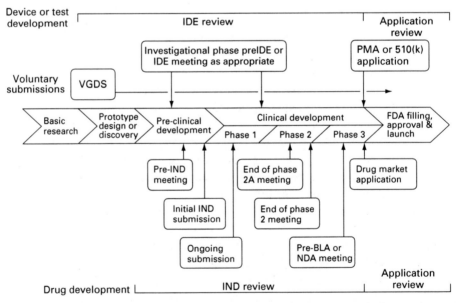

Figure 5.10   Regulatory pathway and timings proposed for co-development of personalized medicines, where a diagnostic test is required before a drug prescription is written. The schematic depicts parallel regulatory actions in submissions, meetings and review towards final approval of co-developed drugs and diagnostics. From a white paper titled *Drug-Diagnostic Co-development Concept Paper*, published by the Department of Health and Human Services (HHS), Food and Drug Administration (FDA), April 2005.

concurrently with the NDA/BLA for the drug and the co-approved, co-developed drug and diagnostic will be launched with co-dependent marketing for concurrent use of both. The timings of meetings with the FDA and review periods are shown in Figure 5.10 for both tracks of development. This proposed conceptual pathway might work once the developers understand better what to expect from the FDA and learn how to adapt their business models towards this type of co-development of two different but synergistic products.

5.8   Combination products, genetic material, and tissues

A combination product includes (Definition from 21 CFR Part 3, Subpart A, Section 3.2 (e)):

- A product comprising two or more regulated components, i.e.; drug and device; biologic and device; drug and biologic; or drug, device and biologic; that are physically, chemically, or otherwise combined or mixed and produced as a single entity;
- Two or more separate products packaged together in a single package or as a unit and comprised of drug and device products, device and biological products, or biological and drug products;
- A drug, device, or biological product packaged separately that according to its investigational plan or proposed labeling is intended for use only with an approved individually specified drug, device, or biological product, where both are required to achieve the intended use, indication, or effect, and where upon approval of the proposed product the labeling of the approved product would need to be changed, e.g., to reflect a change in intended use, dosage form, strength, route of administration, or significant change in dose; or
- Any investigational drug, device, or biological product packaged separately that according to its proposed labeling is for use only with another individually specified investigational drug, device, or biological product, where both are required to achieve the intended use, indication, or effect."

The Office of Combination Products was created in 2002 to help guide manufacturers who are increasingly designing and developing innovative medical products such as drug–device, drug–biologic, and device–biologic combinations that cross over historical FDA review divisions (CDER/CDRH). While this office has broad regulatory responsibilities for these products, primary regulatory responsibilities for, and oversight of, specific combination products remain in one of three product centers – the CDER, the CBER or the CDRH – to which they are assigned.

The Office of Combination Products (OCP) (as described on the FDA website www.fda.gov/oc/combination/faqs.html):

- Does not review marketing applications for combination products,
- Assigns a lead center (CBER, CDER, or CDRH) that will have primary jurisdiction for the pre-market review and regulation of a combination or single-entity product,

- Develops policy for combination product regulation,
- Is also responsible for ensuring timely and effective pre-market review of combination products by overseeing the timeliness of and coordinating reviews involving more than one agency center,
- Ensures consistency and appropriateness of post-market regulation of combination products,
- Is available as a resource to industry and agency reviewers to help facilitate the review process, to help clarify or develop appropriate regulatory pathways, or to provide any other assistance as appropriate to OCP's mission.

When a product submission is made to the OCP, a determination is made for assignment to the lead reviewing agency (CBER, CDER, or CDRH), based partly on the primary mode of action of the combination product. A guidance document on how the FDA and OCP regulate combination products and make designation or primary mode of action decisions was posted on the FDA website in September 2006 (www.fda.gov/oc/combination/innovative.html).

Once a lead review agency is appointed, the OCP continues to organize consultative or collaborative reviews. The process for review of the combination product by the OCP is described on the FDA website (www.fda.gov/oc/combination/faqs.html) and excerpts are reproduced below:

What is the difference between consultative and collaborative reviews of combination products?

When combination products are assigned to a lead center, that center may consult or collaborate with another center as part of the review process. The FDA has a standard operating procedure (SOP) for the intercenter consultative and collaborative review process. The SOP includes the definitions of consultative and collaborative reviews, and sets out the procedures, policies, and processes for Agency staff to use when requesting, receiving, handling, processing, and tracking formal consultative and collaborative reviews of combination products, devices, drugs, and biological products. The SOP is posted at www.fda.gov/oc/combination/consultative.html.

A consultative review, which is the most frequent process used for the review of combination products by a center other than the lead center, is a review activity in which a reviewer in one center requests advice from a reviewer in another center on a specific question or issue raised in the review of a submission. The consultative review is used to assist the requesting reviewer in making appropriate regulatory or scientific decisions.

In contrast, a collaborative review is a review activity in which reviewers in two or more centers have primary review responsibilities, generally for a defined portion of a submission. Regulatory and scientific decisions will be made by the management of each center for that portion of the review assigned to it, including the decision to approve or disapprove the product.

Some recent examples of approved combination products are:

- Bioresorbable hemostat that contains collagen and thrombin,
- Transdermal patch containing drug for ADHD,
- Dental bone grafting material with growth factor,
- Paclitaxel-eluting coronary stent system,
- Dermagraft human fibroblast-derived dermal substitute.

5.8.1 Cellular, tissue, and gene therapies

The Office of Cellular, Tissue, and Gene Therapies was formed in 2002 in CBER with the increase in biological tissue therapeutics, to provide consistent review and develop expertise in this area. This office works with the Office of Combination products. The mission of this office is to regulate, review, and develop policy and education on:

- Tissues,
- Cellular and tissue-based products,
- Gene therapies,
- Xenotransplantation,
- Combination products containing living cells or tissues,
- Unique assisted reproduction (ooplasm transfer).

Finally, this office is responsible for assuring the safety, identity, purity, and potency of all the products listed above.

Cell, tissue, or gene therapy products do not need pre-market approval if:

- There is minimal manipulation,
- There is homologous use,
- They are not combined with a drug or device,
- They exert no systemic effect, or
- They exert a systemic effect, but they are:
  - Autologous,
  - Allogeneic in a first-degree or second-degree relative,
  - For reproductive use.

However, good tissue practices (guidance published by the Office) must be followed, donor eligibility and screening is required, the establishment must register with the FDA and compliance with the rules will be determined on inspection.

Regulations that apply (with some guidance) are available at www.fda.gov/cber/rules/gtpq&a.htm (21CFR Part 1270 and 1271).

For non-tissue products, IND/BLA or IDE/PMA rules apply. The Office goes out of its way to initiate a dialogue with the sponsor in order to understand the technology fully and give appropriate guidance on a case-by-case basis.

Tissue-engineered products are treated as combination products and guided to their independent reviews in their respective divisions. If the primary mode of action depends on the biologic component, CBER will take the lead, whereas CDRH will take the lead if the mode of action is dependent on the device; and each will consult each other with the Office of Combination Product or Cellular Therapies coordinating these consultations and reviews. Finally, it is possible that completely separate reviews will be required for each component.

In general, combination products usually incorporate novel technologies or use existing technologies in novel ways, which often leads to delays or uncertainty in the FDA review, as the published literature may be sparse or the new area of developing technology is not one that FDA staff scientists are familiar with. This lack of familiarity may result in onerous requirements or guidance statements that require multiple or additional tests. The company scientists, who may be more familiar with the new technology may not have seen these tests as necessary and may need to repeat several levels of pre-clinical studies (e.g., prolonged toxicity testing or additional stability testing) or even clinical studies (e.g., increase patient population size, follow patients longer, or make additional measurements) that the company scientists may have thought unnecessary. Box 5.9 illustrates one such story of a combination product that ran into delays because of the uncertainty with the FDA reviews and other issues that eventually caused the company to fail. The case study in Box 5.9 indicates that a company with novel products not only has to work very aggressively in product and technology development, but must work equally diligently on education and passage of regulatory and reimbursement issues.

Box 5.9 FDA issues felled advanced tissue sciences: how a biotech with products on the market still failed

By Andy Stone, June 1, 2003
(*reproduced here with permission from* Genetic Engineering News)

The wound repair industry is littered with defunct, bankrupt companies. Advanced Tissue Sciences (ATS; La Jolla, CA) is but one of the latest victims, a company with good marketed products that nonetheless failed, owing to a complex array of forces, ranging from the difficulties in getting FDA approvals to the vagaries of the investing public.

The company was based on an innovative technology that enabled the 3-D ex vivo growth of human cells. This technology would eventually give rise to products aimed at the treatment of moderate to severe burns and coverings for diabetic foot ulcers, a market with a potential of about half a million users annually in the USA, and other products related to the basic 3-D matrix.

But ATS lost $300 million over its nearly 15-year history, which came to an end with Chapter 11 bankruptcy and liquidation, beginning in the fall of 2002.

Promising beginnings

The beginnings of ATS, originally named Marrow Tech, seemed promising enough. The company raised its first round of investment through a $5-million IPO in 1988. Marrow Tech was formed on the heels of early biotechnology success stories, such as Amgen, Genentech, and Genzyme, and came to life in an environment in which grants and other forms of early funding were all but non-existent but where public markets were eager to jump on the biotech bandwagon.

The original business plan of Marrow Tech was for the storage, cryopreservation, and expansion of a patient's own marrow. The benefit was that a small

Box 5.9 (cont.)

amount of that marrow could be used, instead of the painful normal removal involving 50–100 punch samples from the iliac crest.

It was then shown that the administration of growth factors, such as EPO and SCP from Amgen and Genetics Institute in the late 1980s, could release stem cells into the peripheral circulation, where they could be collected through a simple transfusion and separation process.

As a result, Marrow Tech, based on its core tissue-culturing technology, altered its focus to the development of human skin substitutes and changed its name. Advanced Tissue Sciences' first product appeared in October of 1990. Skin2 was a full-thickness, human-derived skin that was used to test consumer products, replacing, for example, rabbit-eye and skin tests and allowing companies that produced cosmetics and consumer products to avoid some ethical dilemmas.

Regulatory difficulties

The stage was set, though, for ATS' first run-in with the FDA, in a pattern that would repeat itself over the course of the company's history, with disastrous consequences.

"Skin2 was accepted and well published, but the FDA didn't move quickly to approve the product," says Gail Naughton, former vice chair of ATS and current dean of San Diego State University's business school. As a result, ATS had to abandon Skin2. "The company couldn't afford to work on therapeutic products and move Skin2 through the approval process at the same time," Naughton explains.

Despite this early setback, the company labored on and, by 1996, had entered a joint venture with medical device leader Smith and Nephew (Andover, MA) for the development of wound-repair products based on ATS' tissue-repair technology.

The first product, Dermagraft, comprised a 3-D matrix of living human cells that was initially intended as a treatment for medium-thickness to full-thickness burns. "It turned out that healing took longer with Dermagraft than with alternatives, such as cadaver skin," Naughton says.

The company followed up with a new product, Transcyte, which would be manufactured at Dermaquip, the joint venture GMP-manufacturing facility established by the two companies for the manufacture of tissue-engineering products. Transcyte received FDA approval in 1997 as a covering for medium-thickness to full-thickness burns.

The target market for Transcyte was estimated at 40 000 burn victims annually; the actual market potential may have been much lower. "The burn market is not terribly large, with between 5000 and 15 000 burns per year that require skin grafting," says Michael Lysaght, director of Brown University's Center for Biomedical Engineering.

Despite its effectiveness, Transcyte was not an immediate market success, and a confluence of factors, including the product's high price and slow adoption rate, denied ATS revenues needed to fund further company and product development.

Box 5.9 (cont.)

Marketing disappointment

"Transcyte works and is an excellent product that reduces pain and scarring," states Abe Wischnia, former head of investor relations at ATS, "but there were several factors militating against it in the marketplace. The first was cost, and Transcyte was competing with much less expensive gauze bandages, as well as cadaver skin." The price of Transcyte was $1350 for two 5″-by-7½″ pieces of product, about three times the cost of cadaver skin and much more expensive than traditionally used gauze with an antimicrobial agent.

Another important factor was the willingness of doctors to try new technologies. "Smith and Nephew had to call on doctors for a year at the Children's National Burn Center in Washington before the doctors would listen to them," Wischnia reports.

In contrast to the cardiovascular market, adds Naughton, "Wound care in general is very conservative, and doctors don't jump easily to new products." The combination of a lack of innovation and few new revolutionary products severely hampered adoption, and, with sales well below projections, put the company into tough financial straights.

As ATS turned to the development of other products, notably the development of Dermagraft for a much larger diabetic foot ulcer market, the company was forced to return to public markets to fund itself. By the time the company filed for bankruptcy in the fall of 2002, Naughton explains, "We had gone to the public markets at least five times, with over 70 million shares and tremendous dilution."

The fatal blow that befell ATS occurred in 1998, when the company had completed clinical trials for Dermagraft for the treatment of diabetic foot ulcers. In January 1998, an FDA PMA panel approved Dermagraft, by eight to one, and momentarily it looked as though the product would soon go to market.

Then, in an unexpected and eventually disastrous turn of events, the FDA refused approval and demanded an additional clinical trial, to involve 350 patients. This took an additional three and one-half years before approval was finally granted in the fall of 2001. In the meantime, the company continued to burn money at a rate of up to $3 million per month, while gaining disappointing revenues from Transcyte and further diluting its ownership.

Retrospective analysis rejected

"The FDA has been consistent in not allowing a retrospective analysis of a subset of data as the basis for approval," Wischnia notes. What ATS did to perform the additional clinical trials of Dermagraft was, "analyze its clinical data retrospectively, and what the company realized was that Dermagraft had higher viability after ATS had changed to a more effective cryopreservation process, enhancing the bioactivity of the product with a higher percentage of living cells engaging the wound bed, thus enhancing the product's effectiveness."

Box 5.9 (cont.)

"Advanced Tissue Sciences decided to look only at the patients treated after the change in the cryopreservation process," Wischnia said, "and these healing results were what was submitted to the FDA. The FDA said that it couldn't approve retrospectively with only a subset." The result was the delay of approval and huge expenses for ATS, as well as lost revenue.

In the meantime, other market forces had come into play that would increase the difficulty ATS faced in gaining money through capital markets. Another tissue-engineering company, Organogenesis (Canton, MA), had come to the market with a diabetic foot ulcer product, Apligraf, which had several problems, including a short shelf life and the need for patient immobilization, which slowed acceptance.

Organogenesis, which eventually filed for bankruptcy, failed to meet its financial targets. "Many felt that tissue engineering had become a poor investment prospect," Wischnia says. "The companies had made assumptions that everyone with diabetic foot ulcers would use the product and this showed up in their projections, he notes. "The experience colored the view of the investment community, which ATS similarly had to overcome."

Advanced Tissue Sciences finally got FDA approval for Dermagraft at the end of September 2001, and the product received a reimbursement code from Medicare in March of 2002. But sales didn't grow according to forecast, partially because Dermagraft still needed approval from regional care intermediaries for reimbursement.

Smith and Nephew, which handled the marketing for Dermagraft, had only attained coverage for the product in about half of the United States when ATS finally filed a voluntary petition for reorganization under the Chapter 11 bankruptcy code in October of 2002. During the final year of operations, the company's stock plunged from over $4 per share to the $1 range as the public markets took an increasingly sour view on investing in tissue engineering.

On November 13, 2002, ATS decided to undertake an orderly liquidation of assets, a decision based on the difficulty it foresaw in raising additional money to sustain operations, including the $25 million that it would need to match funds from Smith and Nephew for continued operation of the Dermaquip joint venture.

On the eve of the declaration of bankruptcy, the market capitalization of ATS hovered around $14 million, down from approximately half a billion dollars at the peak of expectation in 1996. Since the declaration of bankruptcy, Smith and Nephew purchased ATS' half of the Derma-quip joint venture at a fire sale price of $10 million, while offering employment to about 110 of ATS' 220 employees . . .

By-product Submitted to FDA

As a by-product of the Dermaquip joint venture, ATS developed additional products toward the end of its activities. Dermaquip produced human collagen that was sold to Inamed (Santa Barbara), a marketer of products for esthetic

---

Box 5.9 (cont.)

applications. The product was an injectable collagen used to hide wrinkles and was an alternative to bovine-derived products on the market.

In early 2001, the FDA surprised ATS by requiring skin allergy testing before granting approval for the product. One year and a 400-patient skin trial later, marketing approval was granted, but again, regulatory issues had cost the company badly needed revenues.

Steep learning curve

Overall, it was the steep learning curve in regulatory and reimbursement matters that got the best of ATS. "The company needed to coordinate its regulatory and reimbursement activities," so that both would be optimized and the least amount of time would be lost in getting the products to market, Naughton observes.

5.9   Summary

Devices, drugs, and diagnostics have two general regulatory paths: innovative, novel products (first time in human beings) have a longer regulatory path requiring at least two pivotal clinical trials and more time and money than the process for products (generic drugs, devices with predicates) which are similar to other marketed products. These "similar" products have a shorter, less expensive regulatory path, where they have to show some form of equivalence to the products to which they are most similar. Low-risk or well established products are exempt or waived from FDA reviews, but still have to adhere to some regulations. These products are OTC drugs, exempt devices, and most ASR diagnostics products. The three main divisions in the FDA (CBER, CDER, and CDRH) review market applications and interact with manufacturers in a process that is driven by scientific principles. The goal of the FDA is to ensure the safety of the health of the US public by getting safe and effective products to markets.

Exercises

Assuming a novel product is being developed:

5.1 Select the indication for your product and state the desired product label claims.

5.2 Identify and describe the clinical endpoints for the product clinical trials.

5.3 If your product is a drug, then describe points of contact with the FDA, IRB, and IACUC and specific topics for emphasis and attention in these interactions and submissions.

5.4 If your product is a device, then discuss the rationale for classification and the pathway for marketing approval.

> 5.5 Feedback regulatory pathway information and rethink your product development.
>
> 5.6 Generate a time line showing potential interactions (meetings and submissions) with the FDA mapped onto the product development stages.
>
> 5.7 What data will you submit to the FDA at those interaction points? Describe key data that will verify the mode of action and support the indication for the product, for each submission. Identify the time line for these submissions and review processes.

References and additional reading

Beck, J. M. and Vale, A. *Drug and Medical Device Product Liability Deskbook*, Law Journal Press, 2004.

Coenraads, J., Van Broekhoren, B., Hartmann, S., Tander, H., and, Veldkamp, M. *The CE Mark: Understanding the Medical Device Directive*, Paton Press, ringbound edn., 1997.

Harnack, G. *Mastering and Managing the FDA Maze: Medical Device Overview: A Training and Management Desk Reference for Manufacturers Regulated by the Food and Drug Administration*, ASQ Quality Press, 1999.

Licinio, J. (ed.). *The Pharmacogenomics Journal*, Nature Publishing Group.

Pines, W. L. (ed.). *How to Work With the FDA*, Food and Drug Law Institute, 2nd edn., 2003.

Pisano, D. and Mantus, D. (eds.). *FDA Regulatory Affairs: A Guide for Prescription Drugs, Medical Devices and Biologics*, CRC Press, 2004.

Trautman, K. A. (compiler). *The FDA and Worldwide Quality System Requirements Guidebook for Medical Devices*, ASQ Quality Press, 1996.

Useful websites

www.fda.gov/cdrh/qsr/contnt.html – *Quality systems regulations for devices*
www.raps.org – *Regulatory Affairs Professionals Society of America*

Foreign regulatory agency websites

www.pharmweb.net/pwmirror/pwk/pharmwebk.html – *A list of foreign regulatory bodies and links to their websites*
www.mhra.gov.uk/ – *UK: MHRA (Medicines and Healthcare products Regulatory Agency, UK)*
www.emea.europa.eu/ – *EMEA: The European Medicines Agency*
www.tga.gov.au/ – *Australia: Therapeutics Goods Administration*
www.hc-sc.gc.ca/index_e.html – *Health Canada*
www.mhlw.go.jp/english/index.html – *Japan: Ministry of Health and Welfare*

6   Manufacturing

Plan	Position	Patent	Product	Pass!	Production	Profits
Industry context	Market research	Intellectual property rights	New product development (NPD)	Regulatory plan	Manufacture	Reimbursement

Roadmap of a product commercialization plan. Stage 6

Learning points

- How are products transferred into commercial manufacturing operations successfully?
- When to begin commercial manufacturing planning.
- What determines the commercial scale of manufacturing?
- How is the cost of goods (or the cost of the final product) estimated?
- What controls and systems are needed to comply with regulatory oversight of manufacturing processes?
- What standards apply to manufacturing processes?
- What are the timing and quantity requirements for scale-up of production for drugs, devices and diagnostics?
- What key issues typically arise in the production or scale-up processes for biological or synthetic drugs?
- How does "Design for Manufacturability and Assembly" prepare for device manufacture?

6.1   Introduction

The transition from the new product development environment, of early product versioning and animal testing, to manufacturing environment "operations" is a significant one for a project team. It means that the results to date have shown significant reduction in technology risk and that the product has demonstrated feasibility, safety, and efficacy in living systems.

6.2 Technology transfer to manufacturing operations (drugs, devices, and diagnostics)

Technology transfer is the systematic means of conveying knowledge (product, process, equipment, and method), documentation, and skills between two parties. In manufacturing companies, the term "technology transfer" covers the process of converting small-scale R&D processes or early design and laboratory prototypes to larger-scale bulk manufacturing processes, and specifically involves the transfer of the product and production know-how from the R&D group to the commercial operations group ("Operations"). It is important to note that in the context of intellectual property transactions and in the general business environment of new ventures, "technology transfer" also refers to the process of licensing intellectual property and bringing patented technology in from the university labs to a commercial product development environment.

In scaling up from R&D synthesis processes or from laboratory prototypes, the information that was developed in R&D may not be relevant in this new, larger scale environment, which is concerned about reproducibility and reduction of defects per thousand or million products made, while adhering to the highest degree of regulatory compliance and accountability in highly documented processes. Thus, Operations organizations value compliance, reliability, predictability, and efficiency. In contrast, R&D organizations value scientific innovation, creativity, flexibility, and development speed. There is not only a potential culture-clash in communication between R&D and Operations but also some ignorance about the parameters and boundaries within which manufacturing Operations organizations must operate. These differences have, historically, caused great trouble in the technology transfer process.

Why do "technology transfers" frequently fail?

- "Over the fence" transfer (sharp transfers),
- Lack of respect,
- Lack of engagement of either party,
- Lack of ownership following transfer,
- "Not invented here" syndrome,
- Lack of common goal,
- Too many transfers,
- Incomplete, inadequate documentation.

Three main models of technology transfer are: (1) push (let R&D drive the transfer); (2) pull (let commercial operations participate and share "ownership" early in the product development process); and (3) personnel transfer. Personnel transfers from R&D to Operations are usually the most successful. However, the R&D employees transferred to operations may suffer as their values may be better suited to the R&D organization. Some organizations have adopted a pull model where R&D and Operations co-develop the manufacturing process and product in the final stages. This integrated model embeds Operations technical functions into the product development (NPD) process to learn about integrating the manufacturing technology and the product. The pull model also enables R&D to take the product through approval and Operations successfully to validate and sustain production following launch. Today, thankfully, with integrated, multidisciplinary teams formed early in product development, there is better planning and design for manufacturability than previous historic siloed attitudes of "throw it over the wall to the engineers and let them figure out how to make thousands or millions of products – we're done with our final design and testing and it worked when it left our hands."

6.3   Regulatory compliance in manufacturing

Regulatory oversight and adherence to industry standards are key considerations in the final product development stage of final manufacturing. Most manufacturing sites are visited by the FDA before final approval of a new product (preapproval inspection) and these visits continue post-approval. Most manufacturing companies also seek to bring best practices and efficient, high-quality performance into their organizations through gaining certification under certain standards, such as the International Standards Organization (ISO), which requires a site inspection. These various site inspectors will want to see accurate and detailed record keeping, careful consideration to the maintenance of hygienic or sterile conditions (as appropriate) throughout the process, and most importantly, adherence to ensuring the reproducibility and reliability of the manufacturing process. Compliance with manufacturing regulations and certain standards is, thus, a critical part of getting a safe and effective product through approval to market. The FDA regulations and controls are together referred to as current good manufacturing processes (cGMP).

6.3.1   Current good manufacturing practices

Current good manufacturing practices (cGMP) are defined as "a set of current, scientifically sound methods, practices, or principles that are implemented and documented during product development and production to ensure consistent manufacture of safe, pure, and potent products."

The cGMP regulations are published in the Federal Register in **21 CFR**:

Parts 210 and 211   Drugs,
Part 820   Medical devices,
Part 606   Blood products,
Part 110   Food.

The cGMP regulations:

- Apply to both manufacturing process and facilities,
- Are expected to be in place throughout clinical studies,
- Controls increase as the process progresses to the final commercial stage,

- Include specifically, sterility assurance, and validation
- Include implementation of a quality assurance (QA) or quality control (QC) program,
- Require everyone to document, document, document...

The cGMP controls thus cover the following activities (this is not a comprehensive list):

- Record keeping, documentation,
- Personnel qualifications, training,
- Raw materials selection, purchasing,
- Equipment verification,
- Process validation,
- Specifications and quality control,
- Sanitation, cleanliness,
- Complaint handling.

In particular, over the last few decades, there has been a strong emphasis on establishing quality and design-based systems in pharmaceutical and medical device manufacturing. These quality systems have a bearing on all processes, including management processes. A quality system involves quality control (QC) and quality assurance (QA).

Quality control (QC) usually involves (1) assessing the suitability of incoming components, containers, closures, labeling, in-process materials, and finished products; (2) evaluating the performance of the manufacturing process to ensure adherence to proper specifications and limits; and (3) determining the acceptability of each batch for release. *Quality Assurance* (QA) primarily involves (1) review and approval of all procedures related to production and maintenance; (2) review of associated records; and (3) auditing and performing or evaluating trend analyses.

The cGMP's are constantly being revised to accommodate advances in technology (the discovery of protein A resin for purification of monoclonal antibodies, for example) or to address specific issues that were not know before (e.g., the presence of Hantaviruses in some raw materials used in the manufacturing process). Changes to cGMPs occur through new initiatives from regulatory authorities or from the combined knowledge of the field inspectors who visit each production facility. Their assimilated inspection histories are the basis upon which all facilities are inspected and subsequent changes are recommended.

The CBER and the FDA issued a guidance document, *Guidance for the Industry, Q7A Good Manufacturing Practice Guidance for Active Pharmaceutical Ingredients* in 2001. This guidance document was developed by an expert working group of the International Conference on Harmonization (ICH) of Technical Requirements for the Registration of Pharmaceuticals for Human Use. A final draft of this document is expected to be adopted by the regulatory bodies in the USA, the EU, and Japan. This document will attempt to standardize GMPs across the world.

6.3.2   Validation

Validation is defined as "confirmation by examination and provision of objective evidence that the particular requirements for a specific intended use can be consistently fulfilled (CFR 820.3)" by any process, procedure, equipment, material, activity, or system. Process validation is a part of cGMP and is required in the USA and the EU for a manufacturing license. A validated manufacturing process has a high level of scientific assurance that it will reliably and consistently produce acceptable product. The emphasis on this process (or set of processes, as it can be a multi-stage activity) is a significant part of the activity of synthesizing the product. As an example, the process of cleaning and validating equipment from one batch to the other in biological drug manufacture can sometimes take a few days, and production of one batch can take a similar length of time. The validation process is particularly onerous if a different drug is to be made in the same production facility. Validation in devices includes checking the product characteristics against initial customer and design inputs. Thus "validation" can refer to completely different processes in the diverse context of different types of biomedical technologies.

6.3.3   Drug manufacture regulations – control systems reviewed for compliance

In August 2002, the FDA launched an overhaul of the pharmaceutical GMP regulations with a new focus on integrating quality systems and risk management approaches. This process was called the "Pharmaceutical cGMPs for the 21st Century" Initiative. The goal of this ongoing initiative is to encourage industry to adopt modern and innovative manufacturing technologies. A *Wall Street Journal* article in 2003 (Abboud and Hensley, 2003) reported that the FDA had recorded 354 prescription-drug recalls in 2002, up from 248 in 2001 and 176 in 1998. Most of these recalls were associated with manufacturing-quality issues, indicating the need for improvements and a change in oversight.

Compliance with manufacturing regulations and standards requires that six distinct control processes and systems must be in place at any organization:

(1) Materials system,
(2) Production system,
(3) Packaging and labeling system,
(4) Laboratory systems,
(5) Facilities and equipment system, and
(6) Quality system.

The specific points evaluated by the FDA inspectors for each system are reviewed in excerpts from the FDA Inspectors manual in Appendix 6.1 and makes for informative reading. The six recording and process control systems that are required to demonstrate regulatory compliance are interdependent, with the quality system providing the foundation for other systems within it, as seen in the schematic in Figure 6.1 and as discussed in further detail in Appendix 6.1.

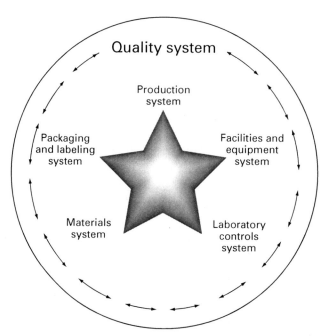

Figure 6.1 The quality system in pharmaceutical GMP controls and systems is the foundation for all other controls. Figure adapted from the FDA document mentioned in Appendix 6.1.

6.3.4 Device and diagnostic manufacture regulations – control systems reviewed for compliance

A quality systems approach to medical device design and manufacture (this also includes diagnostics) was implemented (in 1996) in the Quality System Regulation (21 CFR Part 820) revision to the current good manufacturing practice (cGMP) requirements. The QSR rules for device development (see Section 5.5.6) and the cGMP rules for pharmaceuticals both have a common goal – to ensure that the manufacturer has put a set of reproducible processes in place to make commercial devices, on which people's lives depend, safely and reliably. Documentation, record-keeping and establishment of SOPs are keys to achieving cGMP compliance (described in Box 6.1).

An important component of the revision was the addition of design controls, which have been discussed in Chapters 4 and 5. Design controls are a system of checks and balances that make systematic assessment of the design an integral part of product development.

A Government Accounting Office (GAO) review of medical device recalls during a six-year period in the 1980s found that about 44% of quality problems were attributable to errors or deficiencies in the device design and could have been prevented with proper design controls.[1] Design-related defects have been found

---

[1] US General Accounting Office, *Medical Device Recalls: An Overview and Analysis 1983–1988*, GAO/PEMD-89-15BR, Washington, DC, August 1989.

Box 6.1 Written procedures are essential to compliance with GMP regulations

Contributed by Lawrence Roth, Vice President, Business Development and Operations at Percardia

One central tenet to compliance with GMP regulations is to develop and maintain written procedures. The concept of "document what you do, then do what is documented" is central to the guiding principles of the GMP regulations. Written documentation of the manufacturing process is an integral component of any GMP system. This documentation provides the trained operator with clear instructions on how to perform a process; i.e., the equipment required, the set-up procedures, the step-by-step processing, the components and raw materials to be used, and in-process inspections. This documentation is created during the development of a product and is finalized as part of the device master record (DMR) following design validation prior to transfer to full manufacturing. The objective is to ensure that the product manufactured in volume is equivalent to the product that supported the information submitted to the FDA for approval and that the manufacturer has adequate control over the production to ensure unit-to-unit consistency. Lack of adequately documented written procedures is considered a violation of the GMP regulations.

A search of the CDRH database provides numerous examples of warning letters issued to companies for failure to develop adequate procedures for documenting its manufacturing procedures. A warning letter is issued only for the most serious offenses identified by FDA during a routine inspection of a manufacturer. For example, in September of 2004, Daavlin Distribution Company was issued a warning letter (warning letter CIN-04-22469) for numerous GMP infractions. Daavlin is a leading manufacturer of phototherapy products sold throughout the United States and in over 30 other countries around the world. In addition to offenses related to sale of an unapproved device, the FDA cited the following infractions related to documentation of the manufacturing process:

Failure to maintain device master records (DMRs), as required by 21 CFR 820.181. For example, there are no established and implemented DMRs for any of the medical devices manufactured, which includes the 3 series full body phototherapy device, the Spectra series of phototherapy devices and DermaPal.

Failure to establish and maintain procedures to ensure that the device history records (DHRs) for each batch, lot, or unit are maintained to demonstrate that the device is manufactured in accordance with the DMR and the requirements of this part, as required by 21 CFR 820.184. For example, there are no established and implemented DHRs for any of the medical devices manufactured, which includes the 3 series full body phototherapy device, the Spectra series of phototherapy devices and DermaPal.

Failure to develop, conduct, control, and monitor production processes to ensure that a device conforms to its specifications, as required by 21 CFR 820.70(a). For example, process control procedures for the 3 series full body phototherapy device, the Spectra series of phototherapy devices and DermaPal have not been implemented. Also, the procedures are not signed and approved by management and QA.

> **Box 6.1** (cont.)
>
> Establishing and maintaining written procedures is an important component of systems required for manufacturing a medical device. Failure to comply with the GMP regulations related to manufacturing can have serious effects on the business including loss of goodwill with FDA and customers, loss of sales, and potentially, criminal proceedings.

in such critical products as heart valves, catheters, defibrillators, pacemakers, ventilators, patient chair lifts, and laboratory tests.

As described by the FDA (www.fda.gov/cdrh/devadvice/32.html), "The [Quality System] regulation requires that various specifications and controls be established for devices; that devices be designed under a quality system to meet these specifications; that devices be manufactured under a quality system; that finished devices meet these specifications; that devices be correctly installed, checked, and serviced; that quality data be analyzed to identify and correct quality problems; and that complaints be processed. Thus, the QS regulation helps assure that medical devices are safe and effective for their intended use. The Food and Drug Administration (FDA) monitors device problem data and inspects the operations and records of device developers and manufacturers to determine compliance with the GMP requirements in the QS regulation."

The Quality System regulation can be grouped into seven subsystems and related connected sub-systems (Figure 6.2); however, the following four sub-systems are considered major sub-systems and are the basic foundation of a firm's quality management system: (i) management controls, (ii) design controls, (iii) corrective and preventive actions (CAPA), and (iv) production and process controls (P&PC). The medical device reporting (MDR), corrections and removals, and medical device tracking requirements (where applicable) are satellite systems that are included in the overall CAPA sub-system. The three remaining sub-systems (facilities and equipment controls, materials controls and document, records, and change controls) cut across a firm's quality management system.

Excerpts from the FDA/CDRH's *Quality Systems Inspection Manual* are reproduced in Appendix 6.2 and present an excellent summary of the requirements of various sub-systems needed to establish compliance with GMP regulations.

6.4 Manufacturing standards

6.4.1 What are standards and what is their purpose?

Standards are "a prescribed set of rules, conditions, or requirements concerning: definitions of terms; classification of components; specification of materials,

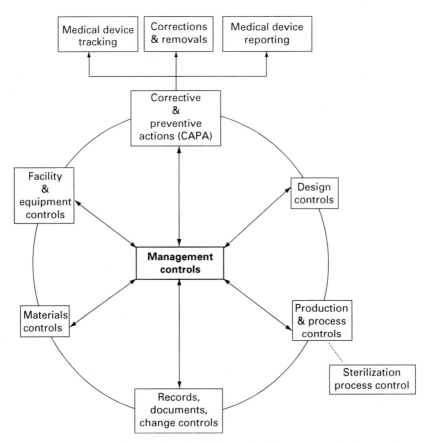

Figure 6.2   Medical device manufacturers have to put several sub-systems and a few satellite systems in place as process controls and documentation controls, to make their facilities and processes GMP compliant. The management controls focus on the quality system which runs through all the main sub-systems shown here.

performance, or operations; delineation of procedures; or measurement of quantity and quality in describing materials, products, systems, services, or practices," (National Standards Policy Advisory Committee; reported on http://ts.nist.gov/ Standards/Conformity/stdpmr.cfm). Standards, if correctly established and tested without bias, are useful tools to communicate between groups and can also be used to set thresholds of acceptance. Standards are important to demonstrate compliance to regulations that reference them and to give a certain comfort to the users who see a certification of having met a recognized standard on the product.

For our purposes, standards can be classified into:

Process standards   These are standards established for validating specific manufacturing processes.

Testing standards   These are methodologies that must be followed to test products or materials – e.g., some standard methods for testing the viscosity of fluids or the compression test for a hip implant are already established by professional societies, and regulatory authorities who have accepted those standards will question the tests if they do not follow the established standard methodologies.

Product or service standards   The product must perform to an established standard, e.g., the purity of a drug compound, the sterility of a device, or the reproducibility of a diagnostic test are also expected performance standards.

6.4.2   Who sets standards?

Various professional bodies in different fields set standards. In the United States alone, approximately 30 000 current voluntary standards have been developed by more than 400 organizations (www.nist.gov). The International Organization for Standardization (ISO) probably produces the largest number of internationally recognized standards. The ISO is a non-governmental organization, and is composed of a network of the national standards institutes of 157 countries, on the basis of one member per country, with a Central Secretariat in Geneva, Switzerland, that coordinates the system. More than 20 000 experts from all over the world participate annually in the development of ISO standards. Two of the more well known ISO standard families are the ISO 9000 and ISO 14000 families, which are "generic management system standards." From the ISO website: "ISO 9000 is concerned with 'quality management' and covers the organization's activities for enhancing customer satisfaction by meeting customer and applicable regulatory requirements and striving continually to improve its performance in this regard. ISO 14000 is primarily concerned with 'environmental management'. This means what the organization does to minimize harmful effects on the environment caused by its activities, and to improve its environmental performance." More information is available at www.iso.org/iso/en/aboutiso/introduction/index.html.

Professional societies have committees that meet regularly to set and update standards. For example the American Society for Testing of Materials (ASTM) has committees of professional engineers who meet to set and update standard methods for testing materials. The CDRH, in particular, references multiple standards from different sources in its guidances for specific classes of products and many of those standards are from the ASTM, defining certain limits or bounds of performance that must be met by the device or by materials used in the device. See www.fda.gov/cdrh/stdsprog.html for further details on how the CDRH evaluates and applies various standards from the organizations listed below to assess quality and compliance from manufacturers

Some examples of organizations that publish standards (this is not a comprehensive list)

AAMI	Association for Advancement of Medical Instrumentation,
ACR	American College of Radiology,
ADA	American Dental Association,
ANSI	American National Standards Institute,
APA	American Psychiatric Association,

ASA	Acoustical Society of America,
ASME	American Society of Mechanical Engineers,
ASQC	American Society of Quality Control,
ASTM	American Society for Testing and Materials,
CENELEC	European Committee for Electrotechnical Standardization,
CGSB	Canadian General Standards Board,
HPS	Health Physics Society,
IEC	International Electrotechnical Commission,
IES	Illuminating Engineering Society of North America,
IEEE®	Institute of Electrical and Electronics Engineers,
INMM	Institute of Nuclear Materials Management,
ISO	International Organization for Standards,
LIA	Laser Institute of America,
NCCLS	National Committee for Clinical Laboratory Standards,
NEMA	National Electrical Manufacturers Association,
RESNA	Rehabilitation Engineering and Assistive Technology Society of North America,
SAE	Society of Automotive Engineers,
UL	Underwriters Laboratories, Inc.®

6.4.3 Which of the thousands of standards apply to my product?

The best practical ways to find the standards that should apply to the product being developed are:

- Check FDA special controls and other guidance documents,
- Check industry association for any offered training courses or seminars,
- Examine existing marketed products and associated literature,
- Talk to people in the business – by asking fellow professionals or attending meetings,
- Hire experienced employees or consultants who have employed standards in product development or organization planning,
- Speak to insurance companies as to their requirements to insure your facility or your products.

6.4.4 What are "clean room" standards?

An important segment of standards apply to the manufacturing environment. Most manufacturing facilities have sterile or aseptic processing areas, which contain "clean rooms" that are used in specific critical processing steps. "Clean rooms" are frequently used in the final manufacture of biomedical products. A clean room is an environmentally controlled area that has a low level of environmental pollutants, such as dust, microbes, aerosol particles, and vapors. Clean rooms have special air-handling systems where outside air is filtered and the air inside is recirculated through special filters (high efficiency particulate arresting; HEPA) to remove internally generated contaminants. The clean-room environment can be a small room or it may be an entire manufacturing plant.

In the USA, clean rooms are defined by US Federal Standard 209. The class of a clean room is determined by measuring the number of particles greater than 0.5 μm in 1 cubic foot of air. The clean room classifications (under the US standards) range from Class 1 (1 particle/ft^3 of air) to Class 100 000 (100 000 particles/ft^3 of air).

The European Union (EU) established a standard in 1997 and it has been widely adopted in Europe as a part of EU GMP. The clean rooms are classified as A through D, with Class A being the "cleanest."

An ISO (International Standards Organization) standard (ISO 14644) for classification of clean rooms was recently introduced. The classifications range from ISO Class 1 (0 particles > 0.5 microns/m^3 of air) to ISO Class 9 (35 200 000 particles).

Most pharmaceutical or device manufacturing processes use clean room technologies that are ISO class 5, class 7, or class 8. For example, tabletting and oral liquid preparation facilities should meet at least ISO class 8 standards, while aseptic filling and manufacture or packaging of implantable medical devices would take place in an ISO class 5 standard facility.

The FDA published a guidance document (www.fda.gov/cder/guidance/5882fnl.pdf) in 2004, which outlines the clean room requirements for aseptic manufacturing facilities.

6.5   Manufacturing in drug development

The biologically active drug molecule is known as the Active Pharmaceutical Ingredient (API) (small molecule or large molecule biologic drug candidate; see Chapter 4).

The final dosage form includes the API and various other excipients that make up the liquid, powder, pill, or capsule that is to be delivered by oral or parenteral route. Many manufacturers make the API in one location and then ship the API to another facility that specializes in final blending, granulation, tabletting, packaging, or filling (in bottles, gels, syringes, etc.) and testing the various dosage forms (e.g., 5 mg, 10 mg, or 25 mg pills; or an injectable fluid formulation). This provides the manufacturer with the flexibility to make multiple types of products (children's medicine, adult dosage form) from one starting point of the active drug moiety. The FDA will evaluate validation data from the final dosage form in addition to validation data of the API production.

Pharmaceutical manufacturing for small molecule (synthetic chemistry) drugs entails different technology and process platforms from those needed for manufacturing large molecule (biologic) drugs. Small molecule drugs need chemical reactors where controlled chemical reactions are used to synthesize the API in a step-wise fashion, whereas biologics need large bioreactor tanks where cells (which produce the biologic API) are grown and harvested under carefully monitored conditions. However, the business risks involved in the investment decision to manufacture in large scale, and the timing of this scale-up and the size of investments are very similar for both types of drugs.

Small molecule drugs are made using large scale (bulk) chemical reactors, filters and dryers in chemical factories. Elements to monitor in the final output are: by-products of the chemical reactions (usually well known), removal of all solvents, and other properties of the API molecule, such as an appropriate chirality or an appropriate mix of enantiomers (which can have an impact on the biological activity of the drug), crystalline forms of compound, and purity of final product, among other parameters.

Biological drugs are typically made using bacterial or mammalian cells, with a selected cell line grown in a tailored and controlled environment. A whole bioreactor is filled with these cellular mini-factories, each cell secreting multiple quantities of the desired protein. A key process step and quality control issue in biomanufacturing is the separation process, to get the API out of the medium that the cells were kept in, while eliminating all other proteins that the cell produces. Other issues also include monitoring the cell phenotype and genotype to make sure that the same protein is reproducibly being made by the cells with the same post-translational modification and initial sterility of the bioreactor. The API protein's function is defined by its composition (linear sequence of amino acids), and its three-dimensional structure. This 3-D structure, and hence the function of the protein, can be altered by a single-point mutation (a change in just one amino acid among hundreds that comprise the protein), by extra crosslinks in the protein (post-translational modifications) or by other subtle changes in the large molecule drug (a protein drug usually contains hundreds, if not thousands, of amino acids). These subtle changes make it necessary to watch closely many parameters of the production process as the biological behavior of the final protein can be strongly influenced by these subtle changes in the manufacturing and final production processes. *Biologics are often said to be defined by their process.* Some of the advanced disciplines that are useful in the complex environment of a bulk drug production facility are given in Table 6.1.

The complex manufacturing process and difficulty in assessing these subtle changes in the final product have been brought up as the main reason that generic

Table 6.1 Disciplines used in biopharmaceutical drug manufacturing

Microbiology
Cell biology
Food science
Analytical chemistry
Mechanical engineering
Biochemistry
Finance and accounting
Chemical engineering
Biochemical engineering
Pharmaceutical chemistry and science
Business management

biological drugs must go through similar development and testing processes as the original innovator product, a much more rigorous and onerous requirement than that required for small molecule generic drugs. The often-quoted example that demonstrates the significance of paying careful attention to the manufacturing process is that of Johnson & Johnson and its biological drug Eprex (see Box 6.2 for more details). A subtle change in the final manufacturing process of Eprex (erythropoietin, which increases red blood cells) led to an increase in serious cases

---

Box 6.2 Case study: small manufacturing changes have a big impact

In 1998, the EU regulatory body directed Johnson & Johnson to stop using human serum albumin (HSA) as a stabilizer in Eprex (human erythropoietin), due to concerns of "Mad Cow" disease. It was subsequently determined over the next few years that an increased number of patients receiving Eprex developed a severe loss of red blood cells (aplasia), which required transfusions. The exposure-adjusted incidence of this aplasia per 100 000 patient years was estimated to be 18 in Eprex without HSA, 6 in Eprex with HSA and 0.2 in Epogen (a product of Amgen, from whom the Eprex manufacturing process was transferred to Johnson & Johnson). Some intense detective work by Johnson & Johnson (the drug was not taken off the market as the benefits to patients outweighed the risks) showed that the replacement stabilizer (polysorbate-80-replaced HSA) reacted with the long-used, uncoated rubber stoppers of the single injection tube in which Eprex was stored, causing plasticizers to leach into the solution. These plasticizers acted as adjuvants, stimulating a very small percentage of patients to mount a strong immune response to the recombinant-injected erythropoietin. These antibodies would then attack the patient's own erythropoietin, leading the body to shut down all red blood cell production and leading to severe anemia. In 2002, Johnson & Johnson switched to PTFE-coated rubber stoppers, which halted the leaching problem and reduced the immune response. This example and the continued difference in incidence of these immune responses is often cited when arguments are made against allowing biosimilars (biological generics) to come on the market without substantial clinical testing to demonstrate biological safety and efficacy, essentially going down the same path of tests as the original drug.

The complexity and subtlety of changes and the difficulty in characterizing biological drugs is apparent in a continuing article on this matter, published in 2006. This article argues that product aggregate formation may in fact be the cause of the differences in behavior between the two products rather than adjuvant-induced immune reaction.

References

Douglas McCormick, Small changes, big effects in biological manufacturing, *Pharmaceutical Technology*, November 2004, (accessed online August 2006).
Schellekens, H. and Jiskoot, W. *Nature Biotechnology*, **24**, 613–614, 2006.

of aplasia (lack of red blood cells). On the other hand, Amgen changed its manu-facturing process for its version of erythropoietin after launching Phase III studies and successfully demonstrated equivalence and efficacy for the new process and product in a series of clinical trials.

6.5.1   Process validation before approval

Pharmaceutical products are approved only after submission of data that validates the manufacturing process. The companies submit data demonstrating that the processes are validatable (often called qualification studies). At the time of the pre-approval inspection (PAI), the companies must have validation protocols written and available for review. Validation data are often submitted as part of the first annual report after approval. The FDA could require production of one or more conforming batches of material and submission of those records and analyses to the FDA prior to approval.

The FDA has defined process validation as "establishing documented evidence that provides a high degree of assurance that a specific process will consistently produce a product meeting its predetermined specifications and quality attributes" (www.fda.gov/cdrh/ode/425.pdf). In addition to process validation, firms must also perform analytical method validation, facility and equipment validation, soft-ware validation and cleaning validation. The final product quality is assured when all these elements are combined with other elements of GMP established by the FDA.

However, advances in process analytical technology (PAT) have resulted in the improved validation of manufacturing processes with real-time feedback and the ability to measure multiple parameters on-line (see Box 6.3 for more details on PAT). The FDA is responding to these technological and engineering advances by issuing new GMP guidelines for batch validation of manufacturing processes.

Some extracts from the 2004 FDA report on "Pharmaceutical cGMPs for the twenty-first century," accessible in full at (www.fda.gov/cder/gmp/gmp2004/ GMP_finalreport2004.htm), and other policy guides are reproduced here:

[The FDA has] ... begun updating ... [its] current thinking on validation under a Cross-Agency Process Validation workgroup led by CDER's Office of Compliance Coordinating Committee with participation from CDER, CBER, [and others]. ... [The] FDA began this process [by] issuing a compliance policy guide (CPG) entitled *Process Validation Requirements for Drug Products and Active Pharmaceutical Ingredients Subject to Pre-Market Approval* (CPG 7132c.08, Sec 490.100).

[The CPG states that] agency drug product pre-market review units may approve applications for marketing before a firm has manufactured one or more conformance batches at commercial scale (also sometimes referred to as "validation" batches). The revised CPG again recognizes certain conditions under which a firm may market batches of drugs while gathering data to confirm the validity of the manufacturing process ... The document clearly signals that a focus on three full-scale production batches would fail to recognize the complete story on validation.

Advanced pharmaceutical science and engineering principles and manufacturing control technologies can provide a high level of process understanding and control capability. Use of

Box 6.3 Process analytical technology

Contributed by Tony Rao, Principal at Stantec Consulting

Process analytical technology (PAT), as defined by the FDA, is a system for designing, analyzing, and controlling manufacturing processes through timely measurements of critical quality and performance attributes of raw materials and processes with the goal of ensuring final product quality. The primary use of PAT is to generate product quality information in real time. This type of real-time quality analysis is most useful in a continuous product manufacturing environment like a chemical manufacturing process – i.e., pharmaceuticals.

Most pharmaceutical facilities are adopting PAT to reduce operating costs and improve manufacturing efficiencies. It is being increasingly utilized in non-complex, though critical, manufacturing steps – like the purification of water and generation of water to be used to constitute products that will be injected into human beings. The introduction of automated TOC analyzers has reduced the cost of water generation tremendously.

The term "analytical" could include chemical, physical, microbiological, mathematical, and risk analysis, all of which must be conducted in an integrated manner, requiring a thorough understanding of the manufacturing process for the best implementation and use of PAT.

Conventional process monitoring often involves taking samples from the production line into the testing (QA or QC) laboratory, whereas PAT relies on in-line testing. Examples of on-line or in-line analytical instrumentation are:

- Spectroscopy (UV, NIR, turbidity, refractivity),
- Chromatography (HPLC),
- Electrochemical (pH, DO, conductivity),
- Chemical,
- Physical (temperature, pressure).

Through the use of strategically placed probes in the process, critical endpoints at specific stages of the process can be pinpointed to a high degree of certainty. Sampling errors (and, more importantly, failed batches) can be minimized.

Process analytical technology is not a regulatory requirement. The FDA guidance documents encourage the use and adoption of risk-based approaches to the development of automated process control systems in the pharmaceutical industry.

Reference

Guideline of General Principles of Process Validation (May 1987, originally published by CDER, CBER, and CDRH and presently recognized by CDER, CBER, and CVM). www.fda.gov/cder/guidance/pv.htm.

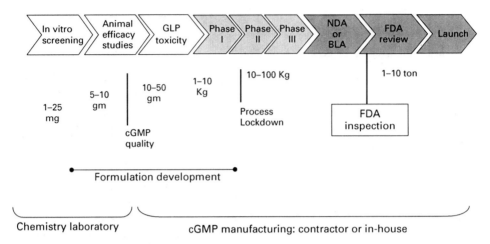

Figure 6.3   Pharmaceutical manufacturing needs and scale-up timing.

these advanced principles and control technologies can provide a high assurance of quality by continuously monitoring, evaluating, and adjusting every batch using validated in-process measurements, tests, controls, and process endpoints. For manufacturing processes developed and controlled in such a manner, it may not be necessary for a firm to manufacture multiple conformance batches prior to initial distribution.

Thus, products manufactured in more innovatively designed, efficient, and updated plants with better process control and analysis technology will benefit from lowered costs of compliance to cGMP.

6.5.2   Bulk drug scale-up and production stages

Figure 6.3 highlights the various scale-up requirements of material used for various tests and stages of product development. The scale-up requirements are similar for biologics and small molecules. The following text puts Figure 6.3 into context.

After the molecule moves into advanced pre-clinical development, the earliest scaled-up material is made for animal toxicological studies to determine safety. Up to this point, a few milligrams of material for in vitro studies or a few grams for animal-efficacy studies are typically produced using lab-bench production techniques in the laboratory. However, in advanced pre-clinical development, from tens of grams to a kilo of material will typically be required (depending on the length of time and range of dosages of the particular drug to be tested). At this stage, the manufacturing process used should yield the product close to (but not necessarily as pure as) the purity ultimately desired. This is the pilot-manufacturing or first-stage scale-up process. While optimizing the scaling-up process, it is critical that the final manufacturing process should not introduce additional contaminants or product variants that would cause a repeat of the toxicology studies. Therefore, the ultimate manufacturing process should yield material that is at least as pure as the material used for the toxicology studies.

At this stage of first scale-up and pilot manufacturing, it is a good idea to test the cost of production and project it onto the final commercial scale of production. This calculation (along with input from reimbursement specialists – see Chapter 7) will allow for; (1) a projection of whether the product can be made cost effectively on a commercial scale or whether alternative manufacturing procedures should be investigated, and (2) the development team to optimize those parts of the manufacturing process that contribute substantially to the overall manufacturing cost.

Another important step at this point of first-stage or pilot production is to establish the characteristics of the ideal product as they apply to manufacturing issues; e.g., how is it packaged, what is its shelf life, what is the formulation? Most small companies typically outsource this part of the manufacturing process.

As the program moves ahead to commercial level manufacture in kilogram or ton quantities, it is essential that the process be scalable and produce material that is comparable to early toxicology testing material in its purity profile, stability, bioactivity, or other characteristics of the molecule. Thus, the process of technology transfer between R&D, pilot manufacturing, and large-scale manufacturing must be carefully and actively managed.

6.5.3 Commercial manufacturing planning

During the initial selection of a product for development, a rough estimate of the cost of goods is made. Revenue estimates are also created, based on the potential market size and early market surveys. In the absence of defined supply chains and commercial manufacturing processes, rough estimates of the cost of goods are made based on experience with similar products.

As the product progresses through proof of concept (Phase I/II), estimates of market size and product dosing significantly improve. With this information, commercial manufacturing plans are developed. A typical commercial manufacturing plan includes:

- Product development; approval timeline,
- Commercial forecast (number of patients, dosages, regional requirements),
- Commercial product definition (marketed package or SKU),
- Target commercial manufacturing concept (processes, scale, batch size),
- Supply chain (including make vs. buy, single or multi source, strategic relations),
- Facility requirements (scope and capital estimate),
- Organizational requirements,
- Cost of goods,
- Commercialization estimate,
- Risk management plan (including mitigation plans for highest risks).

The commercial manufacturing plan is used as a guide for the development of manufacturing processes for Phase III and commercial sales and also for making capital investment decisions. As mentioned above, it is critically important that the Phase III manufacturing process and product are representative of the ultimate commercial process and product. If changes are made to the process or product after Phase III, it is likely that additional clinical trials will be required with an

---

Box 6.4 Case study – Immunex and manufacturing planning

The corporation: biotech and the spoils of success, Business Week Online, Aug 13, 2001.

Immunex' rheumatoid arthritis (RA) drug, Enbrel, was approved in November 1998 as the first biologic to treat the disease. Immunex initial sales estimates focused on the 25% of RA patients who failed traditional therapies, and so when the FDA approved the drug for children in 1999 and then as a first-line defense for RA patients in 2000, the company was unprepared for the demand. Only 75 000 of the 1 million patients who might benefit from the drug could get Enbrel, resulting in lost sales of over $200 million (that is, $500 000 or more lost every day). Immunex had contracted Boehringer Ingelheim Pharma of Germany to manufacture Enbrel – but that wasn't enough. Immunex and its partner American Home Products (now Wyeth) started a new plant in 1999 at the cost of $450M, but the plant would not be ready until the end of 2002. This left the door open to competitors, such as Johnson & Johnson's Remicade, approved a year after Enbrel. The CEO of Immunex said in early 2001 that if he could recreate history, he would have prepared more aggressively.

---

associated delay of the product development time line (and at significant added expense). This is especially true for biologics.

The decision on implementing specific scale of manufacturing is also affected by the cost of goods (COGS or bill of materials) requirements of the product. The COGs includes the cost of materials, labor for manufacturing, testing, release, facilities (depreciation on capital), utilities, and overhead. The typical cost of goods (COGs or bill of materials) for drugs and biologics ranges from 5% to 25% of the sales price.

A major issue arises towards the beginning of Phase III studies, especially when developing biologicals – whether to continue to contract out production or build a production plant? The risk has been reduced with a positive Phase II proof of concept result, and the company has to decide on the best use of its resources on the path forward – an expensive Phase III trial has to be balanced with the investment in building a dedicated manufacturing facility. The key issue here is the large investment needed ($15–$50 million) and the still-lingering uncertainty (the product still has an industry average of 50% chance of success at this point). The build or buy decision is discussed in greater detail in Section 6.8. It is also important at this stage to have strong market research (see Chapter 2) to predict the scale of production needed and either prepare contractors or build out to compensate for that volume, else, as Immunex learned to its chagrin (see Box 6.4), a success can quickly become a bust.

Another important part of planning manufacturing activities is to understand the context of manufacture for drugs – for example, barbiturates must be manufactured in a highly controlled and regulated environment with only a few plants in the world currently configured to make those kinds of drugs. Similarly, for cytotoxic drugs used for chemotherapy, the product must be made in a facility with extremely high levels of protection for personnel, with the physical plant configured to allow for completely closed environments for production, formulation, and final packaging of the toxic product. These special manufacturing considerations will significantly increase the manufacturing cost of the product and could have an unforeseen impact on the profit margins of the business.

The steps of packaging and filling usually require specialized plants and apparatus for these steps, and it is common to outsource these last steps of making the final oral (capsule, gel, tablet) or parenteral preparation to specialized filling facilities.

Finally, the FDA will inspect the manufacturing site before approving the drug for marketing. Typically, this PAI (pre-approval inspection) is announced, giving a company enough time to prepare. The inspectors go over minute details in the operations, evaluating the books of standard operating procedures (SOPs) and training SOPs that are vital for GMP process implementation (section 6.2). Outcomes of an inspection can range from including comments in an inspection report, specific recommendations to change or improve processes, or if the non-compliant process or system is found potentially to affect product quality, the inspector can even issue an injunction or restraining order to close down the plant or to close down the production of that specific product until the situation is satisfactorily rectified and the plant is in compliance again.

6.6 Manufacturing in devices and diagnostics

Owing to the highly varied nature of products in the device sector, the comments here are fairly general but relevant to most device manufacturing processes, as prototypes are scaled up to production level.

After the first few prototypes have been made in machine shops based on early sketches (Figure 6.4) and used for proof-of-concept testing and design optimization, the production needs to turn to pilot manufacture or full-scale manufacturing for in vivo application and testing.

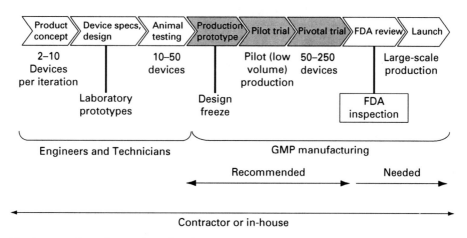

Figure 6.4 Device manufacturing needs and scale-up.

Pre-manufacture planning steps include identifying and selecting suppliers, developing a pilot run plan, a manufacturing strategy (build or buy, see Section 6.8), identifying costs and timelines and other plans to prepare for transfer of the technology from R&D to production. As shown in Figure 6.4, pilot production needs could be met without full GMP processes but a GMP-compliant production facility will need to make validation batches of products before the FDA will approve marketing the device.

At this pre-manufacture stage, the following processes and considerations are useful for the management and development team to review as part of the design process before investment in pilot production or full-scale production:

- Verify and validate (V&V) customer needs,
- Verify and validate (V&V) needs translated to design requirements and performance,
- Material selection,
- Packaging and sterilization,
- Pre-clinical testing,
- Use of engineering analyses for production, assembly and testing planning.

Good engineering analysis at this stage can point the way to a manufacturing prototype and investment in analytical planning and virtual (computer-aided) design can help to:

- Accelerate development,
- Minimize prototype iterations,
- Avoid design mistakes.

However, it is not a replacement for full prototyping and testing.

Material selection is another important iterative pre-manufacturing step that must be considered from multiple perspectives, beginning with the end use and stepping through all the steps and processes used in larger scale manufacturing. This phase of "technology transfer" between R&D prototype product and production prototype is a critical stage where many development failures occur. For example, starting with "medical grade" pure materials does not put an end to the technology transfer issues or the assessment of material quality and characteristics – it is important to consider the overall processing conditions at each step of production, including sterilization and packaging, and also including specific forms of usage possible at the site of delivery. This analysis is partly included in the validation stage mandated in quality systems for cGMP compliance (see Chapter 4 and Appendix 6.2). Certain standards in ISO 10993 also lay out specific paths for materials testing in development stages, including the toxicity testing discussed in Chapter 4 and additional testing (leachables, extractables) for each component used in the manufacturing process.

In this stage of planning final manufacture and final design reviews, the key issues of packaging and sterilization are interconnected as:

- Packaging depends on the product design,
- Sterilization methods depend on product design – e.g., a biological product cannot be sterilized with gas or steam methods,

- Packaging depends on sterilization method – e.g., packaging must allow sterilization to penetrate (gas sterilization) or must not degrade (irradiation sterilization).

6.6.1 Design for manufacturability

Important issues that can derail a product development process in production stages owing to increased cost or time need to be considered in the design phase. Specifically, keeping manufacturing issues in mind assures that a design can be repeatedly manufactured while satisfying the requirements for quality, reliability, performance, availability, and price. The design should be reviewed to make it less costly by the following considerations, wherever possible:

- Simplify design to use fewer parts; eliminate non-functional parts and reduce functional parts,
- Use simple production processes with low defect rates in process,
- Design in higher quality and reliability,
- Make it easier to service.

6.6.2 Design for assembly

The final steps of assembly, packaging, and sterilization can be made easier by specifically keeping requirements of assembly of parts in mind, using the following points:

- Checking overall design concepts, keeping assembly processes in mind,
- Component mounting connections,
- Test points accessible at various stages of assembly,
- Stress levels and tolerances of connections; points well tested,
- Printed circuit boards standardized or component connections clearly identified.

After delivery of the first production batch to the consumer, continue to monitor field performance and correct or improve the manufacturing process or device design. In particular, the case with recall of Sulzer hip implants (Box 6.5) points out the need to monitor field use of the final products for manufacturing or production problems that may have escaped notice in final testing.

6.7 Manufacturing in diagnostics

The following section is adapted from the FDA guidance document: *Guideline for the Manufacture of In Vitro Diagnostic Products* (www.fda.gov/cdrh/comp/918.pdf, published 1994).

Box 6.5 Sulzer Hip implant recall – case of subtle changes in manufacturing causing large problems

In 2000, Sulzer Orthopedics recalled about 17 500 hip replacement acetabular shells. These shells fit into the hip socket and interface with the stem that fits into the femur. These products were part of a batch of 25 000 that had been manufactured between 1997 and 1999. In the fall of 2000, orthopedic doctors began reporting problems with the hip implant. Sulzer voluntarily recalled the implant after researching patient records, surgical techniques, and the product itself. It was found that some mineral oil-based lubricant had leaked into the machine coolant and left an oily residue on the acetabular shell. The shell went through the established cleaning process but that did not remove the oily residue, which went undetected. The acetabular implant was made to snap into the hip socket so that bone would grow into it. The oily residue interfered with the bonding of the bone and allowed the implant to loosen and fail, requiring another surgical procedure to fix the problem.

In February 2002, Sulzer agreed to settle patient's lawsuits for $1 billion.

References

Lefevre, G. Hip replacement patients may face more surgery, *CNN*, January 17, 2001; accessed at www.cnn.com

Sulzer website: www.sulzer.com

In vitro device characteristics are defined during the pre-production process. Apart from parameters such as *physical characteristics*, *chemical composition*, and *microbiological characteristics*, critical performance characteristics such as accuracy, precision, specificity, purity, identity, and sensitivity are also specified. These established specifications will determine the appropriate production and process controls, such as mixing and filling processes, sterilization, or lyophilization needed to manufacture the IVD. The specifications established for the IVD will also determine the appropriate environmental controls needed, in conjunction with the manufacturing process, to ensure that product specifications are consistently met. The consistency of these product attributes is not "tested into" the finished product, but is achieved through the establishment of adequate product specifications; and by ensuring that these specifications are met through product and process design, process validation, process water controls, manufacturing controls, and finished product testing.

The specifications for the product, the manufacturing process, and the environment are maintained as part of the device master record (DMR), as required by CFR 820.181.

Non-compliance to these regulatory requirements can have severe consequences as described in Box 6.6. Small businesses with a single product line are well advised to invest in assuring compliance to quality and testing regulations.

Box 6.6 Seriousness of Non-Compliance to FDA manufacturing and quality regulations

Abbott, a large diagnostics manufacturer (that also makes and sells drugs and devices) had its diagnostics manufacturing plant shut down in 1999 by the FDA when inspections found that they did not comply with cGMP or QSR. The letter from the FDA to the public explaining the reason for this serious step is reproduced here in excerpts: (from www.fda.gov/cdrh/ocd/abbottletter.html)

Dear Colleague:

On November 2, 1999, the Department of Justice, on behalf of the Food and Drug Administration (FDA), entered into a consent decree of permanent injunction with Abbott Laboratories and responsible officials. This action involves the company's diagnostic devices division. We are writing to explain the significance of this action, and how it may affect the healthcare community.

Reason for seeking an injunction

We took this action because of the firm's long-standing failure to comply with the FDA's good manufacturing practices (GMP) regulation, now called the quality system regulation, and its failure to fulfill commitments to correct deficiencies in its manufacturing operations.

These failures go back to 1993, when our inspection of the facilities where Abbott Diagnostics Division manufactures diagnostic products showed non-compliance with the GMP requirements. Areas of non-compliance included process validation, corrective and preventive action, and production and process controls. The company's failure to comply with these requirements increases the likelihood that the diagnostic products produced at these facilities may not perform as intended.

Subsequent inspections, including one as recent as July 1999, showed little improvement in the company's compliance, despite three warning letters from the FDA. Since 1995, the FDA repeatedly encouraged the company to achieve compliance voluntarily. Despite assurances by the company that it would correct the manufacturing problems, the firm failed to bring its manufacturing operations into compliance. Ultimately, in order to protect the public health, FDA sought action by the Department of Justice.

Public health significance of non-compliance

It is important to understand the public health significance of the FDA's quality system regulation. When a manufacturer complies with the regulation, there is a level of assurance that the product has been properly designed and manufactured in a consistent way and will perform as intended. Conversely, a manufacturer who fails to comply is less likely to produce a product that performs as intended. We are especially concerned about Abbott Diagnostic Division's long-standing non-compliance with these accepted manufacturing principles because they represent the minimum requirements for manufacturing quality.

What does the firm's failure to comply with the Quality System regulation mean for the users of its diagnostic products? It does not mean that these products will necessarily fail to perform as intended. It does mean that users have less assurance of successful performance than they would have had if these products had been manufactured properly . . .

6.7.1   Labeling requirements for in vitro devices

Product developers should read the specific guidelines and controls for labeling of the final product, described in 21 CFR 809.10(b) (see Table 5.5 for website links), and summarized here. The label includes the following details:

- Proprietary and established names,
- Intended uses,
- Summary and explanation of test,
- Principle of procedures,
- Information on reagents,
- Information on instruments,
- Information on specimen collection and preparation,
- Procedures,
- Results,
- Limitations of the procedure,
- Expected values,
- Specific performance characteristics,
- Bibliography,
- Name and place of business,
- Date of the package insert.

6.8   Buy or build

In drug or device manufacture, the decision to buy (contract out) or build a manufacturing facility for a new product can get clouded with debates over political, financial, emotional, and strategic issues. However, there are some clear strategic and financial discussion points that should be primary considerations. Figure 6.5 exemplifies one such set of parameters that should be evaluated here.

In manufacturing biomedical products, building one's own facility for a new product is a typically large and high-risk investment. Many companies start by

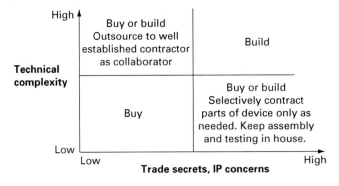

Figure 6.5   Buy or build decision – one set of strategic considerations.

Table 6.2 The buy or build decision – pros and cons of contract manufacturing

Pros	Cons
Cost	
Using a CMO avoids high up-front investment and conserves cash	Must pay a mark-up
The CMO spreads the overheads among many projects and can achieve economies of scale that would not be possible for a small company with only one product	Cancellation of contract carries penalty payment
Time	
Faster to use a CMO – avoid recruitment and building time, improve speed to market	Management must put aside resources, time, and people to manage the CMO process, time line, and objectives
Experience at ACMO might speed up trouble shooting in process	A CMO might not be able to provide capacity whenever needed in the time frame wanted by the company
Capability	
Able to access experienced staff through the CMO for specific needs and time periods	Contracting company is not building the expertise internally for future projects or products
	Proprietary optimized process (trade secret) will be disseminated to industry competitors through CMO, potentially losing competitive edge
Capacity	
Volume required for production can be configured from existing large volume facilities at CMO	Smaller capacity needs may get lower priority in the waiting list with CMOs
Uncertainty in product development success can be restrictive in building large capacity in-house, allowing developers to plan for production capacity with CMO	

using a contract manufacturing organization (CMO) (buying the capacity as needed) and once approval is obtained, start building their facility and transfer the process from the CMO. Some of the other reasons are discussed briefly below, with one set of strategic issues laid out in Figure 6.5. This type of matrix can be used to compare and contrast other parameters that are listed in Table 6.2.

In general, if capacity and capability are available, the discussion focuses on company strategy. For example, if a product that addresses a very large market is being developed right behind a product designed for a smaller market, it is possible that the company will decide to reserve capacity for the product still in development and outsource the current product. If the manufacturing process is very sensitive to minor changes or is very complex, the decision to keep manufacturing in-house may be the right one. Another reason to not use a CMO is if you perceive a risk that your project may get less attention if a much larger project comes up for the CMO. This is always a risk in working with a large CMO that has the capacity flexibility

Table 6.3 Examples of virtual and semi-integrated CMO arrangements

Virtual		Semi-integrated	
Focal, Inc.	Vendors	Focal, Inc.	Vendors
Defines product requirements	Component manufacturing	Defines product requirements	Component manufacturing
Works with clinicians to refine design	Device assembly	Works with clinicians to refine design	Formulation and vial fill
Performs testing to verify performance	Packaging sterilization	Synthesizes polymers Assembles devices Packages system Performs testing to verify performance	Sterilization

small companies are looking for, since the CMO is also looking for the larger projects that take up more guaranteed capacity and thus could assign lower priority to these smaller jobs. There are also other more general transaction costs, such as increased time from management, etc. Some of these considerations and others are discussed in Table 6.2. An example of two device companies that made selective and strategic arrangements with CMOs for their final production illustrates (Table 6.3) that the arrangements can be very flexible to suit the company's strategic needs and capabilities.

6.9　Summary

The manufacturing process requires a rather different mindset in its organization and people than was prevalent through the product development process so far. Compliance to regulations, reproducibility, operational precision, and efficiency all become the center of focus of operations.

Manufacturing organizations must establish standard operating procedures (SOPs) that adhere to international standards and must also have well documented operational processes that show compliance to FDA regulations. Successful scale-up from laboratory prototypes or small-scale production batches requires intense oversight and good management practices.

Exercises

6.1 Project and identify the timing of scale-up of various volumes of product into the overall product development plan.

6.2 Project the total volume needed during peak sales of the product, high-lighting key assumptions. Review the assumptions frequently during further product development activities.

6.3 Develop a manufacturing plan for the product, including a summary discussion and rationale of the decision to build or buy. Identify the level of GMP compliance and the biosafety levels needed for manufacturing and packaging, the projected product life cycle and the need for product diversification from one core manufacturing template (e.g., different dosage forms from one API or diagnostics developed for multiple assay platforms).

6.4 Assess the product for any steps in synthesis, production, or assembly that might be unusually complex or have a high cost of materials. For example, special medical grade rare-metal alloys, specific injection molding techniques, or expensive starting chemicals.

6.5 Decide on final packaging and delivery needs – is it important to keep the item away from light at all times, is it necessary to keep the product at a specific temperature during storage or shipping?

6.6 Get cost and timeline estimates for pilot scale-up and for large-scale/bulk production from suppliers in the industry – this is product dependent and most suppliers/CMOs (contract manufacturing organizations) will sign confidentiality agreements in order to receive product details and give back quotes/proposals.

6.7 Refer to the industry association or to the Drug Information Association (DIA) meetings to which your company belongs, for training courses in GMP and other regulatory issues.

References and additional reading

Abboud, L. and Hensley, S. Factory shift: new prescription for drug makers, *The Wall Street Journal*, (Eastern edn.), September 3, p. A1, 2003.

Bhatia, S. *Microfabrication in Tissue Engineering and Bioartificial Organs (Microsystems)*, Springer, 1999.

Guarino, R. (ed.). *New Drug Approval Process, Accelerating Global Registrations*, Informa Healthcare, 4th edn., 2004.

Levin, M. (ed.). *Pharmaceutical Process Scale-Up*, Informa Healthcare, 1st edn., 2001.

Shuler, M. L. and Kargi, F. *Bioprocess Engineering: Basic Concepts*, Prentice Hall, 2nd edn., 2001.

Signore, A. and Jacobs, T. (ed.). *Good Design Practices for GMP Pharmaceutical Facilities*, Informa Healthcare, 2005.

Vogel, H. C. and Todaro, C. C. *Fermentation and Biochemical Engineering Handbook: Principles, Process Design, and Equipment*, Noyes Publications, 2nd edn., 1996.

Willig, S. (ed.). *Good Manufacturing Practices for Pharmaceuticals: A Plan for Total Quality Control from Manufacturer*, Informa Healthcare, 5th edn., 2000.

Useful websites

http://ts.nist.gov/Standards/Conformity/stdpmr.cfm – *Standards – ABCs of standards in the USA*

www.iso.org/iso/en/aboutiso/introduction/index.html – *ISO website*

www.fda.gov/cder/guidance/5882fnl.pdf – *Clean rooms*
www.fda.gov/cder/guidance/pv.htm – *Process validation guidance*
www.ispe.org – *International society for technical professionals in the healthcare manufacturing industry*

Appendix 6.1 Compliance to pharmaceutical GMP

Extracts from the FDA/CDER inspector's manual for inspection of GMP pharmaceutical facilities are reproduced here. The manual is available in its whole form at www.fda.gov/cder/dmpq/7356-002f-CDER.pdf.

Compliance program guidance manual   Program 7356.002F
Chapter 56 – Drug quality assurance
Appendix E

Quality system

Assessment of the quality system has two phases. The first phase is to evaluate whether the quality unit has fulfilled the responsibility to review and approve all procedures related to production, quality control, and quality assurance and assure the procedures are adequate for their intended use. This also includes the associated record-keeping systems. The second phase is to assess the data collected to identify quality problems and may link to other major systems for inspectional coverage . . .

. . .

For each of the following, the firm should have written and approved procedures and documentation resulting therefrom. The firm's adherence to written procedures should be verified through observation whenever possible. When this system is selected for coverage in addition to the quality system, all areas listed below should be covered; however, the actual depth of coverage may vary from the planned inspection strategy depending upon inspectional findings.

Facilities and equipment system

(1) Facilities:
- Cleaning and maintenance,
- Facility layout, flow of materials and personnel for prevention of cross-contamination, including from processing of non-drug materials,
- Dedicated areas or containment controls for highly sensitizing materials (e.g., penicillin, beta-lactams, steroids, hormones, and cytotoxics),
- Utilities such as steam, gas, compressed air, heating, ventilation, and air conditioning should be qualified and appropriately monitored (note: this

system includes only those utilities whose output is not intended to be incorporated into the API, such as water used in cooling or heating jacketed vessels),

- Lighting, sewage and refuse disposal, washing and toilet facilities,
- Control system for implementing changes in the building,
- Sanitation of the building, including use of rodenticides, fungicides, insecticides, cleaning, and sanitizing agents,
- Training and qualification of personnel.

(2) Process equipment

- Equipment installation, operational, performance qualification where appropriate,
- Appropriate design, adequate size, and suitably located for its intended use,
- Equipment surfaces should not be reactive, additive, or absorptive of materials under process so as to alter their quality,
- Equipment (e.g., reactors, storage containers) and permanently installed processing lines should be appropriately identified,
- Substances associated with the operation of equipment (e.g., lubricants, heating fluids, or coolants) should not come into contact with starting materials, intermediates, final APIs, and containers,
- Cleaning procedures and cleaning validation and sanitization studies should be reviewed to verify that residues, microbial, and, when appropriate, endotoxin contamination are removed to below scientifically appropriate levels,
- Calibrations using standards traceable to certified standards, preferably NIST, USP, or counterpart recognized national government standard-setting authority,
- Equipment qualification, calibration and maintenance, including computer qualification, validation and security,
- Control system for implementing changes in the equipment,
- Documentation of any discrepancy (a critical discrepancy investigation is covered under the quality system),
- Training and qualification of personnel.

Materials system

- Training, or qualification of personnel,
- Identification of starting materials, containers,
- Storage conditions,
- Holding of all material and APIs, including reprocessed material, under quarantine until tested or examined and released,
- Representative samples are collected, tested, or examined using appropriate means and against appropriate specifications,

- A system for evaluating the suppliers of critical materials,
- Rejection of any starting material, intermediate, or container not meeting acceptance requirement,
- Appropriate retesting or re-examination of starting materials, intermediates, or containers,
- First-in–first-out use of materials and containers,
- Quarantine and timely disposition of rejected materials,
- Suitability of process water used in the manufacture of API, including, as appropriate, the water system design, maintenance, validation, and operation,
- Suitability of process gas used in the manufacture of API (e.g., gas used to sparge a reactor), including, as appropriate, the gas system design, maintenance, validation, and operation,
- Containers and closures should not be additive, reactive, or absorptive,
- Control system for implementing changes,
- Qualification, validation, and security of computerized or automated process,
- Finished API distribution records by batch,
- Documentation of any discrepancy (a critical discrepancy investigation is covered under the quality system).

Production system

Training and qualification of personnel:

- Establishment, adherence, and documented performance of approved manufacturing procedures,
- Control system for implementing changes to process,
- Controls over critical activities and operations,
- Documentation and investigation of critical deviations,
- Actual yields compared with expected yields at designated steps,
- Where appropriate, established time limits for completion of phases of production,
- Appropriate identification of major equipment used in production of intermediates and API,
- Justification and consistency of intermediate specifications and API specification,
- Implementation and documentation of process controls, testing, and examinations (e.g., pH, temperature, purity, actual yields, clarity),
- In-process sampling should be conducted using procedures designed to prevent contamination of the sampled material,
- Recovery (e.g., from mother liquor or filtrates) of reactants; approved procedures and recovered materials meet specifications suitable for their intended use,
- Solvents can be recovered and reused in the same processes or in different processes provided that solvents meet appropriate standards before reuse or commingling,
- API micronization on multi-use equipment and the precautions taken by the firm to prevent or minimize the potential for cross-contamination,

- Process validation, including validation and security of computerized or automated process,
- Master batch production and control records,
- Batch production and control records,
- Documentation of any discrepancy (a critical discrepancy investigation is covered under the quality system).

Packaging and labeling system

Training and qualification of personnel:

- Acceptance operations for packaging and labeling materials,
- Control system for implementing changes in packaging and labeling operations,
- Adequate storage for labels and labeling, both approved and returned after issued,
- Control of labels that are similar in size, shape, and color for different APIs,
- Adequate packaging records that will include specimens of all labels used,
- Control of issuance of labeling, examination of issued labels, and reconciliation of used labels,
- Examination of the labeled finished APIs,
- Adequate inspection (proofing) of incoming labeling,
- Use of lot numbers, destruction of excess labeling bearing lot or control numbers,
- Adequate separation and controls when labeling more than one batch at a time,
- Adequate expiration or retest dates on the label,
- Validation of packaging and labeling operations including validation and security of computerized process,
- Documentation of any discrepancy (a critical discrepancy investigation is covered under the quality system).

Laboratory control system

Training and qualification of personnel:

- Adequacy of staffing for laboratory operations,
- Adequacy of equipment and facility for intended use,
- Calibration and maintenance programs for analytical instruments and equipment,
- Validation and security of computerized or automated processes,
- Reference standards; source, purity and assay, and tests to establish equivalency to current official reference standards as appropriate,
- System suitability checks on chromatographic systems,

- Specifications, standards, and representative sampling plans,
- Validation or verification of analytical methods,
- Required testing is performed on the correct samples and by the approved or filed methods or equivalent methods,
- Documentation of any discrepancy (a critical discrepancy investigation is covered under the quality system),
- Complete analytical records from all tests and summaries of results,
- Quality and retention of raw data (e.g., chromatograms and spectra),
- Correlation of result summaries to raw data; presence and disposition of unused data,
- Adherence to an adequate out-of-specification (OOS) procedure, which includes timely completion of the investigation,
- Test methods for establishing a complete impurity profile for each API process (note: impurity profiles are often process-related),
- Adequate reserve samples; documentation of reserve samples examination,
- Stability testing program, including demonstration of stability indicating capability of the test methods.

Appendix 6.2 Compliance to device and diagnostic GMP

This manual was developed by the FDA/CDRH for inspectors of device and diagnostic facilities. It is available in its whole form at www.fda.gov/ora/inspect_ref/igs/qsit/qsitguide.htm. Refer to Figure 6.2.

CDRH: quality system inspection technique (1999)

This guide to inspections of quality systems (QS) provides instructions for conducting medical device quality system and GMP inspections. It is to be used in conjunction with the compliance program entitled *Inspections of Medical Device Manufacturers* (7382.845).

Most device firms are inspected more than once. By probing different sub-systems, different devices or different processes each time, the FDA will eventually have covered most of the firm's quality system ... As a general rule of thumb, one day should be sufficient to cover each sub-system when using the "top-down" approach described within this document.

Management controls

The purpose of the management control sub-system is to provide adequate resources for device design, manufacturing, quality assurance, distribution, installation, and servicing activities; assure the quality system is functioning properly; monitor the quality system; and make necessary adjustments. A quality system that has been implemented effectively and is monitored to identify and address problems is more likely to produce devices that function as intended.

A primary purpose of the inspection is to determine whether management with executive responsibility ensures that an adequate and effective quality system has been established (defined, documented, and implemented) at the firm. Because of this, each inspection should begin and end with an evaluation of this sub-system.

Quality policy

The firm must have a written quality policy. It means the overall intentions and directions of an organization with respect to quality. The firm is responsible for establishing a clear quality policy with achievable objectives and then translating the objectives into actual methods and procedures. Management with executive responsibility (i.e., that has the authority to establish and make changes to the company quality policy) must assure that the policy and objectives are understood and implemented at all levels of their organization.

Management review and quality audit procedures

... the manufacturer has written procedures for conducting management reviews and quality audits and there are defined intervals for when they should occur. The firm's quality audits should examine the quality system activities to demonstrate that the procedures are appropriate to achieve quality system objectives, and the procedures have been implemented.

Quality plan

The firm must have a written quality plan that defines the quality practices, resources, and activities relevant to the devices that are being designed and manufactured at that facility. The manufacturer needs to have written procedures that describe how they intend to meet their quality requirements. Quality plans may be specific to one device or generic to all devices manufactured at the firm. Quality plans can also be specific to processes or overall systems.

Quality system procedures and instructions

The term "quality system"... encompasses all activities ... necessary to assure that the finished device meets its predetermined design specifications. This includes assuring that manufacturing processes are controlled and adequate for their intended use, documentation is controlled and maintained, equipment is calibrated, inspected, tested, etc.

Management controls inspection steps

(1) Verify that a quality policy, management review and quality audit procedures, quality plan, and quality system procedures and instructions have been defined and documented.

(2) Verify that a quality policy and objectives have been implemented.

(3) Review the firm's established organizational structure to confirm that it includes provisions for responsibilities, authorities, and necessary resources.

(4) Confirm that a management representative has been appointed. Evaluate the purview of the management representative.

(5) Verify that management reviews, including a review of the suitability and effectiveness of the quality system, are being conducted.

(6) Verify that quality audits, including re-audits of deficient matters, of the quality system are being conducted.

(7) Evaluate whether management with executive responsibility ensures that an adequate and effective quality system has been established and maintained.

Design controls (discussed in more detail in Chapter 4)

The purpose of the design control sub-system is to control the design process to assure that devices meet user needs, intended uses, and specified requirements. Attention to design and development planning, identifying design inputs, developing design outputs, verifying that design outputs meet design inputs, validating the design, controlling design changes, reviewing design results, transferring the design to production, and compiling a design history file help assure that resulting designs will meet user needs, intended uses, and requirements.

The design control requirements of Section 820.30 of the regulation apply to the design of Class II and III medical devices, and a select group of Class I devices. The regulation is very flexible in the area of design controls.

Inspection of design controls

If design control requirements are applicable to the operations of the firm, select a design project ... that provides the best challenge to the firm's design control system. This project will be used to evaluate the process, the methods, and the procedures that the firm has established to implement the requirements for design controls.

Utilize the firm's design plan as a road map for the selected design project. Plans include major design tasks, project milestones, or key decision points and must define responsibility for implementation of the design and development activities and identify and describe interfaces with different groups or activities. Verification and validation activities should be predictive rather then empiric. Acceptance criteria must be stated up front. Design verification activities are performed to provide objective evidence that design output meets the design input requirements.

Verification activities include tests, inspections, analyses, measurements, and demonstrations.

Review how the design was transferred into production specifications. Review the device master record. Sample the significant elements of the device master record using the sampling tables and compare these with the approved design outputs. These elements may be chosen based on the firm's previously identified essential requirements and risk analysis.

Corrective and preventive actions (CAPA)

The purpose of the corrective and preventive action sub-system is to collect information, analyze information, identify and investigate product and quality problems, and take appropriate and effective corrective or preventive action to prevent their recurrence. Verifying or validating corrective and preventive actions, communicating corrective and preventive action activities to responsible people, providing relevant information for management review, and documenting these activities are essential in dealing effectively with product and quality problems, preventing their recurrence, and preventing or minimizing device failures. One of the most important quality system elements is the corrective and preventive action sub-system.

Inspection objectives for CAPA

(1) Verify that CAPA system procedures that address the requirements of the quality system regulation have been defined and documented.

(2) Determine if appropriate sources of product and quality problems have been identified. Confirm that data from these sources are analyzed to identify existing product and quality problems that may require corrective action.

(3) Determine if sources of product and quality information that may show unfavorable trends have been identified. Confirm that data from these sources are analyzed to identify potential product and quality problems that may require preventive action.

(4) Challenge the quality data information system. Verify that the data received by the CAPA system are complete, accurate, and timely.

(5) Verify that appropriate statistical methods are employed (where necessary) to detect recurring quality problems. Determine if results of analyses are compared across different data sources to identify and develop the extent of product and quality problems.

(6) Determine if failure investigation procedures are followed. Determine if the degree to which a quality problem or non-conforming product is investigated is commensurate with the significance and risk of the non-conformity. Determine if failure investigations are conducted to determine root cause (where possible). Verify that there is control for preventing distribution of non-conforming product.

(7) Determine if appropriate actions have been taken for significant product and quality problems identified from data sources.

(8) Determine if corrective and preventive actions were effective and verified or validated prior to implementation. Confirm that corrective and preventive actions do not adversely affect the finished device.

(9) Verify that corrective and preventive actions for product and quality problems were implemented and documented.

(10) Determine if information regarding non-conforming product and quality problems and corrective and preventive actions has been properly disseminated, including dissemination for management review.

Medical Device Reporting (MDR) – CAPA satellite system

The Medical Device Reporting (MDR) regulation requires medical device manufacturers, device user facilities, and importers to establish a system that ensures the prompt identification, timely investigation, reporting, documentation, and filing of device-related death, serious injury, and malfunction information. The events described in medical device reports (MDRs) may require the FDA to initiate corrective actions to protect the public health. Therefore, compliance with medical device reporting must be verified to ensure that CDRH's surveillance program receives both timely and accurate information.

Reports of corrections and removals – CAPA satellite system

The corrections and removals (CAR) regulation requires medical device manufacturers and importers to notify the FDA promptly of any correction or removal initiated to reduce a risk to health. This early notification improves the FDA's ability to quickly evaluate risks and, when appropriate, initiate corrective actions to protect the public health.

Medical device tracking – CAPA satellite system

The purpose of the medical device tracking regulation is to ensure that manufacturers and importers of certain medical devices can expeditiously locate and remove these devices from the market or notify patients of significant device problems.

Production and process controls

The purpose of the production and process control sub-system is to manufacture products that meet specifications. Developing processes that are adequate to produce devices that meet specifications, validating (or fully verifying the results of) those processes, and monitoring and controlling the processes are all steps that help assure the result will be devices that meet specifications.

Inspection objectives for production and process controls

(1) Select a process for review based on:
  (a) CAPA indicators of process problems,
  (b) Use of the process for manufacturing higher risk devices,
  (c) Degree of risk of the process to cause device failures,
  (d) The firm's lack of familiarity and experience with the process,
  (e) Use of the process in manufacturing multiple devices,
  (f) Variety in process technologies and profile classes,
  (g) Processes not covered during previous inspections,
  (h) Any other appropriate criterion as dictated by the assignment.
(2) Review the specific procedures for the manufacturing process selected and the methods for controlling and monitoring the process. Verify that the process is controlled and monitored.
(3) If a review of the device history records (including process control and monitoring records, etc.) reveals that the process is outside the firm's tolerance for operating parameters or rejects or that product non-conformances exist:
  (a) Determine whether any non-conformances were handled appropriately,
  (b) Review the equipment adjustment, calibration, and maintenance, and
  (c) Evaluate the validation study in full to determine whether the process has been adequately validated.
(4) If the results of the process reviewed cannot be fully verified, confirm that the process was validated by reviewing the validation study.
(5) If the process is software controlled, confirm that the software was validated.
(6) Verify that personnel have been appropriately qualified to implement validated processes or appropriately trained to implement processes which yield results that can be fully verified.

Sterilization process controls – process control satellite system

The purpose of the production and process control sub-system (including sterilization process controls) is to manufacture products that meet specifications. Developing processes that are adequate to produce devices that meet specifications, validating (or fully verifying the results of) those processes, and monitoring and controlling the processes are all steps that help assure the result will be devices that meet specifications. For sterilization processes, the primary device specification is the desired sterility assurance level (SAL). Other specifications may include sterilant residues and endotoxin levels.

7 Reimbursement, marketing, sales, and product liability[1]

Plan	Position	Patent	Product	Pass!	Production	Profits
Industry context	Market research	Intellectual property rights	New product development (NPD)	Regulatory plan	Manufacture	Reimbursement

Roadmap of a product commercialization plan. Stage 7

Learning points

- Who are the purchasers and who are the payers in the health system in the USA?
- What is the flow of products and payments for devices and drugs in the US healthcare system?
- What are technology assessments and who uses them?
- What steps can a biomedical product company (drugs, devices, diagnostics) take to maximize revenues in the US healthcare system?
- What specific payer perspectives should be taken into account during product development?
- How can product development be planned for maximum reimbursement benefit?
- What factors influence pricing and revenue projections?
- How do new products gain recognition and reimbursement in the healthcare payment system?
- What is the role of marketing and how can it improve product acceptance?
- What product liability risks exist for manufacturers?

7.1 Introduction

The healthcare system of payments and reimbursements in the USA is a complex system and causes much confusion for those who are not familiar with the processes and the various players. Most other countries have a simpler single-payer system,

[1] This chapter has been significantly improved by the insights and editorial feedback provided by Parashar Patel, currently Vice President of reimbursement at Boston Scientific and past Director at CMS; and Jayson Slotnick, Director of Medicare Reimbursement and Economic Policy at the Biotechnology Industry Organization (BIO).

where the government is the dominant payer and the provider. A careful reading of this chapter along with active reference to other texts and the Centers for Medicare and Medicaid Services (CMS) website will help the reader gain the fundamental understanding required before launching a product in the USA.

Two commonly used terms in this chapter are: *providers* (healthcare providers, such as hospitals, clinics, pharmacies, physicians, etc.), who give services and administer products and are also the primary purchasers of biomedical products; and *payers* (private insurance companies, government), who reimburse the providers.

This chapter also emphasizes the role of reimbursement planning, which typically begins before clinical development of the biomedical product. This planning is used (1) to determine if the product can deliver appropriate returns, (2) to develop specific clinical data on performance and benefit, for differentiation of the product for payers and hospital and clinical customers, and (3) to identify possible strategic business relationships for product launch.

7.2   Healthcare system in the USA

7.2.1   Economic impact of the healthcare system

Healthcare spending has been increasing faster than the Gross Domestic Product (GDP, an aggregate figure that is used to assess the overall economy of a country) and is projected to reach 17% of GDP by 2011 (Table 7.1 and Figure 7.1; data from CMS). The rise over the last four decades threatens the stability of the US economy, as healthcare spending is now at about 15% of the overall economy and demographic trends indicate that this trajectory is likely to continue.

7.2.2   Insurance coverage of the US population

Most people (59.5% of the population) were covered by a health insurance plan related to employment for some or all of 2005, 9.1% purchased private insurance

Table 7.1 National healthcare costs – part of GDP and per capita

	1965	1980	2000	2004
National healthcare spend ($ billions)	$41	$246	$1359	$1878
Percentage of GDP	5.7%	9.1%	13.8%	16.0%
Per capita amount	$205	$2821	$4739	$6280
Source of funds		*Percentage of total*		
Private	75.1%	59.6%	55.7%	54.9%
Public	24.9%	40.4%	44.3%	45.1%

Source: CMS, office of the actuary, US Dept of Commerce, Bureau of Economic Analysis, US Bureau of the Census

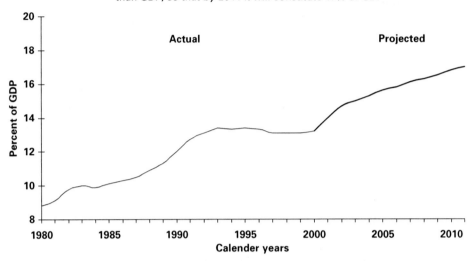

National health expenditures as a share of
gross domestic product (GDP)

*Between 2001 and 2011, health spending is projected to grow 2.5% per year faster
than GDP, so that by 2011 it will constitute 17% of GDP*

Source: CMS, Office of the Actuary, National Statistics Group.

Figure 7.1   National healthcare spending is increasing faster than the GDP and will reach 17% of
the GDP by 2011. Data and chart from the CMS. For current data and graph, visit
www.commercializingbiotech.com.

directly, and 27.3% were covered by public health insurance (Medicare, Medicaid,
or other programs) in 2005 (Figure 7.2 and Table 7.2; data from CMS and US
Census). A large percentage (15.9%) of the population was uninsured for at least a
portion of the year in 2005, as reported by the US Census Bureau (Figure 7.2). The
various public programs are described in more detail in 7.1.3.

7.2.3   Who pays for the national healthcare costs?

Eventually, we all pay for healthcare, one way or another. However, in the US
healthcare system, the payments to providers of services and goods are made by
third parties – public and private payers.

Public payers include the US government's Department of Health and Human
Services (DHHS), and the main agencies, the Centers for Medicare and Medicaid
Services (CMS), whose programs (Medicare and Medicaid, described below)
account for about one third of all payments in the healthcare system. If the
Veterans' Administration and other programs are included, the state and federal
governments pay almost half of the healthcare bills (Figure 7.3).

Medicare is a federal insurance program that covers most individuals over the
age of 65, the disabled (who satisfy certain statutory requirements) and end-stage
renal disease sufferers (totaling over 38 million people in 2005). Medicare is an
important trend setter and has a large impact on many providers because its

Table 7.2 Public and private coverage by age and other economic groupings

Age or other grouping	Dominant form of insurance coverage
65 and older	Predominantly *public* insurance with private self-purchased or employer paid
Needy and indigent and other select groups who would not be able to buy private care (end-stage renal disease patients, children)	*Public* insurance cover
Below 65 years of age	Predominantly *private* insurance through employers or direct purchase plus some public coverage (if in above groups)

Note: A significant percentage of the population is uninsured in the USA.

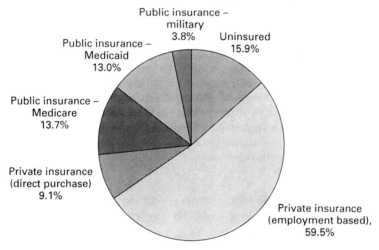

Insurance coverage in US population 2005

Public insurance – military 3.8%

Uninsured 15.9%

Public insurance – Medicaid 13.0%

Public insurance – Medicare 13.7%

Private insurance (direct purchase) 9.1%

Private insurance (employment based), 59.5%

Figure 7.2 Analysis of the health insurance coverage of the US population in 2005 shows that the majority of the population is covered by employer-based private insurance. Data from DeNavas-Walt, et al. (2006). For current data and graph, visit www.commercializingbiotech.com.

national decisions affect 38 million beneficiaries. Medicare has several parts (programs) that have evolved over time. Each part has a different annual deductible and co-insurance structure. Parts A and B reimburse the provider based on a prospective payment system, having evolved from an original fee-for-service payment structure (see Section 7.4.3 for details on payment system structures). Medicare coverage and payment policies are made at the national level. Administration (and in many cases, decision for coverage) is left to locally contracted entities. Legislation passed in 2003 will reduce the number of these local and regional Medicare carriers and fiscal intermediaries from over 50 to approximately 10 Medicare Administrative Centers (MACs). This process should be closely monitored because of its possible effect on local coverage decisions for new products (see Section 7.4.1).

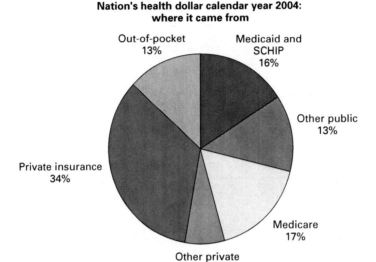

Nation's health dollar calendar year 2004: where it came from

Out-of-pocket 13%
Medicaid and SCHIP 16%
Other public 13%
Private insurance 34%
Medicare 17%
Other private 7%

Figure 7.3   The distribution of payments across various payers in the US healthcare system shows that the government pays for almost half of the healthcare bill. "Other public" includes programs such as worker's compensation, public health activity, Department of Defense, Department of Veterans Affairs, Indian Health Service, state and local hospital subsidies, and school health; "Other private" includes industrial in-plant, privately funded construction, and non-patient revenues, including philanthropy. Data and figure source: CMS, Office of Actuary, National Health Statistics Group. For current data and graph, visit www.commercializingbiotech.com.

Part A (Hospital Insurance) – most people do not pay a premium for Part A because they or a spouse already paid for it through their payroll taxes while working. Medicare Part A (Hospital Insurance) covers inpatient hospital care; including critical-access hospitals, and skilled nursing facilities (not custodial or long-term care). It also helps cover hospice care and some home healthcare. Beneficiaries must meet certain conditions to get these benefits and pay certain deductibles and co-insurance for each separate site of care. Under Medicare Part A, hospitals and other facilities are paid by Medicare fiscal intermediaries.

Part B Medical Insurance – beneficiaries, if they choose to enroll in Part B, pay a monthly premium for Part B. Medicare Part B covers doctors' services (in all settings), durable medical equipment, clinical laboratory services and outpatient care, and intravenous and injectable drugs. Medicare carriers pay doctors, durable medical equipment (DME) suppliers, ambulatory surgical centers, and other suppliers.

Part C: also known as Medicare Advantage – provides beneficiaries the choice of enrolling with private health plans to receive Medicare benefits. These private health plans must provide the same coverage as traditional Medicare (Parts A and B) and can also offer additional benefits, such as prescription drug coverage. Beneficiaries may pay an extra premium to cover additional benefits.

Part D: Outpatient Prescription Drug Coverage – individuals must pay a monthly premium, co-insurance, and annual deductibles for this coverage. As of January 1, 2006, new Medicare prescription drug insurance coverage is available to everyone with Medicare. Beneficiaries can choose either a stand-alone drug plan from a private company or a comprehensive benefit (Parts A, B, and D) from a private company.

Medicaid is a state-administered assistance program that covers people below the poverty level, in specific eligibility groups, and a large managed care population (the total number covered was about 45 million in 2005). The Medicaid program is administered by state Medicaid agencies and each state sets its own guidelines regarding eligibility and services. The federal government sets broad policies and shares in the cost (from 50% for higher-income states to over 70% for lower-income states).

Private insurers, who are paid premiums by employers and individuals, include companies like Blue Cross Blue Shield of Massachusetts, Anthem, Aetna, Cigna, Wellpoint, and HMOs (Health Maintenance Organizations) like Kaiser Permanente. These private insurers usually dominate regionally and cover all contracted healthcare services. Insurance policies have gone beyond their original intention and use, which was to safeguard against high-cost hospitalization events, and now cover routine medical care as well. Coverage is provided using a range of plan types that offer varying degrees of provider choice. Preferred provider organizations (PPO) and health maintenance organizations (HMO) are the two most common plan types.

This mix of private and public insurance coverage in the USA, with private insurance and Medicaid or private insurance and Medicare (for those above 65) is a unique system among industrialized countries as discussed further in Section 7.8. Figure 7.3 shows the source (payers) of the nation's healthcare spending dollars.

Medicare is often the most important payer for medical procedures in the patient population who are 65 years or older. This trend will only strengthen as the US population demographic shifts towards a more aged population. Additionally, Medicare reimbursement policies greatly influence the private payers.

7.3 Flow of payments and distribution models for products and services

In the US third-party payer system, the flow of funds from multi-party payers is described schematically in Figure 7.4. Wholesalers, who buy and stock products, sell these products to the providers – the hospitals, clinics, and other healthcare providers. The government and private insurance payers reimburse the providers, and the patients pay their assigned co-pay, unless they are uninsured. Thus, the payment system for healthcare products and services is a third-party payment system. The (insured) patient who receives the services does not directly pay the full payment for the services and in most cases does not know the true cost of healthcare products and services. Medicare is the predominant payer for patients above 65. Private insurance payers are the predominant payers for patients under 65 unless the patient falls into one of a number of special category groups (e.g., low income; veteran, end-stage kidney disease).

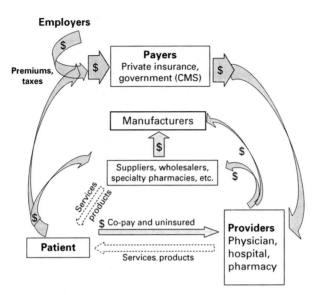

Figure 7.4   Flow of payments in the third-party payer US healthcare system.

An important conclusion from this schematic (Figure 7.4) describing the flow of payments is that the purchasing and payment decision is influenced by a variety of stakeholders, and so *most biomedical product companies will have to market their product and its context-specific benefits to different groups at the same time.* For example, an insurance company needs to be shown how the innovative product can reduce the overall costs of healthcare for a given health problem; a hospital, pharmacy, or physicians' clinic needs to know how the innovative product can increase efficiencies or operating margins compared with the total reimbursement they are given by the payers; and the patients must understand why the new product is better for them, especially if they can influence the usage decision. Physicians are the most important influencers of the purchasing decision for drugs, devices, and diagnostics, but in some instances, patients also have significant influence, as seen by drug companies' efforts to drive drug product purchasing or usage decisions by direct-to-the consumer (DTC) marketing.

While drugs are typically purchased from the manufacturer by wholesalers, devices are usually purchased from the manufacturers by hospitals or physicians directly or through group purchasing organizations (which negotiate discounts). The end providers the hospitals, the clinics, the hospital pharmacies, the retail pharmacy organizations – get reimbursed by the public or private insurers. *Given this flow of payments, most manufacturers' reimbursement and sales efforts are driven towards making sure that the hospitals and providers or direct purchasers get adequately reimbursed for purchasing the drugs or devices.*

Figure 7.5 shows the various groups in the healthcare systems to which the US healthcare dollar gets paid out – the providers of services and products and the intermediary distributors and wholesalers.

Nation's health dollar calendar year 2004: where it went

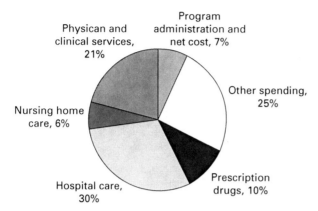

Figure 7.5 Percentage of healthcare payments to specific groups of service and good providers in 2004. Other spending includes dentist services, other professional services, home health, durable medical products, over-the-counter medicine and sundries, public health, other personal healthcare, research and structures and equipment. Source: CMS, Office of the Actuary, National Health Statistics Group. For current data and graph, visit www.commercializingbiotech.com.

7.4 Distribution and payment flow for biomedical product types

7.4.1 Drugs and biologics: product payment and distribution model

Drugs are distributed to the patient by two means: (i) self-administered drugs delivered through pharmacies, (ii) provider-administered or infused drugs (most biologics) delivered through hospital inpatient or outpatient settings, or a physician's office (Figure 7.6). Pharmaceutical manufacturers typically sell drugs in bulk to either wholesalers or large pharmacy groups. In the case of infused drugs, the purchasers are specialty pharmacies or pharmacies at care-provider institutions or physician's offices (Figure 7.7).

Thus, the payments flow as shown in Figure 7.6, from the payers through the providers or retail outlets (pharmacies, hospitals) and through the wholesalers to the manufacturers. When a prescription is filled at a pharmacy, the pharmacy collects any co-pay and then bills the insurance company or payer to get reimbursed for the drug.

Manufacturers offer discounts and rebates to the pharmacy benefit manager (PBM) companies that manage formularies and drug reimbursement programs for many different payers. These PBMs emerged in the period 1995–2006 as discount formulary negotiators, and now influence the providers and payers (hospitals and private insurers) to select specific drugs into a formulary. The various discounts and rebates (discounts for early payments, volume discounts, pre-negotiated rebates, etc.) offered to the supply chain parties (wholesalers, pharmacies, PBMs) make drug pricing a complex field. Large institutional pharmacies or chains of pharmacies

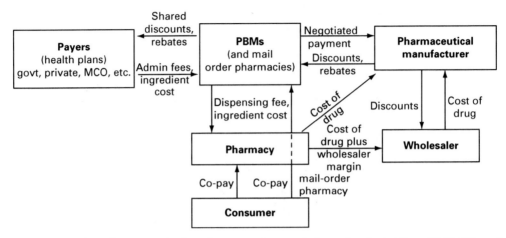

Figure 7.6   Flow of payments back to drug manufacturer (schematic adapted from CMS Office of Research Development and Information).

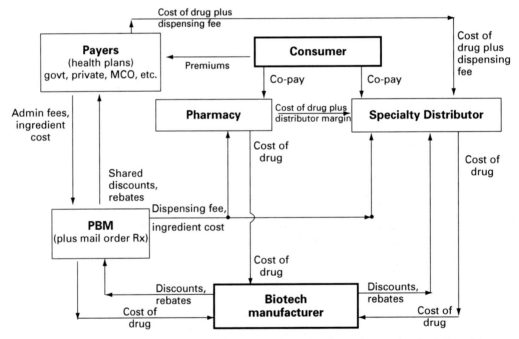

Figure 7.7   Payment flow for infused drugs (biologics and other drugs that need to be delivered by caregiver) through a specialty distributor. The PBM does not play a major role in this process.

and specialty pharmacies that have their own warehousing logistics can order direct from the manufacturer and thus pay the manufacturer directly. This specific flow of payments from pharmacy direct to manufacturer is also shown in Figure 7.6.

A *formulary* is a select menu of drugs that a managed care organization or insurer (Medicare, private insurers) will cover under its plan. The drugs are selected by a Pharmacy and Therapeutics (P&T) Committee in a hospital or through insurance plans. The P&T committee is composed of physicians, pharmacists, and administrators. The formulary not only lists drugs, but can also contain additional prescribing guidelines. The P&T committee reviews drugs based on parameters such as clinical safety and efficacy (compared with other products in that class), indications for use, dosages, method and route of administration, net cost, physician demand, and impact on total care costs and quality of life (pharmacoeconomic data).

Formularies are effectively used today as a formal system that assures the selection of cost-effective, affordable medications in quality patient care. If a physician wants to prescribe a drug outside the formulary, either the patient has to pay full price at the pharmacy, or the physician has to call in or write in to the health plan to obtain prior authorization, a time-consuming process that has to be repeated each time a refill is required. Two main types of formulary are those that will only pay for drugs on the formulary list ("closed formulary") and those that may vary the co-pay required for different drugs depending on a tiered system established in the formulary ("open formulary"). Drug manufacturers collect data and exert efforts to get their drugs positioned correctly in the "preferred" (lowest co-pay) tier. As an example of the importance of the formulary positioning, when Merck's Zocor drug went off-patent (patent expired) it agreed to drop its price to that of the generic medications. If it had kept its original price, Zocor would probably have been substituted or moved to a higher co-pay on formularies, as cheaper generics were now available. Merck could still retain its brand name recognition and use that to cross-sell other products to the formulary and the patients.

On the other hand, drugs that are infused through an intravenous catheter directly into the patient's blood or that need specific provider interaction for delivery *are reimbursed to the care-provider organization, as part of the procedure of administering the drug, in the same manner as devices.* Most of these infused drugs are biological drugs (proteins) or chemotherapy drugs that need special handling or care-provider monitoring and are infused in hospital settings or clinics. The biologics are typically distributed and sold through specialty distributors that also educate the patient and provide home-based services if needed (Figure 7.7). More details on the differences between infused and self-administered drugs (pills) are discussed in Sections 7.6 and 7.7.

7.4.2 Devices and diagnostics: product payment and distribution model

The flow of payments and distribution of product is similar for devices and diagnostics (and for provider-administered infused drugs). For devices, infused drugs, and diagnostics, the provider (the hospital if in the hospital, or the physician's office if outside) purchases the product and submits a claim to the payer charging for the services and the product. The service costs are derived as a combination of effort and facilities costs, making the site of delivery a major variable in the reimbursement payment. Thus, *device reimbursement is usually bundled with the overall procedure reimbursement and payment level is dependent on the site of delivery*, creating different dynamics in sales and product pricing for this product type, compared with self-administered drugs.

Medical devices are typically sold through specialized distributors or through a direct sales force to hospitals or clinics or to their purchasing consortia. The device and related procedures are delivered in the hospital or clinic and payments from the insurers or the patient are collected by both, the hospital, and the physician. The hospitals and clinics pay for the devices at purchase and typically hold the inventory, getting discounts that have been pre-negotiated through group purchasing organizations or directly with the manufacturer. The insurers and government payers typically reimburse the care provider (who purchased the device; usually the hospital) or the specialized distributor, or else the payers reimburse the customer directly (this is not common) if the patients themselves paid entirely for the product or treatment (e.g., for home medical products or out-of-network costs). Care providers can try to get expensive devices reimbursed separately from the all-inclusive cost of the specific procedure, but have to meet specific criteria (as per Medicare guidelines) for their product to be considered for "add-on" payment. Most payers will want to bundle the cost of the device with the cost of the procedure or other billing group. In this situation, not getting reimbursed adequately for an expensive device will result in pressure from the finance division of the hospital to discontinue or reduce use of the new device that was chosen by the physicians. This will, obviously, impact sales significantly. For cases where there is no reimbursement, the hospital or clinic bills the patient directly.

Clinical diagnostic tests that are cleared through the 510(k)/CLIA process, or approved via the PMA process, are usually sold to large centralized laboratories or to one of thousands of local clinical or hospital-based diagnostic labs. These products (reagents, diagnostic kits, etc.) are purchased by the laboratory or service provider organization within which the laboratory is housed (e.g., a hospital) and reimbursement is claimed directly from the insurers or payers per use as part of a procedure claim for the specific test or panel of tests based on the patient condition diagnosis (see Figure 7.8). The Deficit Reduction Act of 1984 required independent laboratories to bill Medicare directly, created a fee schedule (which is different for each local region) for lab services that capped payments, and eliminated beneficiary co-payments for laboratory services. This Medicare lab fee schedule was set based on what local labs were charging for tests in 1983 and has been periodically updated for inflation. The newer genomic diagnostics (nucleic acid tests or NAT) that are sold directly to certified labs as analyte specific reagents (ASRs) or as home-brew kits are also dealt with similarly. The outdated fee schedule for diagnostic laboratory tests is a disincentive for innovative new diagnostics that enter the market and is further discussed in Section 7.8.

7.5   Components of the reimbursement process

The previous sections gave a brief overview of the flow of payments and the distribution structure for the industry. *Reimbursement* is the key to healthy sales revenues in the biomedical marketplace, as most purchasers will buy more of your

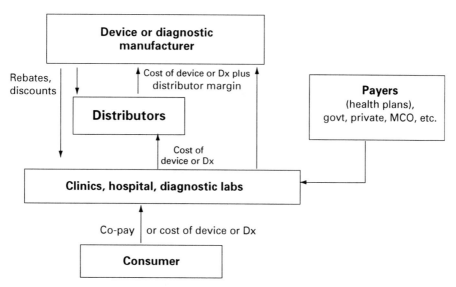

Figure 7.8   Payment flow for devices and diagnostics sold through distributors or directly through service providers to consumer.

product if there is an adequate third-party (insurance) reimbursement available to those purchasers (hospitals, individuals, care-providers) for those products. A few key questions that drive and control sales revenues underlie this section:

- Is the control on prices influenced more by the manufacturer, the third party payer or the purchasers?
- How does one get agreement for reimbursement for a newly approved drug or device from the various payers? In other words, how does a newly approved biomedical product get adopted and accepted into the reimbursement system?

The three components that must be in place for adequate reimbursement are discussed below – *coverage*, *coding*, and *payment*. Will the payer cover the product? Is there an appropriate code that the provider can use to bill the payer? Is the payment rate in reimbursement adequate for the provider?

Of these components, the manufacturer can influence the coverage decision by appropriate product development planning (clinical trial design and data collected) and by payer education; the manufacturers can influence the payment rates, as they set the price they wish to receive for their products and can use their collected data and payer education to achieve the right amount of reimbursement which will incentivize the purchasers. All three components must be in place for adequate reimbursement.

However, it is important to note that even if all three components are not in place, approved products may still be sold. In the case that the product does not fit into the standard process for reimbursement, the sales will not achieve their full potential, as each caregiver will either have to pay for the product themselves and then risk collecting full payments from patients, or they will have to struggle and do more work than normal to convince a payer to reimburse the product under the applicable insurance policy. These and other revenue ramp-up challenges can derail a company even after FDA approval for its products. The decision to use and order specific products is generally influenced by the physicians, but if finance departments in the hospitals or other purchasing organizations see that the cost of the product is not being recouped through the reimbursement process, they may intervene and sales will slow.

7.5.1   Coverage

This term refers to a payer's decision to provide program or plan benefit for a specific product or service. The process of making the decision to offer coverage is typically one of clinical, technical, and economic evaluation of an FDA-approved product or technology. Most payers will not accept a product into full review before it is approved by the FDA (see Box 7.1 for a discussion on this subject).

Since CMS/Medicare is the largest single healthcare payer for most patients over 65 (the most medically needy population) and because their review process

---

Box 7.1 Can a new device be covered for reimbursement before FDA clearance or approval?

A new device can achieve reimbursement before it gets FDA approval, but only after it has passed an IDE (see Chapter 5 for details of an IDE). The device must also be categorized as a non-experimental or investigational (Category B) device by the FDA:

A category B device refers to a device believed to be in Class I or Class II, or a device believed to be in Class III for which the incremental risk is the primary risk in question (that is, underlying questions of safety and effectiveness of that device type have been resolved), or it is known that the device type can be safe and effective because, for example, other manufacturers have obtained FDA approval for that device type [as in 42 CFR 405.201].

Once the device is categorized as a Category B non-experimental or non-investigational device by the FDA, this categorization is reported to CMS. Care-providers who are using this device in a clinical trial can appeal for coverage and reimbursement to the local Medicare insurance provider. Coverage evaluation will be made using standard criteria of "reasonable and necessary." If a positive coverage decision is made, the manufacturer could get paid for the use of the device in the clinical trial as the provider will get reimbursed, albeit the reimbursement will be at the rate established for previously approved similar devices and related procedures.

For further details, see FDA guidance document at www.fda.gov/cdrh/d952.html and related article from Device Link Online at www.devicelink.com/mddi/archive/03/05/018.html.

is public, the coverage decision by the CMS can have a significant impact on the coverage decision by other payers in the industry.

The FDA is a *regulator* and principally puts weight on safety and efficacy (see Chapter 5). Historically, the FDA and CMS have not communicated with each other. Obtaining coverage is usually a sequential process that follows FDA approval. Drugs (self-administered and provider-administered) are usually covered and reimbursed for their FDA-approved indication, mainly on the basis of the high quality of data generated during the clinical trials with placebo and randomized groups. However, if the clinical study did not cover specific patient groups that are a large component of a prescription drug plan, some insurers could drop the drug from their formulary. Over 85% of devices are usually cleared through the 510(k) process (see Chapter 5 for details) and the data required for clearance may not be rigorous enough to satisfy payers, whereas a device approved through the PMA process (Chapter 5) may have more rigorous clinical trial data.

The CMS is a *purchaser* that pays for services and products and heavily weighs the outcomes of clinical usage when making coverage decisions. Specifically, the Social Security Act [Section 1862(a)(1)(A)] mandates that the government agency (CMS) should only make payment if the treatment is "*reasonable and necessary* for the diagnosis or treatment of illness or injury or to improve the functioning of a malformed body member." The CMS applies the criteria of "reasonable and necessary" and evaluates whether there is adequate evidence to conclude that the item or service (1) improves net health outcomes, and (2) is applicable to the Medicare population.

There are three main routes to coverage:

(1) If a drug, or a procedure associated with a new device or diagnostic and the indication for which it is approved, falls under existing payment categories or codes, it will be covered by Medicare and can be covered simply by billing it under the existing payment category for the specific diagnosis or condition for which the technology is approved.

(2) A local coverage decision (LCD) by the Medicare Administrative Contractor (MAC), which holds authority for processing Medicare reimbursements in each specific region. Most coverage decisions (more than 90%) are local and the manufacturer must work with each region in turn to gain coverage.

(3) A national coverage decision (NCD) by Medicare/CMS is usually a route taken by the manufacturer or initiated by Medicare if the new technology represents a significant medical advance or if local coverage policies are inconsistent.

There are many benefits (e.g., a possibility to appeal a negative coverage decision) for companies to work through such local coverage decisions (LCD), even though it is more work than getting a single national coverage determination (NCD).

Currently, the CMS is not required formally to take cost-effectiveness into consideration while making coverage decisions. However, with the rising costs of healthcare weighing on the US economy and on its budget, the CMS is informally considering the impact of coverage decisions on healthcare costs (Box 7.2).

Box 7.2 Cost considerations and health economics

Payers do consider cost in making a reimbursement decision

In 2004, the CMS was faced with a difficult choice: two drugs, recently approved by the FDA were up for coverage and reimbursement decision: Bexxar from GlaxoSmithKline and Zevalin from Biogen Idec. The drugs, which cost about $28 000 for a single dose (also the entire course), were approved as a third-line treatment for non-Hodgkin's lymphoma, only after other treatments had failed. However, some physicians were using these expensive drugs as first-line medicines in "off-label" or unapproved indications. In a New York Times article ["US weighs not paying for all uses of some drugs" by Gardiner Harris, *New York Times*, 30 January 2004], Medicare officials were quoted as saying that cost was the program's primary concern in reviewing its reimbursement policy for Bexxar and Zevalin when they were used in non-approved indications (off-label use). Until then, Medicare was paying for all uses of approved drugs. It was apparent that the increased costs of these expensive drugs, which were being used by physicians in settings where their utility had not been proven by randomized clinical studies, led to a review by Medicare of its policy against these and other new expensive drugs used off-label in diseases such as cancer. A long review in early 2004 ended up with no change in national coverage policy for the use of these drugs and passed the problem to the local coverage decisions. In general, as long as the drugs were approved for one indication, the reimbursement decision for off-label uses was left to the individual local contractors. In their written decisions (accessed on the CMS website), the CMS declared that cost was not a consideration.

In the UK, the National Institute for Health and Clinical Excellence (NICE) is an independent organization, responsible for deciding which medicines are paid for on the National Health Service (NHS). The NICE has been issuing recommendations for taking drugs off the NHS list based largely on cost-effectiveness evaluations. These recommendations have generated significant public and industry discussion in the last few years, as many drugs which are being reimbursed in the USA and other European countries have been rejected as not being cost-effective enough by NICE.

Health economics
Health economics is a branch of economics concerned with the allocation and distribution of health and healthcare and covers the various types of analyses and sub-disciplines discussed below. Specific examples of health economic analyses are cost-minimization analysis, cost-benefit analysis, cost-effectiveness analysis and cost-utility analysis.

Cost effectiveness, healthcare economics and pharmacoeconomics
Cost-effectiveness (or cost-utility) is a measure of cost per unit of effective outcome ("effective outcome" varies with context and perspective) of a therapy,

Box 7.2 (cont.)

procedure, program, etc. For example, a common measure of effectiveness of a medical intervention is through quality-adjusted life years, or QALYs, based on the number of years of life that would be added by the intervention. The cost per QALY is typically used as a comparator or threshold to review a novel medical treatment or new intervention against the existing treatment paradigm. The UK agency (NICE) is typically said to use about US $30 000/QALY as the threshold to decide whether a new therapy is worth paying for by the National Health Service, whereas the general consensus in the USA is that a QALY figure of US $50 000/QALY or less is "cost effective" (i.e., if a medicine costs more than $50 000 and only increases the life of a patient by 1 year on average, it may be judged to be not cost effective enough and either the QALY count should increase or the cost must decrease for it to be covered for reimbursement). Various measures of cost effectiveness are typically used by private payer organizations to make decisions on coverage. The CMS does not formally include cost effectiveness in its decisions on coverage.

Cost effectiveness is only one factor considered by a broader field of study called health economics, which is a branch of economics concerned with issues related to scarcity in the allocation of health and healthcare.

Healthcare economics (as distinct from "health economics") is a term usually used in the industry to refer to cost considerations for the purchasers and an assessment of economic benefit afforded to the purchasers and users through adoption of the new products or services. These calculations usually integrate facilities and other costs and typically cover the entire referral chain up to discharge of the patient or resolution of the illness, assessing the economic impact to the entire healthcare system and particularly to the purchaser or payer. Healthcare economic data is collected by the manufacturer of the product and is typically used to help influence decision-making for purchasers or payers. For example, Smith and Nephew (a large medical device firm) states on its website in its 2005 report: "Healthcare economic considerations are integrated into the product development process to ensure that the benefits from the company's new products and line extensions not only seek to improve patient outcomes and, provide better treatment and procedures for both clinician and patient, but also contribute more cost-effective solutions for healthcare services … we also aim to deliver overall cost savings through such benefits [as] improvements in efficiency, such as reduced frequency of dressing changes, shorter operating theatre times, reduced length of time spent in hospital and overall faster patient recovery rates. Healthcare economic benefits are a primary focus in our product development and marketing." In recent studies with Lipitor (a cholesterol-reducing atorvastatin drug), Pfizer has explicitly referred to the reduction in hospitalization costs that result from the use of Lipitor, showing the economic value of prescribing that drug for the patient groups studied. Baxter's department of healthcare economics "has expertise in assisting healthcare

---

Box 7.2 (cont.)

providers, patients and payers with a variety of economic, insurance, and reimbursement-related issues." An increasing number of product development clinical trials are, a priori, including the collection of economic data in the trial design.

Pharmacoeconomics is a specific sub-discipline of *health economics* that compares the value of one drug therapy with another, considering costs and effects (discussed above). Pharmacoeconomic data are now regularly collected by manufacturers during clinical trials of their drug product and submitted to payers to help make the case for a positive coverage and formulary decision. Appropriate reimbursement planning processes have to be integrated into product development to make this part of the trial protocol, in addition to data collected for FDA approval.

See reading list at end of chapter for more details on these topics.

References

Smith and Nephew: www.smith-nephew.com/sustainability2005/rep-45.html

A website with ratios used in cost-utility analysis publications is at: www.tufts-nemc.org/ CEARegistry/

www.wikipedia.org

Private insurers may include economic analysis of the resultant change in overall healthcare costs for their own coverage decisions.

A key step in the coverage process for a new technology can be the *technology assessment* review. However, most devices (over ~95%) *do not* go through a formal coverage review process (technology assessment) as they are usually introduced and used as part of an already covered process. Most drugs also do not go through a formal coverage process, as the rigorous FDA approval process establishes the efficacy of the drug with pertinent endpoints. Private insurers or payers in other countries (e.g., the UK) are more likely to conduct technology assessments. In the USA, the private payers either follow CMS' lead in coverage decisions or perform a technology assessment.

The following criteria could be used by a technology assessment panel at an insurer or CMS (these are paraphrased here with permission from the Blue Cross Blue Shield Technology Evaluation Center (TEC)).

- The appropriate governmental regulatory bodies must approve the technology.
- Scientific evidence must permit conclusions about the effect on health outcomes.
- The technology must improve the net outcome.
- The technology must be as beneficial as any established technology.
- The improvement must be attainable outside the investigational setting.

However: (1) a positive technology assessment from a technology assessment organization like the Blue Cross Blue Shield TEC is no guarantee of coverage from different insurers, and (2) a negative technology assessment may occur even with an FDA-approved product, and insurers may still decide to cover the product. An example of an evaluation from the Blue Cross Blue Shield Technology Evaluation Center is in Appendix 7.1. This evaluation rejects a product that has passed FDA approval.

The rare technical assessment step to determine coverage for new technologies, either done internally at CMS or through one of several external technology review panels, is probably the most important reimbursement process step that can be directly influenced by the product development program and clinical study design. In particular, the quality of the data given by the manufacturer to the payer will dictate the coverage decision. The value of a product development plan that includes multiple inputs in planning becomes apparent here.

The data must address the above described technology assessment criteria. Frequently, the clinical trial design that is sufficient for approval (for example, a trial for 510(k) clearance) may not have sufficient rigor or strength of evidence to convince CMS or other private insurers or commercial payers. Additional data to prove cost-effectiveness of the product should also be collected (including the cost of ancillary services, radiological exams, lab and pathology tests, etc.) during the clinical trials as all payers will want to see some such data before offering coverage.

In general, the strength of the evidence decreases in order with the following designs of clinical trials (see Box 4.13 for a discussion of trial designs):

- Large double-blind, multi-center randomized control trial (patients are assigned randomly to treatment or control group, without the patients or the caregivers knowing which group is which – typical design for drug trials),
- Large, multi-center randomized control trial (patients randomly assigned with identification of control and treatment groups – typical in device trials),
- Meta-analysis of grouped data,
- Smaller, single-site RCTs,
- Prospective cohort studies,
- Retrospective cohort,
- Poorly controlled studies (historical controls),
- Uncontrolled studies (case series or reports).

A manufacturer designs trials to gain FDA approval and the various meetings with the FDA – pre-IND or pre-IDE meetings and pre-PMA or pre-Phase III meetings – are important points at which clinical trial design is discussed and agreed on (see Chapter 5). Similarly, the manufacturer could also meet with CMS's Coverage and Analysis Group or other payers, early during product development to receive input on trial design and the data to be collected based on the projected coverage requirements. However, the decision to meet with payers should be a carefully considered decision and is not necessary for most products.

The threshold for coverage varies among the private and public payers and the *value proposition* that is important for a coverage decision may be very different among these payers and may vary even more between countries. For example,

Avastin and Erbitux are two cancer (infused) drugs that are approved and reimbursed in the USA by most payers but are not covered for payment in the UK health system (as of August 2006).

7.5.2   Coding

Alphanumeric codes assigned to products and services allow for uniform and efficient processing of payments. Codes are used on insurance claim forms by purchasers or providers to get reimbursed. Codes are important for healthcare providers as they facilitate submission of claims and the use of codes enables payers to process and pay claims efficiently. However, getting a code is not a guarantee of coverage, nor is there any guarantee that the payment rate assigned to the code will be reasonable.

Although manufacturers do not use these codes (they do not normally seek reimbursement from the payers), knowledge of which codes apply to their products is critical to helping position their products and to help purchasers obtain adequate reimbursement. Therefore, many manufacturers provide education material to their customer to assist in billing appropriate codes for the procedures used with manufacturers' technologies. However, it should be kept in mind that the use of specific codes on claim forms is always at the sole discretion of the provider.

Two different types of codes are described briefly below:

- Codes that identify specific procedures or products: CPT, HCPCS, and ICD-9 procedure codes,
- Codes that identify diagnosis or disease: ICD-9 diagnosis codes.

CPT or HCPCS codes: The Current Procedural Terminology codes (CPT codes: a numeric coding system maintained by the American Medical Association (AMA)) *identify specific services carried out by physician*. The CPT codes are also synchronously published by the CMS, and in their system, CPT codes are called Level 1 HCPCS (Healthcare Common Procedure Coding System) codes. *Products and services* not included in the Level I HCPCS codes are identified in a group of Level II HCPCS codes. Some level II HCPCS code groups relevant to this book are:

B codes: Enteral (oral or through the gastrointestinal system) and parenteral (such as through intramuscular or intravenous injection) therapy,
C codes: Transitional pass-through codes for reporting new technologies that are used in outpatient settings,
D codes: Dental codes,
E codes: Durable medical equipment (DME),
G codes: Procedures or professional services,
J codes: Drugs and solutions (infused or injected; delivered by a caregiver),
L codes: Orthotics, prosthetics, and implant procedures,
P codes: Pathology and laboratory services,
Q codes: Temporary codes,
S codes: Temporary local codes (used locally; non-Medicare).

The International Classification of Disease Ninth Edition, Clinical Modification (ICD-9-CM) numeric codes classifies disease diagnoses (volumes 1 and 2) and procedures (volume 3). All hospitals and ambulatory care settings use this classification to capture diagnoses for administrative transactions. The ICD-9 codes are used by the hospitals on their inpatient claim forms. The USA is moving towards adoption of the enhanced ICD-10 classification. The ICD codes are managed by the World Health Organization (WHO) and in the USA, the American Hospital Association (AHA) and CMS act as clearing houses and consultants on this international standard.

- The ICD-9 diagnosis coding is matched up with and supports the CPT codes used for reimbursement of services or devices; these have to be consistently and correctly applied on claim forms.
- For almost all medical services and procedures there is a corresponding CPT code.
- Combinations of CPT and ICD procedure and diagnosis codes are packaged into the various context-dependent payment groupings (discussed in Section 7.5.3).

Other coding systems:

CDT-2: Current Dental Terminology (CDT) is used for reporting dental services. CDT-2 codes are also included in alphanumeric HCPCS with a first digit of D.

NDC: National Drug Codes (NDC) are used for reporting prescription drugs in pharmacy transactions and claims by health claim professionals. The NDC is a ten-digit code that is generated by the FDA, and identifies the labeler, product, and trade package size.

Drugs that are self-administered (pills or self-dosed solutions) are usually claimed for reimbursement through their NDC codes by pharmacies. Drugs that have to be administered by the caregivers are also assigned HCPCS level II J-codes or C-codes that must be used on the claim forms for reimbursement.

Diagnostics and devices get CPT or HCPCS codes for a procedure associated with the diagnostic test or devices. If the procedure associated with the product is not described by any of the existing codes, a new CPT or HCPCS code might have to be obtained – this is not an easy task and can take up to several years. This delay (depending on the timing of submissions and committee meeting dates) can really hurt a smaller company that was planning on a rapid uptake to generate sales revenue immediately after FDA approval or clearance. Assistance of the specialty physician group involved in the treatment is critical to getting approval for launching a new code (if one is needed) and manufacturers must work with the appropriate medical society from an early stage in the process. A written request is made by the specialty society to the appropriate American Medical Academy (AMA) committee detailing the need for a new code, along with a complete description of the procedure or service and with a full list of references to peer-reviewed articles published in US journals showing the safety and effectiveness of the procedure. The following website has more details on getting a new CPT code: www.ama-assn.org/ama/pub/category/3882.html.

7.5.3   Payment[2]

Note: the payment processes discussed here are assumed to be under CMS or Medicare, unless specifically mentioned otherwise.

Manufacturers set the price and get paid for their new technology by wholesalers, providers, or distributors as appropriate for each product type. However, understanding the system by which these purchasers get paid is critical to ensuring good sales and revenue growth. While not discussing pricing strategies here (pricing is a complex consideration that follows thorough review of not only reimbursement status, but also many market conditions and parameters), it is clear that an inadequate reimbursement level for a high-priced item will keep the new product from reaching its potential maximum market penetration and revenue. The manufacturer can influence the reimbursement payment levels by strategically planning the product development in the context of a reimbursement strategy (see Section 7.6). Further discussion on payment is split into two parts – one focusing on payment for drugs and the other focusing on payment for physician or provider-administered products (infused drugs, devices, diagnostics, etc.).

Payment levels (reimbursement to pharmacies) for drugs (for self-administered drugs; prescription pills, etc.)

These are based on pricing communicated by the manufacturers and negotiated by the payers (insurance companies, CMS) and providers (pharmacies, hospitals), and payments are calculated from either the average wholesale price (AWP), the average sales price (ASP) or other set formulas (drug acquisition costs to the retailer) reported by the manufacturer. Section 7.7 and Box 7.3 have more details on drug sales price terms. Other steps in the distribution chain may change the prices paid by insurers and retailers, such as rebates and discounts given through wholesalers and group purchasing organizations, pressure by state formularies, and negotiated discounted pricing or rebates to pharmacy benefit managers (PBMs). Physician-administered drugs (infused drugs) are usually reimbursed based on ASP data (Medicare reimbursed at 106% of ASP in 2005).

If the drug is not covered by the formulary or has not got "preferred" status, and the doctor has not been able to get prior authorization (a process within each health plan) for coverage, the patients may have to pay the full price for the drug at the pharmacy. Therefore, the bulk of efforts by manufacturers relate to positioning their drug in the preferred group in the formularies. These efforts may take several months after approval depending on the payer mix. Matching pricing and reimbursement levels for drugs is a complex issue, as different rebates and discounts offered to various parties affect the actual cost of the drug to the purchasers, as illustrated in Figures 7.6 and 7.7. Payers use their own standards to calculate reimbursement rates and various pricing calculations are described in Box 7.3. See Section 7.4.1 for some discussion on payment pathways for drugs.

---

[2] Some text in this section is reproduced from the MedPac documents on www.medpac.gov.

Box 7.3 Using drug pricing for payment or reimbursement

Average manufacturer price (AMP):   the average price paid to a manufacturer by wholesalers, for drugs distributed to retail pharmacies. Section 1927(b)(3) of the Social Security Act requires a participating manufacturer to report quarterly to CMS the average manufacturer price (AMP) for each covered outpatient drug. Section 1927(k)(1) defines AMP as the average price paid to the manufacturer by wholesalers for drugs distributed to the retail pharmacy class of trade, after deducting customary prompt pay discounts. The AMP data are not publicly available.

Average sales price (ASP):   defined in the Social Security Act (42 USC 1395w-3a), the ASP is reported by the manufacturer as the weighted average of all non-Federal sales to wholesalers net of chargebacks (see below for definition), discounts, rebates, and other benefits tied to the purchase of the drug product, whether it is paid to the wholesaler or the retailer. The basis for reimbursement for products covered under Medicare Part B changed under the Medicare Modernization Act of 2003 from AWP to ASP.

Average wholesale price (AWP):   the average price at which wholesalers sell drugs to physicians, pharmacies, and other customers. It is a figure reported by commercial publishers of drug pricing data and is used by payers to make reimbursement payments (AWP minus some percentage). The AWP is sometimes referred to as a "sticker" price and is not reflective of the true market price as it does not include the discounts or rebates given by the manufacturers. The basis for reimbursement for products covered under Medicare Part B changed under the Medicare Modernization Act of 2003 from AWP to average sales price (ASP).

Chargeback: when the manufacturer has negotiated discounts with PBMs or large pharmacies that bring the price to be paid by the pharmacies to the wholesaler lower than the AMP (the price paid by the wholesaler to the manufacturer), the wholesaler charges the manufacturer to make up the difference in payment – this is called a chargeback.

Wholesale acquisition cost (WAC):   the price paid by a wholesaler for drugs purchased from the wholesaler's supplier, typically the manufacturer of the drug. Publicly disclosed or listed WAC amounts may not reflect all available discounts.

Thus, the actual price paid by a provider for a particular drug product can be difficult to measure accurately, giving rise to fairly complex averaging calculations carried out by various payers.

Reference: Various webpages and glossaries at www.cms.org

Payment for products delivered with physician administration or in a provider facility (devices, diagnostics, physician-administered drugs):

Reimbursement for services and products are mainly composed of two or three parts:

(1) Payment to the facility for services and supplies provided (includes product cost), by Medicare Part A.
(2) Payment to the physician for services provided, paid by Medicare Part B.
(3) Sometimes, a specific payment is made for (a very few) new products that are deemed to result in "substantial clinical improvement," by Medicare Part B.

The payment process for these provider-administered products starts with the physician's notes in the medical record. The billing and coding department of a provider facility (hospital, physicians' office) reviews the notes and selects the appropriate diagnosis and procedure codes. Virtually all public and private payers require ICD-9 diagnosis codes in claim filings, to document the patient's illness and the reason for the treatments. The ICD-9 diagnosis codes help justify the medical necessity for a given procedure or product (identified by CPT or HCPCS codes). Accurate coding is a complex task for which compliance is critical and coders are trained on a regular basis.

The billing or claim form is then submitted to the payer (Medicare contractor), who reviews the coding and documentation for medical necessity and enters the various codes into grouping software. A group code is assigned by the software based on the location of service (see Figure 7.9), the base payment rate is looked up, and adjustments are made on the basis of the provider's charges and local pricing in each market area. The operating and capital payment rates are adjusted to account for facility and case-specific factors. If the procedure is deemed medically necessary based on the ICD-9 diagnosis codes, the calculated payment is sent to the provider facility and physician. All these steps are carried out through electronic data forms in computing systems. However, if the product is not covered or has been assigned a temporary procedure code, the provider is required to send a printed form, which is processed manually by the payer, resulting in significant delays in receiving payments and the documentation required to justify the charges can be burdensome to the provider.

How are payment levels for facilities and physicians set for given provider-administered procedures and products?

As shown in Figure 7.9, the combination of codes submitted in the claim form (usually electronically) to the payer describes procedures at a specific site of delivery for treatment of a given health problem (diagnosis code). The codes shown in Figure 7.9 are compiled by the payer's software into specific payment groups (e.g., DRG, APC, or ASC) based on recognition of the site of service – e.g., hospital inpatient locations, hospital outpatient locations, ambulatory surgical centers, or other clinics or doctors' offices. Each payment group or site of service has a different set of parameters applied to calculate the payment level, typically comprising capital payment rates that cover depreciation, interest, rent, insurance, and taxes, and operating payment rates that cover labor and supplies. The final calculated

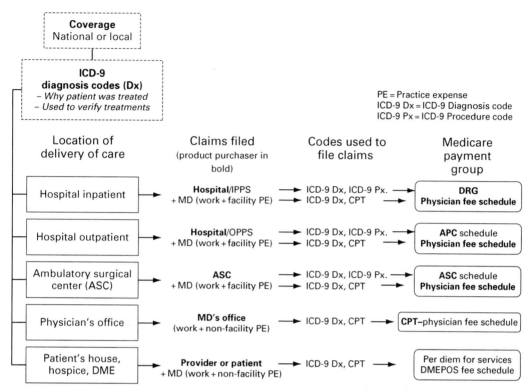

Figure 7.9 Payment codes and calculations of reimbursement amount vary by setting of healthcare delivery. DRG – diagnosis related groups, APC – ambulatory procedure classifications; DME – durable medical equipment, DMEPOS – durable medical equipment, prosthetics, orthotics, and supplies. Adapted, with permission, from original schematic by Parashar Patel, Boston Scientific.

reimbursement level thus depends largely on the setting in which the product or service is applied (Figure 7.9) and then on other case-specific factors, such as the complexity of procedures. This reimbursement is a lump-sum (or bundled) payment that includes the cost of the product. The cost of the product may be a large or very small part of the overall payment, depending on each product and associated procedures. For example, the cost of an artificial hip joint might be about $6500, which is a large portion of say, a $9500 average Medicare reimbursement payment to the hospital for the entire treatment until discharge of patient. This does not leave much room for increasing the price of the artificial joint unless a significant improvement in clinical outcome (e.g., savings to the hospital from a shorter stay) can also be shown. On the other hand, a catheter used in the same surgery may cost about $50 and may face less pressure from the hospital for increases in price.

Prospective payments are prices (calculated from formulas and processes laid out by law) that Medicare uses to reimburse hospitals for inpatient and outpatient services, as well as skilled nursing facilities, rehabilitation hospitals, and home health services. Most insurers work with this type of payment process. Payments to hospitals for inpatient services are made in the *inpatient payment system* (IPPS), using the Diagnosis Related Groups (DRG) codes. The DRG coding is based on the diagnoses for which the patient is admitted. The DRG codes work by grouping the 20 000 or more ICD-9 diagnosis and procedure codes into a more manageable number of meaningful patient categories (~500). Patients within each DRG category are similar clinically and in resource use. The payment amount is the same regardless of the length of the stay. Payments for medical devices and other physician-administered products are covered under DRG payment groups, and this has significant implications on revenue, marketing, and pricing considerations. Hospitals can also receive additional payments in the form of outlier adjustments for extraordinarily high-cost services or payments for qualified new technologies in the form of add-on ICD-9 procedure codes for the given DRG.

Another prospective facility payment system is the *outpatient payment system* (OPPS), based on the Ambulatory Payment Classifications (APC), which cover groups of procedures or services provided in outpatient settings. The unit of payment under the OPPS is the individual service as identified by HCPCS codes. The CMS classifies services into ambulatory payment classifications (APCs) on the basis of clinical and cost similarity. The OPPS sets payments for individual services using a set of relative weights, a conversion factor, and adjustments for geographic differences in input prices. New technologies that meet the CMS criteria become eligible for "transitional pass-through" payments. New services remain in these pass-through APCs for two to three years while the CMS collects data necessary to develop payment rates for them, after which they are bundled into an APC payment rate. More than one APC payment may be made during one episode of care, depending on the services required. The CMS pays separately for professional services, such as physician services.

The physician's payment is based on a relative value assigned to the specific procedure code and is based on the location and the physician's specific practice. Medicare refers to the Physician Fee Schedule, which is an elaborate price list that Medicare uses to pay physicians for their services (and also to pay other healthcare providers for items and services that are not bundled into prospective payment systems). Physicians are paid separately from the hospital for the procedures they perform. After a product is approved or cleared by the FDA for a specific indication, and a procedure code (or codes) is assigned or established, a relative value is assigned to that procedure code by an AMA sub-committee, starting from the recommendation of the medical society representing that practice or therapeutic area (e.g., American Academy of Dermatology, American Academy of Otolaryngology, and others). The manufacturer thus works collaboratively with the medical society from an early stage to establish the appropriate detailed procedures and costs involved with using that product, including establishing the clinical benefits to the various stakeholders in the process. The relative value of a physician's service is calculated based on (1) the cost to provide service–practice expenses, professional liability insurance, etc., (2) the physician's labor, effort, skill, and time, and (3) practice expenses based on rent, supplies and equipment, and other staff costs.

This value is then passed on to the CMS, which usually accepts the AMA committee's recommendation. A recent abrogation of this process, when Johnson & Johnson got the CMS hospital payment review started before FDA approval was obtained for their drug-coated stent (Cypher^{TM}), gained kudos from industry rivals but also raised a lot of controversy.

If a procedure for which the device is used cannot be described by an existing CPT code, a "not otherwise classified" (NOC) or other similar generic code is used and pricing and reimbursement has to be worked out each time a procedure that uses the device is billed. If coverage is denied, either the provider will have to work with the insurer's process to help obtain some level of payment from the insurer or the patient may have to pay out of pocket (there are several more complicating issues in this patient liability, depending on the benefit package and contractual arrangements). Therefore, not having a CPT code assigned can hamper device sales, preventing a product from reaching its market potential. However, the case in Box 7.7, later in this chapter, is an interesting example of a company that successfully got a higher reimbursement level for their new product by working the system aggressively with a temporary CPT code.

For *diagnostic products*, the clinical laboratory payment environment is largely based on Medicare-published schedules that use CPT codes for each diagnostic step or set of processes. The CMS has established the laboratory fee schedule, which is a schedule of CPT codes and corresponding payment rates. Each CPT code could cover individual components of laboratory tests or a panel of tests together as one bundle. This schedule is used as a benchmark for reimbursement and contracts between laboratories and private insurers. More details on pricing and payment for specific product categories are discussed in the following sections.

It is important to remember that when Medicare relative value units are assigned to procedure codes (CPT codes and ICD-9 procedure codes), the payment levels calculated in various payment systems (Figure 7.9) are fixed for a given year, with annual adjustments influenced by new data, grouping changes, or policy changes. Because government policies may have a major influence on payment rates set by other insurers, powerful manufacturers', hospitals', and physicians' lobby groups work to provide input to CMS and to exert pressure through Congress when changes in payment rules are proposed by CMS. In general, manufacturers should stay aware of specific policy changes (see Box 7.4) that could completely change market conditions, open new markets or close an existing product market.

Private insurers do not have to follow the CMS relative values and can assign their own values to the procedures and services associated with the new product. Other types of payment systems used by other payers are:

Capitation fee structures are used by private insurers who contract with a healthcare provider to pay a fixed fee for all care furnished by the provider, but unpredictable increases in costs are turning many groups away from this method of payment. *Carve-outs* are payment contracts built to avoid the risk associated with capitated contracts, allowing for specific separate payment for new technologies or procedures.

Box 7.4 Policy changes can affect reimbursements and revenues

The healthcare industry is highly regulated through all aspects of the value chain.

Regulations are laid down in response to laws that are passed by elected representatives. These representatives are sensitive to political pressures and public opinions.

As seen by the example below, laws and regulations can affect payment and reimbursement for many products and services, as the government (Center for Medicare and Medicaid Services, Veteran's Administration, and others) is the largest single payer for healthcare in the country.

Case example: Amgen, Epogen, and the government in April 2007

The drug: Amgen has been selling Epogen (erythropoietin; a stimulant of red blood cell production), a protein drug that stimulates the production of red blood cells in the body, reducing the need for transfusions.

The application: The major market for this drug is dialysis patients who need regular transfusions. Epogen was approved for the reduction of transfusions in patients undergoing dialysis. Physicians titrate Epogen by more frequent or higher doses to get patients' hemoglobin content to 10–12 mg/dl (normal range) or slightly higher for some, to 13 mg/dl. Recent data have shown that dialysis patients with a hemoglobin target of 13 mg/dl or more are at higher risk for heart attack, stroke, or death.

The market: The 2006 world-wide sales of Aranesp and Epogen (EPO drugs) for dialysis and chemotherapy induced anemia were $6.6 billion.

The payers: The US government (CMS) is the largest customer for Amgen as 93% of dialysis patients qualify for the Medicare End-Stage Renal Disease program.

The story: A *Wall Street Journal* article on April 10, 2007 reported that private dialysis centers made high profits from buying a lower-priced drug and getting higher reimbursement from Medicare as the drugs are reimbursed separately. These doctors and centers potentially had financial incentives to over-prescribe the use of Erythropoietin drugs and a House Ways and Means committee meeting in December 2006 noted that 40% of dialysis patients had hemoglobin counts greater than 12 mg/dl.

The politics: The House Ways and Means committee wants the CMS to eliminate separate payment for erythropoietin drugs, bundling this payment into the overall cost of dialysis, thus forcing clinics to focus on overall profit margins and removing financial incentives to over-use erythropoietin drugs. The chair of the committee said (as reported in the article) that Congress would have to act to safeguard the public from abuse from profit-seeking centers, if CMS did not change the payment schedule, a gross demonstration of how politicians and regulation influence the biomedical market.

> **Box 7.4** (cont.)
>
> *Note:* While the Erythropoietin drugs are an unusual case in terms of government focus on a drug, elected representatives in particular are very conscious of their constituents' complaints on the high cost of healthcare and manufacturers of biomedical products (drugs, devices, and diagnostics) must engage with their representatives and industry associations to make sure that appropriate information is delivered to the decision makers who can influence the healthcare markets.

7.6   Reimbursement planning activities

Reimbursement planning activities begin in the very early stages of product development when market assessments are made (Figure 7.10). Most smaller companies do not explicitly consider reimbursement planning, as it is a complex area of analysis, but implicitly look at it through market research, potential pricing and revenue forecasts, and competitive assessments of the market. Most start-up device companies focus on approval of the device and do not have the resources to engage a full-time reimbursement professional or spend the $500 000 or more required to launch a complete reimbursement program that addresses all three pillars of reimbursement – coverage, coding, and payment. However, there is a clear value and need emerging for active and explicit reimbursement planning, as healthcare costs increase and pricing pressures affect reimbursement, which can no longer be taken for granted once approval or clearance is achieved for a device. These smaller companies that do not have experienced reimbursement personnel in-house are best advised to consult reimbursement and regulatory experts at an early stage to assess the specific steps (and timing of those steps) of reimbursement activities to achieve maximum value of their products. An option for start-up device companies would be to focus on only one specific issue among the three, the most inexpensive being the coding aspect.

The first review of reimbursement issues arises when a patient population is identified as being the most appropriate (target) for the new product (Figure 7.10). Based on the population demographics, identify the payer mix and start planning the reimbursement strategy to target a specific payer. During the product development phase of clinical trials, collect data related to FDA approval and also cost and economic data (see Box 7.2) related to reimbursement. The reimbursement data should typically satisfy the value proposition that will be evaluated by the payers and should be able to meet at least the technology evaluation criteria discussed in 7.5.1. However, it is useful to reiterate that most devices and diagnostics can be described by existing codes, are covered, have appropriate payment, and will not go through a detailed and formal technology evaluation by the payers.

As explained further in section 7.11, reimbursement planning can be valuable to the marketing function of a company. Market research is used during product development to assess market perceptions of pricing, acceptance, awareness of product, and the possibility of reimbursement or coverage by payers. Marketing

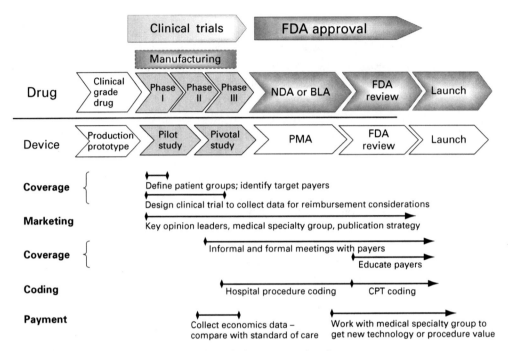

Figure 7.10   Timing of activities related to reimbursement planning.

efforts at the early product development stages are focused around awareness, aiming to influence the coverage decisions by increasing awareness of the product technology or novelty and its value proposition (see Section 7.11). Educating payers is also another vital component of marketing efforts.

Just as there are meetings with the FDA during product development, companies can meet payers in informal and formal meetings to convey information and data on clinical usage of their products and to get guidance on development parameters or product characteristics. In particular, economic usage data requested by payers, if collected during clinical trials (Figure 7.10), may increase the development costs, but these costs may be recouped in the faster rise in sales due to quicker acceptance of coverage, coding, and appropriate pricing. Economic and clinical outcome data could also help in achieving a suitable pricing level for the product. *Note*: these efforts must be done with some advanced understanding of the field, otherwise there is a risk that the product could end up with more scrutiny than needed and greater burden; the company might do better in some cases not to be too aggressive in these efforts, and the judgement needs to be made thoughtfully and with some consultation among people experienced in reimbursement.

7.7   Reimbursement path for self-administered drugs (mostly pills)

Drugs that are taken directly by the patients have a fairly straightforward reimbursement path. The manufacturer has to approach the various providers (payers, hospitals, etc.) with the FDA approval letter and then demonstrate, with existing or additional clinical trial data, the value proposition of their drug and establish a price point for their drug. On approval, the drug is automatically assigned a NDC code and coverage for approved indications is almost automatic. Most FDA-approved drugs are covered and paid for by insurers as the clinical trials required for drug approval are more rigorous than for devices, and the efficacy and safety balance is usually clearly established by the FDA approval and label. However, patients may have one or more levels of co-payment and pharmacies or providers may have different reimbursement levels, depending on the tiers in the formulary (see Section 7.4.1). In the process of reimbursement planning, once an indication is chosen for the new product, the patient demographics can be determined and subsequently the specific insurer mix is identified. Since private payers and Medicare Part D and Medicaid/VA payers have different approaches to managing their formularies and pricing, the company can start to bring this reimbursement feedback into the portfolio planning discussions. In particular, once the specific insurers are identified, various points of emphasis in the clinical trial – from the data to be collected, to trial design or patient recruitment strategies – become clear and a reimbursement strategy can be developed hand in hand with the product development plan (Figure 7.10). Pharmacoeconomics is the discipline that calculates and demonstrates the effectiveness of drugs (Box 7.2) to payers and formulary committees. Most large companies have specific personnel who are trained in collecting this data.

7.8   Reimbursement path for devices and infused drugs

In many cases, early stage biotech drug or device companies whose product has reached this stage and who plan to take their product to the market themselves, will want to contract with a third-party logistics provider or consultant to help navigate these complex steps. Clearly, the providers or consultants need to be hired at an early stage of development, as seen in Figure 7.10.

- Reimbursement planning begins in the pre-clinical phase, where the target patient population affected by the disease and treatment or diagnosis is identified.
- The mix of patient demographics affected by the targeted disease will dictate the mix of payers. For example, product A targets a patient population with the following demographics (payer mix):
  10% – Medicare,
  70% – Under 65 years of age, private payers (e.g., Cigna, United Health Care, Blue Cross, Blue Shield),
  10% – Medicaid.

- As public and private insurers pay differently for the same treatment, the information about payer mix expected for a particular product could be used as a component input into the portfolio selection process and also into product pricing and development planning activities.

- The manufacturer could approach representatives from the payers to discuss the planned clinical benefit from their technology and also familiarize the payers with the novelty and advantages offered by the technology. *Note that: most products will not need to approach the payers*, as payments can be generated by simply selling the approved product to the buyers (care providers or patients) with a matching code that fits into the existing reimbursement plans. Meeting the payers could create additional (negative) ramifications and this decision should be made in consultation with someone familiar with the reimbursement systems and processes.

The path diverges here between physician-administered drugs and devices or diagnostics.

7.8.1   Reimbursement path for physician-administered drugs (continued)

- While drug marketing approval is being obtained from FDA, meet payers to familiarize them with technology, benefits, etc. (see cautionary note above).
- When a drug is approved by the FDA, reimbursement coverage for the approved use is usually assured as soon as it is sold. Reimbursement levels can be influenced by the manufacturer as described in Section 7.7. Physician-administered drugs are typically reimbursed under a J-code in the CPT (procedure codes), or could get one of the temporary J-codes, such as J9999.
- The growth in sales will be hindered with a temporary code, because a temporary code requires a physician or provider to purchase the drug up front, fill out a paper form, send it in to the insurance company or payer, address any specific questions from the payer, and finally receive payment a few weeks later. On the other hand, an established code can be entered electronically and payment is received rapidly once the payment amount is established.
- Getting a permanent J-code for the physician-administered drug is a process that can take from 8 to 18 months, depending on the timing of FDA approval and the CPT panel bi-annual meeting date. A submission that does not get in for the first panel meeting at mid-year will take 18 months to be assigned a new permanent code.
- The submission can be made with some assistance from the medical specialty group, but the involvement of the medical specialty group is not as important to this process as it is for the devices, which typically involve much more procedural work by the medical specialty group.
- Payment for physician-administered drugs provided in a physician's office is primarily based on the price of the drug as the work component of the procedure is a small part of the total reimbursement. Drugs administered in the hospital to inpatients are paid (reimbursed) under a DRG (IPPS system) payment which reflects the total cost of administering the drug in the inpatient system. Similarly, payments for drugs administered in the outpatient setting are paid through the APC (CPT J-codes) schedule in the OPPS system. If the drugs are administered in an ambulatory surgical center, the payments are based on the prospective ASC fee schedule. The different types of reimbursement pathway for a drug can influence the value of the project, the marketing strategy, and other development considerations (see Box 7.5).

Box 7.5 Same disease, similar drugs, different reimbursement
paths and planning

*Written with assistance from Jayson Slotnik, JD, MPH, currently Director of Medicare
Reimbursement and Economic Policy at the Biotechnology Industry Organization (BIO).*

Differing reimbursement structures affect reimbursement planning, clinical trial
design, marketing strategies, and patient assistance programs. The example
discussed here shows how differing reimbursement paths between two competing drugs can impact drug development and clinical decision making.

Etanercept (Enbrel) and infliximab (Remicade) are protein therapeutics that
bind to TNF-alpha (a naturally-occurring protein) and inhibit the inflammation
caused by the release of TNF-alpha at sites of rheumatoid arthritis or other
pathologies. The drugs are both approved for treatment of rheumatoid arthritis
but are administered differently, creating distinct reimbursement issues and
considerations. Both drugs are expensive, with 100 mg of each costing ≈$650
to $700 and with an annual cost of $10 000–$16 000 to treat a patient with
rheumatoid arthritis.

Etanercept is a protein that mimics the receptor of TNF-alpha and inhibits
TNF-alpha. This drug is self-administered by the patient with a single injection
below the skin twice every week and is therefore covered by either the patient's
pharmacy benefit or Medicare Part D. In this case, the specialty pharmacy or
regular pharmacy gets reimbursed by both the insurance company (or
Medicare), under drug prescription benefits, and the patient's co-pay.

Infliximab is a monoclonal antibody that is part human and part murine,
requiring co-administration with methotrexate. The drug must be administered
in a physician's office or hospital setting by intravenous infusion over 2 hours
every 6–8 weeks with the provider buying the drug and receiving reimbursement
under either the patient's medical benefit or Medicare Part B. The physician's
office or hospital charges the insurer using procedure codes covering the work
done for the infusion and cost of drug.

Because of the differing reimbursement structures, each therapy must overcome certain challenges to gain market share and manage pricing pressures. For
example, because Infliximab is intravenously administered by a provider and
covered under Medicare Part B, the hospital or doctor's office (provider) must
first purchase the therapy and then collect part of the payment from the
government and the remaining part from the patient. The expense of this drug
obviously hinders cash flow for the provider as they have paid for the product
but may have to wait for reimbursement. The payment situation also poses
certain cost challenges for both the patient and the provider. This dynamic
creates pricing pressure on the manufacturer. On the positive side, since there
is no formulary in this outpatient setting for the physician-administered drug,
coverage is essentially guaranteed.

Etanercept has contrasting positives and negatives. Because Etanercept is
self-administered, it is generally covered under Medicare Part D. However, the

Box 7.5 (cont.)

manufacturer must negotiate for formulary placement with each of the hundreds of Medicare plans and the other private insurers. On the positive side for the sales environment, the provider is not involved in the cash flows and the patient liability is capped at their annual deductible, reducing the pricing pressure on the manufacturer.

Both companies probably have to make different types and levels of investment in patient assistance programs and would also probably adjust their marketing mix to the specific purchase-influencers (physicians or patients) for each drug, based on the mode of administration. Reimbursement planning in this case offers significant insight into pricing pressures and issues around market acceptance or sales projections.

This example shows that an understanding of the reimbursement dynamics, in addition to studying potential product competition and market acceptance issues, should be used to make better decisions or plan better early on in the manufacturer's drug development process. Drug developers should ask the following questions as part of their early product and reimbursement planning:

- What is the targeted population (demographics, etc.) and resulting payer mix?
- Do we want to focus on CMS or private plans for coverage and reimbursement?
- Are the patients healthy enough to self-administer?
- Do we want to market to patients or physicians?
- What is our pricing and discounting strategy?
- What is our patient assistance strategy?

7.8.2   Reimbursement path for devices (continued)

- While device marketing approval is being obtained from the FDA, meet with payers to familiarize them with technology, benefits, etc. However, as noted above, a sophisticated understanding of the overall process should be used to decide on the need or timing of such meetings to make sure that they do not create additional hurdles to coverage and payment.
- A major difference between approved infused drugs and marketed devices is that FDA approval or clearance for marketing a new device does not always mean that reimbursement will be provided by the payers.
- Describe the procedure and the caregiver setting (inpatient, outpatient, physician's office) in which the device will be used or delivered. Identify if an existing CPT code will apply to this procedure (if applied in the inpatient setting, identify an ICD-9 procedure code as well). Simultaneously, determine the ICD-9 diagnosis code used to describe the patient indication or problem. Combinations of these various codes will point to the specific payment grouping code that will be

used to pay the providers in the various payment systems (see Figure 7.9 and Section 7.5.3). The various groupings are discussed separately below.

IPPS: inpatient payment system

- The combination of the diagnosis code and the procedure codes will be used by the payers' grouping software to determine the DRG group code. From the DRG code, the manufacturer can determine the specific payment that the hospital will receive for carrying out the procedure. Payment for the device is included in the DRG payment level, bundled as a single payment that includes hospital costs. Thus, if the DRG for a new device is not adequate to cover the increased cost of a new improved device (i.e., cuts into hospital operating profit margins), there is a disincentive for the hospital to purchase and continue to use the device unless the device helps in improving efficiency and increases savings in some part of the overall procedures covered under that DRG. For example, if a new and improved device leads to a reduced hospital stay, the hospital might be able to save enough (the current DRG pays for the longer hospital stay in its bundled single payment) to justify the higher purchase price of the new device.
- On the other hand, if the procedure for the device falls into a DRG that does not pay adequately then the manufacturer has a couple of options (outlined below), but these options will take time to be implemented and revenues will probably suffer in the meantime (a few years). Therefore, the reimbursement assessment must be made at an earlier time so that the manufacturer can make appropriate portfolio investment decisions or cash flow adjustments.
- Insurers carry out annual reviews using past data on claims submitted for similar procedures and set appropriate payment levels for a procedure or group of procedures. The manufacturers can inform the providers or hospitals that placing a charge for the new device on the claim forms submitted to insurers may eventually register in the system as a DRG that needs increased payment. The hospital charges will initially be reimbursed at the set DRG group rate, but if a significant number of sites start using a more expensive new technology, then after a couple of years, the annual reviews will show that this grouping code needs to be raised to account for these consistently higher charges. The problem is that several years could pass before a higher payment is recognized for that DRG. During that time hospitals will probably progressively reduce the purchase of items for which they lose money due to inadequate reimbursement and the product never gets used by enough sites to show up in the national review of DRG charges, leaving the payment rate unchanged. However, if the technology has clear benefits and is a physician-preferred item, there is a possibility that the hospital will continue to purchase the device and may even increase purchases over time.
- An argument could be made to CMS for higher-valued payment by grouping into a new DRG –this is done by an initial appeal (with assistance from the medical specialty group) to the CMS, followed by review by CMS – and could take several years for them to collect the data to justify the right level of payment

and the new grouping. The manufacturer might speed up this assessment if they can present relevant economic data collected in a clinical trial (see reimbursement planning notes above).

- In the interim, in the DRG (inpatient) setting, if the device meets CMS criteria (or other payers' criteria), an add-on payment may be made to the hospital. Evaluation is based on criteria of newness, clinical benefit, and cost.
- If neither of these options work under an existing set of codes, then a new set of ICD-9 procedure codes must be applied for.

OPPS: outpatient setting

- The CPT codes are grouped into the appropriate APC codes (see Figure 4.9).
- The CPT codes for the procedures involving the device are used to identify the APC group code and thus determine the APC payment level. If the payment is not adequate to cover the new device, and the device qualifies as a new technology with significantly improved clinical outcomes or benefits, an add-on payment at cost of the new device may be approved as a "transitional pass-through" payment. The additional reimbursement is based solely on CMS's estimate of the cost of the new device based on hospital charges for the device. This is a transitional code, which is used to collect claims data and in a couple of years this payment level is rolled into an existing or new APC.

Physician's fee schedule: based on CPT procedure codes

Payment is made by accounting for specific physicians' work in the procedure and their practice fees (facility practice fee if carried out in a hospital and non-facility practice fee if in their own offices).

- If no suitable CPT code currently exists to pay the physician for performing additional services with the new technology, collaborate with the appropriate Medical Specialty society and file an application for a new code with appropriate data, with the AMA (American Medical Association) CPT Editorial Committee (see Section 7.5.2 above). Work with the appropriate medical specialty society or AMA committee to get a value assigned to the CPT code for reimbursement basis. Assistance from a medical specialization association is critical at this stage. A reimbursement relative value scale is used to assign values to the new CPT code depending on the complexity of the procedure (attested to by the professional specialty association). For clarity, note that the cost of the device to the hospital is covered under the DRG or APC payments if the procedure is performed in the facility setting.
- Wait for 18–24 months for a new permanent code to become active. Until that time, a temporary procedure code or transitional or add-on code can be applied for as described above. Without permanent codes and approved coverage, the risk of the payer refusing reimbursement or extra efforts required by the physician to get reimbursement could reflect in their choice to recommend purchase or use of new devices.

Final steps

- Set up customer service at the company to assist providers or patients with the reimbursement process. Publish educational materials describing appropriate billing codes, coverage rules, and payment rates and policies. This educational material and any such services must have content that adheres to federal guidelines on appropriate educational activities by manufacturers and must not violate federal laws specifically relating to false claims.

What is clear from this write-up is that reimbursement planning can help redefine product value and specific steps to be taken in development (see Box 7.6 for further discussion and a case example).

Box 7.6 Case example – plan for device reimbursement early in the development process

Written with assistance from Mitchell Sugarman, Director of Health Economics, Policy and Payment at Medtronic Vascular, and fellow associates.

During a surgical procedure known as angioplasty, a balloon is inflated inside an artery at the site of occluding plaque deposits to re-establish the lumen and increase blood flow through the artery. These procedures are usually performed on patients in hospital operating rooms or catheterization imaging labs by interventional cardiologists. To get the balloon into the artery (typically the coronary arteries) a guide wire has to be put into the artery at a distant site, such as the groin or arm, and the guide wire has to be worked past the site of the lesion. Then a catheter with the balloon is threaded on this guide wire to reach the site. The biggest risk during this process is that part of the plaque could get loose as an embolus or thrombotic plaque and flow into the circulation, potentially occluding a smaller vessel completely and causing a heart attack, or flowing into the brain and causing a stroke.

Medtronic, a large medical device maker, acquired a company (PercuSurge Inc.) that had just gotten FDA approval for the first emboli-protection device that would work with these interventional procedures (1999). The only indication approved for use of this device was in angioplasty procedures in saphenous vein grafts (which would frequently get occluded after transplantation). The PercuSurge device was a hollow guide wire with a balloon at its tip. When initially positioned past the lesion, the small balloon at the end was inflated distal to the lesion site, blocking the lumen completely and preventing any loose emboli from flowing further. The angioplasty catheter could be threaded onto the guide wire as usual, and after angioplasty, the occluded pool of blood between the lesion site and the distal occluding balloon would be suctioned up and irrigated, removing all emboli or loose debris from the plaque that had entered the blood stream. The balloon at the end of the PercuSurge guide wire was then deflated, resuming blood flow, and the guide wire could be withdrawn. This device was the first one on the market that would reduce the significant risk associated with the angioplasty procedure, with other solutions

Box 7.6 (cont.)

following at least two years behind (today, in 2007, most companies market mesh
baskets at the end of guide wires that allow blood but not emboli to flow instead of
completely blocking blood flow). The device had the potential to be a high revenue
product as it was the first solution on the market addressing a grave problem with
an increasingly popular interventional procedure. The Percusurge device was priced
significantly higher than the existing guide wires that were being used.

However, the device did not have adequate reimbursement. The small company that Medtronic bought (for $225 million in December 2000) had been
focused only on getting FDA approval and there had been no reimbursement
planning put in place during product development.

In the inpatient setting (payment system – *IPPS*), where almost all angioplasty
procedures were done, Medtronic assessed the specific existing ICD-9 procedure
codes and ICD-9 diagnosis code for saphenous vein graft angioplasty and ascer-
tained the payment DRG group code. Looking up the current payment level, it was
clear that this payment would not allow for adequate reimbursement to cover the
hospital costs and a higher price for the enhanced PercuSurge guide wire device.
Medtronic could appeal for a new DRG to be created to reflect the new procedure
and device. To do that, they would have to collect additional clinical data and
outcome data and then appeal to the CMS. Medtronic assessed that their chances
of getting a new DRG created were low even after this process. At that time (1999),
DRG add-on payments were not yet implemented (these were only available after
Oct 2001) where an extra payment for this device might have been available to a
new technology used under an existing DRG. The outcome of this review meant
that the hospital would have to bear the costs of the new technology ($1500) under
the existing level of DRG payment, creating a significant disincentive for a hospital
to purchase and use this PercuSurge device.

Reviewing the outpatient setting (payment system – *OPPS*) for the outpatient
setting (where very few angioplasty procedures were performed), a similar
situation existed with inadequate APC group payment available (see
Figure 7.9). However, in the APC groups, a transitional pass-through code
that covered the cost of the device could be obtained. Medtronic applied for
and received approval for a pass-through transitional code that would reimburse adequately for use of the device in the outpatient setting. While a good
outcome, it would have negligible impact on the overall sales of the device.

The *physician fee schedule*, based on CPT codes was also reviewed by
Medtronic. Current CPT procedure codes for the use of guide wires in angioplasty were assigned relative values (used for payment calculation by payers)
based on two main components – the physician work and the practice fee. The
work fee component of the existing CPT code did not recognize the extra work
that the PercuSurge device required, as inserting the guide wire past the lesion
site was a difficult and risky process. Therefore Medtronic worked with the
physician specialty group (vascular interventional cardiologists at the American

Box 7.6 (cont.)

College of Cardiology – ACC) to apply for a new CPT code to reimburse them adequately. However, the ACC learnt that to review this petition, the committee would probably have to review all the existing codes for these associated interventional cardiology procedures. Not wanting to risk a reduction in reimbursement value levels that might result from additional reviews of existing codes, the ACC preferred to withdraw the new CPT code petition for the procedure associated with the PercuSurge device. Physicians could use a temporary 99 code for this device to get reimbursed for the extra time it took them to use the PercuSurge, but no values were defined for this code and each usage would have to be followed by extensive discussion with payers to get the physician appropriate reimbursement for their extra effort. Medtronic put together a template to help physicians with forms and information to guide them through this process.

These steps resulted in a less than optimum outcome for reimbursement for the device. There was little that could be done in this situation except continue to educate the payers.

The device is still available and the price has come down significantly to allow it to compete with existing new technologies (mesh baskets that open like umbrellas at the end of the guide wire to catch emboli larger than the mesh openings) but the device has never quite reached its potential revenues. Medtronic had the first such device on the market two years before its competitors, but inadequate planning for reimbursement early on by the start-up company certainly hampered the revenue growth for this device.

In hindsight, if the start-up company had started the reimbursement planning before starting clinical trials, they might have realized the reimbursement challenges ahead. They might have tried a few things listed below.

Physician fee Begin dialogue with the physicians early on, who might have helped to get the procedure cost bundled into the physician CPT codes or ICD-9 procedure codes as they have now done with carotid stenting. When carotid stenting started becoming popular in recent years, the ACC obtained two codes, one for the procedure with embolic protection devices and one without embolic protection devices (the difference between the two reimbursement levels was only $50).

Indication expansion The PercuSurge device was approved with indication only for use with occluded saphenous vein grafts in 2000, not in native carotid arteries, and the company might have also started planning to expand its indications early on as it would have ensured high sales volume and possibly a better reimbursement review.

Collect appropriate clinical data and educate payers early The start-up company could also have lobbied CMS and the CPT committee early on to educate them about the value of using this embolic protection device, and built support by collecting data on the significance of this advancement in care and the resultant reduction in post-operative complications.

7.9   Reimbursement pathway for in vitro diagnostics (IVDs)

Diagnostics are generally reimbursed in a similar way to infused drugs and devices – the primary purchaser is the service provider (central laboratory services, hospitals, physician's offices) – and reimbursement is claimed using an ICD-9 procedure code or CPT code for the test. Diagnostics that have emerged in the last decade, such as molecular diagnostics (or nucleic acid testing, NAT), have a particularly difficult time getting reimbursed at appropriate levels (see Box 7.7 for a case study), because of the outdated Laboratory Fee Schedule used by Medicare to set payment rates. In particular, the procedures for reimbursing new NAT tests have been reported as the main detriment to innovation and application of new innovations to patient care.

The CMS has established the *cross-walk and gap fill processes* to determine payment amounts for new codes added to the fee schedule. *Cross-walking* is the mapping of new codes to technologically or clinically similar codes on the fee schedule: payments are made based on the existing fee schedule. Cross-walk determinations are made internally at the CMS with no formal process for correction currently (2007) in place, leading to protests from manufacturers. The other process, called *gap-fill*, requires local determination of payment rates for new codes, with no formal process in place to help make that determination, leading to confusion and variation in the first year of payment for the new code. In the second year of a new code, the CMS adopts a national limitation amount (NLA) in its fee schedule for the new code, based on the local carrier rates. The lower of the local rate or the NLA is then used to pay for the newly coded test.

To prepare for reimbursement, the diagnostics manufacturer has to:

- Collect appropriate clinical effectiveness data,
- Work with main regional or local bodies of CMS to obtain coverage,
- Approach major identified private payers for coverage determination,
- Identify procedure codes;
  - CPT-4 (level I HCPCS codes) – physician procedure codes,
  - level II HCPCS codes – material, device, or procedure codes,
  - ICD-9 procedure codes (hospitals' procedure code).
- Pick existing applicable procedure codes (preferred) or establish new code (1–3 years) through American Medical Association – CPT board,
- Identify Medicare benefit category – "diagnostic test,"
- Submit application to HCPCS working group at CMS for coverage and reimbursement level determination,
- Wait for determination by CMS in 3–6 months by cross-walk or approach local carriers by gap fill method,
- Work with other major third party payers (Blue Cross, Cigna, etc.) dependent on patient demographics.

Box 7.7 Case study – meeting a reimbursement challenge for new nucleic acid diagnostic tests

Written with assistance from Dr Kim Popovits, currently Chief Operating Officer and President of Genomic Health.

Genomic Health case study

Genomic Health has developed a novel cancer diagnostic test that predicts the likelihood of recurrence of breast cancer by genomic analysis of breast cancer biopsy samples. To gain market acceptance and establish clinical validity of their test, they used over $50 million (invested up to 2005) since inception in 2000 and carried out retrospective clinical trials with good statistical rigor. The studies were successful and results showed that physicians and patients could use the results of their OncoTypeDX test to make decisions in management of their breast cancer, by giving people some quantifiable risk of recurrence and the likelihood that they might benefit from chemotherapy treatment. Their OncoTypeDX Test was qualified under home-brew or ASR diagnostic testing (not requiring to be passed through either 510(k) or a PMA process) and their central reference laboratory, which received samples from around the nation, was granted a CLIA certification with rating sufficient to carry out the most complex tests.

The business model for Genomic Health challenged the existing diagnostic business model of high-volume, (relatively) low-margin operations of most successful companies like LabCorp or Quest Diagnostics. The biggest challenge the company faced (and that was the biggest impedance to getting further investment into the company to continue to develop new diagnostic tests) was the lack of adequate reimbursement based on existing CPT codes. Stacking up all existing CPT codes that could apply to their multi-step test, a cross-walk approach would get them a reimbursement level of about $1300 which was less than half of the target amount for the company to sustain its model of investing in intensive R&D for new tests. It was imperative for the future survival of Genomic Health to establish a higher price point for their test, closer to a therapeutic rather than a diagnostic. They chose to break ground by classifying their product under a miscellaneous CPT code category. This CPT code on a reimbursement request would prompt a manual review of each request, requiring appeals to the payer and submission of validation data for the test. Genomic Health took another inventive step of organizing a reimbursement support team that made appeals on behalf of the patient, who had to sign an authorization for Genomic Health to carry out the appeals. If the payer did not agree to the pricing, Genomic Health would eventually have to bill the patient. This process could potentially create significant delays of 6–14 months in collecting revenues from a given test, creating another level of risk, but thus far Genomic Health has seen good success in this strategy, getting full reimbursement at the right level. This example points to a creative and aggressive approach to the current reimbursement hurdle faced by developers of new diagnostic tests.

7.10   Major differences among selected national healthcare and reimbursement systems

A few national healthcare systems are profiled here in brief (see references at the end of this section).

Canada has a publicly financed, privately delivered healthcare system, which provides universal comprehensive access to healthcare. Hospitals are operated as private non-profit entities run by community boards or provincial health authorities. Doctors are private practitioners paid on a fee-for-service basis. About 9.8% of the GDP is spent on healthcare (2005).

The French healthcare system provides universal coverage to all citizens through a model that integrates public and private insurance. Healthcare expenditures were 10.4% of GDP in 2003. The public system is financed by employer payroll deductions and federal tax. End users are covered with a fee schedule based on socioeconomic status. Private plans reimburse treatment costs above the public system level for out-of-plan expenses. Although the government owns and operates most of the hospital beds, most ambulatory and outpatient care is provided by private professionals who are paid on a per-diem basis. Prescription drugs are reimbursed at prices set nationally.

The German public–private healthcare system covers about 90% of the population and private healthcare insurance covers the rest. Primary funding comes from payroll taxes and is augmented by federal matching funds for certain costs. Employers organize sickness funds, the primary purchasers of government healthcare and the unemployed and indigent are provided membership in sickness funds by the government. The government relies on negotiated spending caps on ambulatory care and pharmaceuticals with individual target hospital budgets. Germany spends about 10.8% of its GDP on healthcare (2005).

China has a two-pronged healthcare system that distinguishes rural versus urban healthcare. About 10% of the rural population is covered by the cooperative medical system, while the remainder is financed by out-of-pocket payments in a fee-for-service system. In the urban healthcare system, about 60% of the population is covered by a nationally paid, regionally administered system. However, out-of-pocket fees remain the predominant mechanism of payment for healthcare through most of the countryside. Healthcare spending is about 6% of China's GDP (2005).

India relies on the private sector to finance nearly 80% of its healthcare system. The central government plays a limited role in the financing and delivery of healthcare with widespread regional variations in health status and outcomes due to varying abilities of state and municipal governments. The central government provides some insurance coverage through the Employees' State Insurance Scheme which covers healthcare for organized labor and is funded through mandatory employer and employee contributions; the scheme covers some 28–30 million workers and retirees. The central government also runs the majority of rural hospitals and clinics that offer ambulatory, neonatal, family planning, and maternal services. The government spending covers 25% of healthcare spending with the remaining 75% coming from household out-of-pocket expenditure. Expenditures for healthcare are about 6% of GDP.

Australia offers both public and private health insurance, achieving universal coverage under a two-pronged system. Public insurance covers about 75% of the population and private insurance covers the rest. Free access to public hospitals is provided through the public system (Medicare) and patients who opt to go to private hospitals pay out-of-pocket or through private insurance. Strict regulations on private healthcare keep private fee rates low and the healthcare provision across public and private resources is not too different. Healthcare expenditures were 9.2% of GDP in 2003.

References used for this section

Blanchette, C. and Tolley, E. *Public- and Private-Sector Involvement in Health-Care Systems: a Comparison of OECD Countries*, 2001, http://dsp-psd.pwgsc.gc.ca/Collection-R/LoPBdP/BP/bp438-e.htm.

Dixon, A. and Mossialos, E. *Health Care Systems in Eight Countries: Trends and Challenges*, The European Observatory on Health Care Systems, The London School of Economics and Political Science.

Ernst & Young. *Report for the World Economic Forum, Health Care Systems and Health Market Reform in the G20 Countries*, 2003.

www.oecd.org *OECD Health Data*, 2006.

Frost & Sullivan. *Report on Economic Analysis for Chinese Healthcare Industry*, 2007.

7.11 Marketing

The purpose of marketing is to convince people to buy a product and once they have bought it, to keep them buying it again. The four key parameters used by marketers, known as the four Ps of marketing, are also called the "marketing mix." These four Ps are used to create a marketing plan and strategy.

The four Ps of marketing are (from http://en.wikipedia.org/wiki/Marketing)

- *Product* The product management and product marketing aspects deal with the specifications of the actual good or service, and how they relate to the end-users' needs and wants.
- *Pricing* This refers to the process of setting a price for a product, including discounts.
- *Promotion* This includes advertising, sales promotion, publicity, and personal selling, and refers to the various methods of promoting the product, brand, or company.
- *Placement* or distribution refers to how the product gets to the customer; for example, point of sale placement or retailing. This fourth P has also sometimes been called *Place*, referring to "where" a product or service is sold, e.g., in which geographic region or industry, to which segment (young adults, families, business people, women, men, etc.).

In a technologically complex environment, such as healthcare, where patients are not fully informed about choices, it is difficult to communicate and market the products accurately with full disclosure, as the general public may not know how to use the information. In fact, mass marketing to consumers of pharmaceuticals is banned or restricted in every Western country except the USA and New Zealand. The US FDA does oversee marketing messages by reviewing advertising materials and regulates the specific claims that can be made while marketing a product or service.

Marketing and reimbursement go hand in hand, as perception of value over the risk can drive demand and can also drive reimbursement. A clear example of this was seen in the Johnson & Johnson Cordis stent case (mentioned in Section 7.5.3). According to an industry reimbursement executive, "Demand makes reimbursement challenges go away." If you can create a strong perception of value in the consumer, then the demand from the consumer can drive positive decisions on reimbursement. An example of the use of this strategy is described in Box 7.8.

The marketing mix in the USA is complicated by the multi-payer system, as each stakeholder needs different information to make purchasing decisions or selections for healthcare. For the large part, marketing efforts from pharmaceutical and device companies are focused around the need to educate all the stakeholders about the benefits and applications of the new product. Adoption of a new technology in the existing healthcare paradigm is a key problem, owing to the conservative nature of the practice of medicine among the bulk of practitioners. Examples of various efforts made by a medical device company, Aspect Medical Systems, to improve adoption of a cutting edge technology, are summarized in Box 7.9.

In the biomedical industry, marketing is involved fairly early in the product development stage. The role of marketing is to ensure rapid growth in market adoption, as quickly as possible after approval, not just by the early adopters and cutting-edge teaching hospitals, but by the larger group of practitioners who make up most of the market. Marketing efforts also include reimbursement specialists who advise on strategies and timing to educate the various payer groups. Product positioning efforts thus focus on different stakeholders throughout the development process. Key opinion leaders can greatly influence early and widespread adoption. Typically, the company will want to involve the opinion leaders in carrying out and publishing results of the clinical studies. Marketing efforts also include developing a publishing and presentation strategy. Key scientific results of clinical studies are used to influence a broader segment of potential prescribers as the product gets close to approval. As the product (e.g., a drug) moves to patent expiration, patients exert more influence on the decision to purchase the branded drug over the generics and the focus of marketing efforts shifts in concert, as shown in Table 7.3.

Market research (see Chapter 2) specifically serves an important and useful role in product development, as described in Chapters 2 and 4. Marketing efforts to position the product can help steer the clinical trials of the product, just as reimbursement considerations influence clinical trial design. As an example, Pfizer's marketing department saw a new market possibility in the side effects of Viagra (sildenafil) when it was being developed in early clinical trials for

> **Box 7.8** Diagnostic company's novel market strategy ramps sales rapidly
>
> Excerpts from "Marketing diagnostic tests directly to the consumer," an article by Sue Auxter in Clinical Laboratory News, **26**, no. 4, 1, 5, 2000, reproduced here with permission.
>
> A new Pap test for cervical cancer, called the ThinPrep test, was approved in 1996 by the FDA. The manufacturer, Cytyc (Boxborough, MA), invested heavily in evaluating the new test against the standard Pap smear, and got FDA approval for a label stating that the ThinPrep test "was significantly more effective" than the conventional Pap smear. The company initially marketed the test to physicians, labs, and managed care companies as typical diagnostic tests are marketed. In the markets where the new test was well accepted by payers and providers, the company then proceeded to launch a direct-to-consumer marketing campaign using advertising in women's magazines and TV spots. This campaign resulted in many women asking for this improvement in their annual Pap testing. "We gained a 10% market share during the time we ran the DTC campaign, over and above what we would have expected to increase the market share without DTC," said Levangie [Dan Levangie, senior vice president of Cytyc Corporation]. "We've been fairly successful in directly educating *payers* [emphasis added] about the value of a better Pap test but I don't think there is any question that consumer pressure also gets their attention," explained Levangie, "and to some extent, a direct-to-consumer campaign by a company like us is indirectly influencing the insurance coverage for the test. The cost of the ThinPrep test varies considerably because of the complex laboratory contracts and regional differences, but the test generally costs $15 to $20 more than a traditional Pap smear ..." The combination of astute regulatory, reimbursement, and advertising strategy helped the company succeed in gaining rapid sales and record over $140 million in revenues in 2000.

blood pressure reduction. Similarly, Glaxo SmithKline's Paxil (paroxetine) was originally developed as an antidepressant but marketing saw more indications of interest and it has subsequently been approved for social anxiety disorder and panic disorder indications.

7.12   Sales

Depending on the route of distribution to the marketplace, sales people are hired to approach buyers and close a purchase contract for the goods. When dealing with wholesalers or PBMs or with payers such as private insurers, the sales people use a combination of incentives or discounts to the buyers, usually depending on the

Box 7.9 Aspect Medical Systems climbs the adoption curve

Reference: Naomi Atkins and Richard Bohmer. Aspect Medical Systems. Case Study no. 9-600-076, Harvard Business School Publishing, 2000.

Aspect has developed a controversial device that measures electrical signals from the brain during anesthesia to evaluate some measure of consciousness – the BIS device. Clinical use of this device has shown that anesthesiologists who use this device are better able to judge optimal dosage, frequently resulting in reduced dosage of drugs and faster functional recovery of patients after surgery, sometimes reducing the length of post-operative hospital stay.

However, after early adopters accepted the device, its sales stagnated (even after FDA approval and reimbursement assignment) as anesthesiologists felt their judgment and skills were being questioned by a machine and many did not want to take chances on a machine or to change their established practice. To increase market adoption, the company undertook the following multiple approaches:

- Get the BIS endorsed as a standard of care by the medical society (American Society of Anesthesiologists),
- Carry out multiple studies in various groups of patients to generate more data,
- Recruit key opinion leaders to use the device,
- Create public awareness of consciousness during surgery; manage public and professional relations during this process,
- Obtain coverage and reimbursement from most major payers,
- Obtain FDA approval for more indications so as to increase applications of equipment – thus making it more economical for hospitals,
- Innovative sales strategy to encourage hospitals to put one in every surgery room in the hospital – thus facilitating widespread usage,
- Capture market channels of distribution to keep off competition,
- Going through the PMA approval process created barriers to entry for others.

The adoption of a new technology can be rapid at first but typically slows down once the "early adopters" are won over. The BIS device had not been accepted by the second tier of end users, the (typically) larger base that makes up 50–70% of the "mass" market. Pushing the BIS device into that market would see the device gain "blockbuster" status, but it also required a significant change in practice of anesthesiology. Thus the determinants that would sway the larger audience had to be carefully understood and market acceptance issues approached on multiple levels for the device to truly attain blockbuster status. The above elements had to be put in place almost simultaneously.

Table 7.3 The focus of marketing changes during development

Phase of development	Purchase influencer targeted
Clinical development	Key opinion leaders
Pre-launch	Physician stakeholders, payers
New indication	Prescribers, payers
Patent expiration	Patients

volume of sales expected. Sales to the patient are rare and sales people are almost always dealing with other institutional purchasing departments (materials management department in a hospital) or third party payers to ensure coverage and inclusion in formulary or inventory.

In the *drug industry*, sales personnel are extensively trained by the company and are expected to be able to explain complex clinical results to physicians. Another tier of salesperson in the drug industry called the Medical Science Liaison (MSL), typically a trained physician or scientist, engages thought leaders. A MSL is hired to explain the benefits of the new drug by discussing the data and clinical relevance, usage, patient concerns, etc., with the practicing physician at a scientific and practical level. These MSLs play an important role in between marketing and sales.

Sales positions in the *device industry* are also highly specialized jobs and most salespeople have a bachelor's degree in sciences or engineering and many have master's degrees in biomedical engineering or related fields. Many sales personnel will need to have intimate knowledge of human anatomy and physiology in addition to product information (depending on their specific roles and the product itself). These salespeople often serve as consultants for the physicians or surgeons, standing by to address questions or problems and offer tips in the surgical suite as the surgeon is implanting or using the new device, until the surgeon is comfortable with the new device and associated procedure. Often the sale of a new device will include one or more training sessions, as *a sound procedure of usage of the device is at least as important as the quality of the device* itself. In the device industry in particular, salesforce feedback can play a vital role in new product design and development as they come back with insightful observations from their complete participation in the product application and usage process.

7.13 Product liability

Once a medical product is approved by the FDA for sale in the market, the company is generally protected against wrongful use of the product – e.g., physicians who use or prescribe the product for any indication other than the one approved are putting themselves at risk for a lawsuit from the patient if something goes wrong, but the manufacturer cannot generally be sued in this instance. For example, if a surgeon implants a device incorrectly, it is the surgeon at risk for malpractice or negligence rather than the device manufacturer. As long as the product is used in the manner and indication for which it is approved, and it works as claimed, the manufacturer in general is not liable for faulty usage.

Specifically, product liability lawsuits have as their basis one of three claims – *negligence*, *strict liability*, or *breach of warranty*. Lawsuits against biomedical product manufacturers typically claim one or more of these legal causes as the basis for recovery of damages.

Negligence is based on the following fact: manufacturers have a duty to care for the patients who are the end users of their products; negligence occurs if the standard for carrying out the duty is breached, and as a result a compensable injury results to the plaintiff.

In these *negligence cases*, the burden is on the plaintiff (patient) to prove negligence. However, manufacturers of products that can have serious risk to the patient should be even more careful during product development than manufacturers of products that may carry lower risk.

Strict liability or product liability cases focus on the product. Does the inherent design of the product have a defect that makes it unreasonably unsafe? Did the product leave the manufacturer's factory in a condition that causes unreasonable danger to the user or consumer? The critical focus in a strict liability suit is whether the product is defective and unreasonably dangerous or whether the manufacturer failed to warn adequately of hazards. The latter is then also a case of negligence, and the majority of cases are of this nature (failure to warn). The criterion of "unreasonably dangerous" is based on a risk–benefit analysis.

Breach of warranty cases assert that the manufacturer breached the warranty or representations made about the product.

Recent lawsuits against drug manufacturers based on *negligence and liability* include those against Glaxo Smith Kline's Plavix (a claim that GSK did not report studies that showed the drug increased suicidal tendencies), American Home Products' Fen-Phen (a diet drug that led to heart valve problems; AHP set up a trust fund to settle class action lawsuits without admitting wrongdoing), Merck's Vioxx (lawsuits claim that Merck did not reveal an increased risk of heart attacks found in early studies) and Bayer's Baycol (a cholesterol-lowering drug caused rare muscular disease; all cases were settled after Bayer won the first two cases). Recent lawsuits against medical device manufacturers include those against Guidant (who covered up knowledge of defects that would cause its Ventak defibrillator to short and fail) and its recently acquired subsidiary Endovascular Corp (who misled the FDA and did not report the majority of malfunctions in its Ancure stent-graft device). In cases involving gross negligence, where the manufacturers have been shown to have been at fault, the manufacturers usually settle the case with payments made to the plaintiffs. The FDA marketing application approval and FDA inspections of the manufacturing facilities provide no protection against these types of lawsuits. All of the lawsuits above had claims involving millions of dollars of payments (reaching billions in many cases).

Along with these product-liability lawsuits and claims, companies usually have to face shareholder lawsuits that claim damages for fall in share price due to mismanagement.

Some of these cases are driven by a product recall announced by the company or the FDA, rather than on specific proof of wrongdoing or misconduct. In one of the most famous cases of this type, after the FDA issued a recall of silicone-filled breast implants, the large number of ensuing lawsuits and claims led the Dow Corning company to file for bankruptcy in order to reorganize and settle the claims through a trust fund. However, subsequent analysis of the medical data has shown no clear link between the reported health problems (silicone adjuvant disease where silicone was claimed to trigger some unknown factor in the immune system) and the silicone breast implants.

In the *product liability cases* that typically blame faulty or unsafe design, the cases have to be introduced into the state judicial system, and often come up against the fact that state law cannot pre-empt (a device approved under) federal law, thus providing some liability protection for FDA-approved devices. In a recent case, Thorn vs. Thoratec, Mrs. Thorn alleged that a defect in the design of HeartMate (a ventricular heart assist device) caused the device to fail in her husband and led to his death. A suture that was required to position a tube came off and a resulting embolism traveled to the brain causing a fatal brain hemorrhage. The judges in the US 3rd Circuit Court of Appeals rejected her bid as the ruling would conflict with the federal law and PreMarket Approval (PMA) regulated process, and state law cannot conflict with federal law under which products were approved for sale.

However, the position that FDA approval provides some shield to manufacturers from certain types of product liability lawsuits is shifting. Several ongoing court cases and proposed bills attempt to address this issue, arguing for consumer protection over manufacturer protection.

Exercises

7.1 What is the patient mix for the product?

7.2 Who are the payers for these types of patients?

7.3 What are the settings in which your biomedical technology will be used? Based on that answer, in which payment group (DRG, APC, etc.) will it be categorized? What are the implications?

7.4 What is the coding (CPT, ICD-9) for your technology and its applications? (If a drug product, what determines whether it needs a CPT code?)

7.5 How will your product be distributed to get it to its proper setting for use?

7.6 Prepare a distribution and reimbursement flow chart for your product.

7.7 Highlight the key issues that will deliver a positive coverage decision for your product, showing value over the competition. Have you planned to collect economic data for analysis in your clinical trials?

7.8 Using Figure 7.10 as a guide, chart out the reimbursement planning time-line for your product/project.

7.9 Most approved innovative products capture an initial lead user group (also known as early adopters) but then revenues stall as acceptance and adoption in the larger market groups proves elusive. What are the key hurdles among the various stakeholder groups for widespread adoption of the product? Are the hurdles based on cost, reimbursement coverage, competitors, or alternative products, or is there inadequate understanding of the risk-benefit ratio? What are the tools you can use to address these hurdles?

7.10 What is the value proposition of your product for insurers? For physicians? Can you summarize the risk vs. benefits of your product?

7.11 Do you need to rethink your product characteristics based on the above questions?

7.12 What levels of payment can you expect right after approval and then over time for your product?

7.13 Based on your answers to the above questions, you should be able to plan the reimbursement path and predict possible revenue cash flows for your product.

References and additional reading

Bingefors, K., Pashos, C. L., Dix Smith, M., *et al. Health Care Cost, Quality, and Outcomes: ISPOR Book of Terms*, International Society for Pharmacoeconomics and Outcomes Research (ISPOR), 2003.

Campbell, J. J, *Understanding Pharma*, Pharmaceutical Institute, 2005.

De Navas-Walt, C., Proctor, B. D., and Lee, C. H. *Income, Poverty, and Health Insurance in the United States: 2005*, US Census Bureau, Current Population Reports, P60-231, US Government Printing Office, 2006.

Drummond, M. F., Sculpher, M. J., Torrance, G. W., O'Brien, B. J., and Stoddart, G. L. *Methods for the Economic Evaluation of Health Care Programmes*, Oxford University Press, 3rd edn., 2005.

Folland, S., Goodman, A. C., and Stano, M. *The Economics of Health and Health Care*, Prentice Hall, 4th edn., 2003.

Folland, S., Goodman, A., and Stano, M. (eds.). *Economics of Health and Health Care*, Prentice Hall, 2007.

Ohsfeldt, R. L. and Schneider, J. E. *The Business of Health: The Role of Competition, Markets, and Regulation*, AEI Press, 2006.

Phelps, C. E. *Health Economics*, Addison-Wesley, 3rd edn., 2003.

Walley, T., Haycox, A., and Boland, A. *Pharmacoeconomics*, Churchill Livingstone, 2004.

Useful websites

www.cms.gov – *CMS Centers for Medicaid and Medicare Services*
www.medpac.gov – *MedPAC – advise Congress on Medicare (summary documents on Medicare processes; look under "other publications" link)*

www.cms.hhs.gov/mcd/search.asp – *Medicare coverage database (search for national and local coverage decisions)*
www.cms.hhs.gov/MedHCPCSGenInfo/ – *HCPCS codes at CMS*
www.ama-assn.org/ama/pub/category/3882.html – *How a new CPT code is created*
www.cms.hhs.gov/apps/acronyms/ – *Useful list of acronyms used in healthcare and by CMS*
www.hrsa.gov/opa/glossary.htm – *Glossary for drug pricing terms*
www.cms.hhs.gov/HospitalOutpatientPPS/ – *Outpatient Prospective Payment system at Medicare*
www.cms.hhs.gov/PhysicianFeeSched/ – *Medicare physician fee schedule*
www.kff.org – *Kaiser Family Foundation*
www.upenn.edu/ldi – *Leonard Davis Institute of Health Economics*
www.nber.org – *National Bureau of Economic Research (has many working papers on health-related topics)*
www.nhs.uk/ – *National Health Service (United Kingdom)*
www.cdc.gov/nchs/ – *National Center for Health Statistics (USA)*
www.who.int/whosis/ – *WHO (World Health Organization) statistical information system*

Appendix 7.1 Technology assessment center for coverage determination

The following summary is used with permission from the Blue Cross and Blue Shield Association. All rights reserved by Blue Cross Blue Shield © *2006, www.bcbs.com/ betterknowledge/tec/.*

This example from the Blue Cross Blue Shield Technology Evaluation Center gives an insight into the process of decision making at major payers across the USA, where FDA approval is no guarantee of reimbursement coverage.

Vagus nerve stimulation for treatment-resistant depression

Assessment Program
Volume 21, No. 7
August 2006
www.bcbs.com/tec/vol21/21_07.html

Executive summary

Background

Depression is a serious psychiatric condition that sometimes does not respond to standard treatments such as medication or psychotherapy. Vagus nerve stimulation (VNS) therapy is administered through an implanted pulse generator and bipolar lead and has been studied in patients with treatment-resistant depression. Vagus nerve stimulation was previously evaluated by the Technology Evaluation Center (TEC) for this indication in 2005 and did not meet TEC criteria. Since the last TEC assessment, the same studies evaluated in the prior assessment have now been published in peer-reviewed journals, and there have been some re-analyses of the same data also published.

Objective

This assessment will review the available evidence to determine if VNS therapy is effective for treatment-resistant depression. This assessment updates the prior TEC assessment of VNS for the same indication.

Search strategy

A search of the Medline® database was completed for the period up to June 2006. The search strategy used the terms "depression" and "vagus [or "vagal"] nerve stimulator/stimulation" as text words or subject terms. Articles were limited to those published in the English language and enrolling human subjects. The Medline® search was supplemented by an examination of article bibliographies and relevant review articles, which were searched for citations.

Selection criteria

Articles were case series, randomized trials, or observational studies evaluating clinical outcomes of VNS therapy. In the prior TEC assessment, results were available only from documents posted to the US Food and Drug Administration (FDA) web site. At this time, the same studies have now been published in peer-reviewed journals, almost unchanged from the FDA documents. New publications analyze the same data in various ways examining duration of benefit.

Main results

The relevant clinical evidence evaluating VNS consists of a case series of 60 patients receiving VNS, a short-term (i.e., 3-month) randomized, sham-controlled clinical trial (RCT) of 221 patients, and an observational study comparing 205 of the RCT patients on VNS therapy with 124 patients receiving usual treatment for depression. Patients who responded to sham treatment in the short-term randomized, controlled trial (approximately 10%) were excluded from the long-term observational study.

Patient selection was a concern for all studies. Vagus nerve stimulation is intended for treatment-refractory depression, but the entry criteria of failure of two drugs and a 6-week trial of therapy may not be a strict enough definition of treatment resistance. Treatment-refractory depression should be defined by thorough psychiatric evaluation and comprehensive management. It has been documented that apparent treatment resistance is common, owing to inadequate medication or trial durations and that, for clinical trial purposes, treatment resistance should be established prospectively, not historically. Patients with clinically significant suicide risk were excluded from all VNS studies.

The case series data show rates of improvement, as measured by a 50% improvement in depression score of 31% at 10 weeks to greater than 40% at 1 to 2 years, but there are some losses to follow-up. Natural history, placebo effects, and patient and provider expectations make it difficult to infer efficacy from case series data.

The randomized study that compared VNS therapy with a sham control (implanted but inactivated VNS) did not show a statistically significant result for the principal outcome (50% reduction in depression score or Hamilton Rating Scale for depression) at 3 months. Fifteen percent of VNS subjects responded, versus 10% of control subjects ($p = 0.25$). Two out of three secondary outcome measures were also non-significant.

An observational study comparing patients participating in the randomized clinical trial and a separately recruited control group evaluated VNS therapy to 1 year. This observational study showed a statistically significant difference in the rate of change of depression score. However, issues such as unmeasured differences between patients and non-concurrent controls, differences in sites of care between VNS therapy patients and controls, and differences in concomitant therapy changes raise concern about this observational study. Analyses performed on subsets of patients cared for in the same sites, and censoring observations after treatment changes, generally showed diminished differences in apparent treatment effectiveness of VNS and almost no statistically significant differences. Given these concerns about the quality of the observational data, these results are insufficient to support the effectiveness of VNS therapy.

Additional reanalyses of these same data to evaluate persistence of response show that among those who achieve a response at 3 or 12 months, 60–75% of such patients are judged to remain a responder at 1 year later. In the context of relatively low overall response rates, these data do not provide evidence of efficacy.

Adverse effects of VNS therapy include voice alteration, headache, neck pain, and cough, which are known from prior experience with VNS therapy for seizures. Regarding specific concerns for depressed patients such as mania, hypomania, suicide, and worsening depression, there does not appear to be a greater risk of these events during VNS therapy.

Author's conclusions and comments

Since the last TEC assessment, there have been no studies reporting clinical outcomes on any new or different patients. Data from the case series and clinical trials have been reanalyzed to show what proportions of patients who respond at one time are still responders at a subsequent time. However, this information by itself does not provide evidence of the efficacy of VNS beyond that provided by the original observational comparison of VNS versus treatment as usual.

Based on the available evidence, the Blue Cross and Blue Shield Association Medical Advisory Panel made the following judgments about whether vagus nerve stimulation (VNS) for the indication of treatment-resistant depression meets the Blue Cross and Blue Shield Association Technology Evaluation Center (TEC) criteria.

(1) *The technology must have final approval from the appropriate governmental regulatory bodies.*

The NeuroCybernetic Prosthesis System (NCP®, Cyberonics, Inc.) received approval of its Pre-market Application (PMA) to market from the US Food and Drug Administration (FDA) on July 16, 1997, for treatment-refractory seizures. The device was approved for use in conjunction with drugs or surgery "as an adjunctive treatment of adults and adolescents over 12 years of age with medically refractory partial onset seizures."

On July 15, 2005, the VNS Therapy System received final PMA approval by the FDA for "adjunctive long-term treatment of chronic or recurrent depression for patients 18 years of age or older who are experiencing a major depressive episode and have not had an adequate response to four or more adequate antidepressant treatments."

(2) *The scientific evidence must permit conclusions concerning the effect of the technology on health outcomes.*

The clinical trials reviewed above report weak evidence that does not demonstrate efficacy.

(3) *The technology must improve the net health outcome*; and

(4) *The technology must be as beneficial as any established alternatives.*

The available evidence does not permit conclusions regarding the effect of VNS therapy on health outcomes or its effect compared with alternative therapies.

(5) *The improvement must be attainable outside the investigational settings.*

Whether VNS therapy for treatment-related depression improves health outcomes has not yet been determined in the investigational setting.

For the above reasons, VNS therapy for the indication of treatment-resistant depression does not meet the TEC criteria.

Glossary and acronyms

Abbreviated New Drug Application (ANDA)
An Abbreviated New Drug Application (ANDA) contains data that, when submitted to FDA's Center for Drug Evaluation and Research, Office of Generic Drugs, provides for the review and ultimate approval of a generic drug product. Generic drug applications are called "abbreviated" because they are generally not required to include pre-clinical (animal) and clinical (human) data to establish safety and effectiveness. Instead, a generic applicant must demonstrate scientifically that its product is bioequivalent (i.e., performs in the same manner as the innovator drug). Once approved, an applicant may manufacture and market the generic drug product to provide a safe, effective, low-cost alternative to the American public (text from www.fda.gov/cder/drugsatfda/Glossary.htm).

ADMET
Acronym for the parameters used to understand drug behavior in a living system: absorption, distribution (among the tissues), metabolism, excretion, and toxicology.

antisense
A nucleic acid sequence that is complementary to the coding sequence of DNA or mRNA.

API
The active pharmaceutical ingredient in a drug (biological or synthetic chemical): any substance or mixture of substances intended to be used in the manufacture of a drug product and that, when used in the production of a drug, becomes an active ingredient in the drug product. Such substances are intended to furnish pharmacological activity or other direct effect in the diagnosis, cure, mitigation, treatment, or prevention of disease or to affect the structure and function of the body – as defined by the FDA.

ASP
Average sales price: a calculation method created by federal and state government prosecutors in settlements with pharmaceutical manufacturers TAP and Bayer to ensure more accurate price reporting. The ASP is the

weighted average of all non-federal sales to wholesalers and is net of chargebacks, discounts, rebates, and other benefits tied to the purchase of the drug product, whether it is paid to the wholesaler or the retailer. Text from the HRSA website.

ASR   Analyte specific reagents (also known as home-brew tests): an analyte specific reagent (ASR) is the active ingredient of an in-house diagnostic test. The FDA defines ASRs as: "antibodies, both polyclonal and monoclonal, specific receptor proteins, ligands, nucleic acid sequences, and similar reagents, which, through specific binding or chemical reaction with substances in a specimen, are intended for use in a diagnostic application for identification and quantification of an individual chemical substance or ligand in biological specimens."

AWP   Average wholesale price: a national average of list prices charged by wholesalers to pharmacies. The AWP is sometimes referred to as a "sticker price" because it is not the actual price that larger purchasers normally pay. For example, in a study of prices paid by retail pharmacies in eleven states, the average acquisition price was 18.3% below the AWP. Discounts for HMOs and other large purchasers can be even greater. Information about AWP is publicly available. Text from the HRSA website.

bioinformatics   The use of extensive computerized databases to solve information problems in the biological sciences. These databases generally contain protein and nucleic acid sequences, genomes, etc. Bioinformatics also encompasses computer techniques such as 3-D molecular modeling, statistical database analysis, data mining, etc.

biologics   Biological macromolecules or large molecular (weight) entities (proteins such as monoclonal antibodies, or enzymes and other molecules, such as glycoproteins, hormones, etc.) developed through biotechnology for therapeutic intervention as drugs for specific diseases. Counterparts are synthetic chemical small molecule drugs that make up the traditional pharmaceutical industry.

CFR   The Code of Federal Regulations (CFR) is the book in which all regulations are codified. The CFR is the codification of the general and permanent rules published in the Federal Register by the executive departments and agencies of the Federal Government. Title (volume) 21

	contains regulations pertaining to food and drugs. The latest text is available at www.gpoaccess.gov/cfr.
CMO	Contract Manufacturing Organization (note: when referring to personnel, CMO = Chief Medical Officer)
CMS (previously HCFA)	The Centers for Medicare and Medicaid Services administer the Medicare and Medicaid programs, which provide healthcare to about one in every four Americans. Medicare provides health insurance for elderly and disabled Americans. Medicaid, a joint federal-state program, provides health coverage for low-income persons, including children, and nursing home coverage for low-income elderly persons. The CMS also administers the State Children's Health Insurance Program. Established as the Health Care Financing Administration (HCFA) in 1977. Headquarters: Baltimore, Md. Websites: www.medicare.gov, www.cms.gov. The CMS had 4943 employees and a budget of $489 billion in 2005.
CPT	Current procedural terminology – a coding system that is maintained by the American Medical Association and is used to describe *services and procedures* provided by physicians. The CPT codes are also known as level I of HCPCS (Health Care Procedure Coding System) codes and make up about 90% of total HCPCS codes.
CRO	Contract research organization: a CRO could range from a one-person biostatistical consultant to a large multinational organization that coordinates all aspects of the clinical trial. Contract research organizations also work on pre-clinical research, most commonly on GLP toxicology studies.
device	Any product that achieves its primary functions in the body through mechanical or physical action (rather than chemical).
DME	Durable medical equipment (DME). Medical equipment which: can usually withstand repeated use, is useable at home, and is not beneficial to a person without an illness or injury. Examples include hospital beds, wheelchairs, and oxygen equipment.
DMEPOS	Durable medical equipment, prosthetics, orthotics and supplies, typically including those medical equipment and supplies that are used outside the physicians' office.
drug	A product that achieves its primary functions in the body by chemical action. In this book, this term covers small molecular weight chemical compounds and also biologics.

enantiomers	Enantiomers are stereoisomeric compounds that are non-superimposable mirror images of one another. Enantiomers can have very different biological properties and a mix of enantiomers in the manufacture or synthesis of chemical compounds needs to be monitored and measured carefully. For more details and implications of enantiomers in pharmaceutical product development see http://en.wikipedia.org/wiki/Enantiomer.
evidence-based medicine	Evidence-based medicine is a principle of making individual treatment decisions by considering the results of many scientific studies.
EMEA	European Agency for the Evaluation of Medicinal Products. In 1993, the European Economic Community (EU) Council established the EMEA to channel product approval through a "centralized procedure."
FDA	The Food and Drug Administration assures the safety of foods and cosmetics, and the safety and efficacy of pharmaceuticals, biological products, and medical devices – products which represent almost 25 cents out of every dollar in US consumer spending. www.fda.gov. Headquartered at Rockville, MD, the agency had 10 446 employees and a budget of $1.8 billion in 2005.
FISH	Fluorescent in-situ hybridization (FISH) is a process that vividly paints chromosomes or portions of chromosomes with fluorescent molecules. A fluorescent hybridization probe is created for the DNA segment of interest. The probe, and attached fluorescent molecule, will combine with any complementary DNA or RNA it encounters (from www.wikipedia.org). This technique is useful for identifying chromosomal abnormalities and gene mapping. It can also be used to identify micro-organisms.
formulary	A formulary is a select menu of drugs that a managed care organization or insurer will cover under its health plan.
GCP	Good clinical practice is an international quality standard for clinical trials involving human subjects. The GCPs are provided by the International Conference on Harmonization (ICH) and issued as regulations by the FDA. The GCP guidelines include standards on how clinical trials should be conducted, define the roles and responsibilities of clinical trial sponsors, clinical research investigators, and monitors.

gene   A gene is the fundamental physical and functional unit of
                        heredity that is made up of tightly coiled threads or
                        polymers of deoxyribonucleic acid (DNA). A DNA
                        molecule consists of two strands that wrap around each
                        other to resemble a twisted ladder or double helix. The
                        DNA molecule is an informational molecule and is made up
                        of four distinct nucleotides: deoxyadenosine (A),
                        deoxyguanosine (G), deoxythymidine (T), and
                        deoxycytidine (C). It is the non-random order of these
                        individual "bases" that results in DNA being an
                        informational molecule. However, in and of itself, DNA has
                        no functional property. It is a chemical that, when placed in
                        an appropriate environment, will direct the synthesis of
                        particular and specific proteins, which make up the
                        structural components of cells, tissues, and enzymes
                        (molecules that are essential for biochemical reactions). This
                        environment is found within the cell. Organisms, from
                        single-celled protozoans to far more complex human beings,
                        are made up of cells containing DNA and associated
                        protein molecules. The DNA is organized into structures
                        called chromosomes, which encode all the information
                        necessary for building and maintaining the organism. A
                        DNA molecule may contain one or more genes, each of
                        which is a specific sequence of nucleotide bases. It is the
                        specific sequence of these bases that provides the exact
                        genetic instructions that give an organism its unique traits.
                        (Taken verbatim from www.bio.org/ip/primer)

gene therapy   Treatment that alters gene expression or introduces new
                        genetic material in the body. In early studies of gene
                        therapy for cancer, researchers were trying to improve the
                        body's natural ability to fight the disease or to make the
                        tumor more sensitive to other kinds of therapy. This
                        treatment may involve the addition of a functional gene or
                        group of genes to a cell by gene insertion to correct a
                        hereditary disease.

generic drug   A generic drug is the same as a brand-name drug in
                        dosage, safety, strength, how it is taken, quality,
                        performance, and intended use. Before approving a
                        generic drug product, the FDA requires many rigorous
                        tests and procedures to assure that the generic drug can be
                        substituted for the brand name drug. The FDA bases
                        evaluations of substitutability, or "therapeutic
                        equivalence," of generic drugs on scientific evaluations.

By law, a generic drug product must contain the identical amounts of the same active ingredients as the brand-name product. Drug products evaluated as "therapeutically equivalent" can be expected to have equal effect and no difference when substituted for the brand name product. (Text from www.fda.gov/cder/drugsatfda/Glossary.htm)

genomics   The identification and functional characterization of genes.

GLP   Good laboratory practice – guidelines on record keeping and procedures to be followed in conducting non-clinical studies. These guidelines are regulations issued by the FDA. Non-clinical data required by the FDA as part of product approval applications must be carried out under GLP.

GMP   Good manufacturing practices (Also, cGMP = current GMP). Guidelines that are developed by the World Health Organization (WHO) and the ICH are incorporated into the FDA regulations. Good manufacturing practices regulate the manufacturing and laboratory testing environment and processes. An extremely important part of GMP is documentation of every aspect of the process, activities, and operations involved with drug and medical device manufacture.

HCFA   See CMS.

HCPCS codes   The Healthcare Common Procedure Coding System (HCPCS) is divided into two principal sub-systems, referred to as Level I and Level II of the HCPCS. Level I of the HCPCS comprises Current Procedural Terminology (CPT) codes, which are used to describe and identify services and procedures furnished by physicians and other healthcare professionals. Level II of the HCPCS is a standardized coding system that is used primarily to identify products, supplies, and services not included in the CPT codes, such as ambulance services and durable medical equipment, prosthetics, orthotics, and supplies (DMEPOS), when used outside a physician's office.

HHS   The Department of Health and Human Services is the principal US agency for protecting the health of all Americans and providing essential human services. The department includes more than 300 programs, including the NIH, FDA, CMS. Many HHS-funded services are provided at the local level by state or county agencies, or through private sector grantees. It administers more grant dollars than all other federal agencies combined (representing nearly a quarter of all federal outlay). The HHS' Medicare program is the nation's largest health insurer, handling more than 1 billion claims per year. Medicare and Medicaid together provide healthcare insurance for one in four Americans. The HHS programs are administered by 11 operating divisions. See details at www.hhs.gov/about/whatwedo.html/. HHS had 67 444 employees and a budget of $698 billion for the financial year, 2007.

Home-brew tests   See ASR for more details.

HRSA   The Health Resources and Services Administration (HRSA), an agency of the US Department of Health and Human Services, is the primary Federal agency for improving access to healthcare services for people who are uninsured, isolated, or medically vulnerable.

IACUC   Institutional Animal Care and Use Committee – this committee reviews and approves all experimental work that involves animals with a view to preventing unnecessary animal experimentation.

ICH   International Conference on Harmonization. A unique project that brings together the regulatory authorities of Europe, Japan, and the United States and experts from the pharmaceutical industry in the three regions with the goal of making the international regulatory processes for medical products more efficient and uniform.

ICD-9; ICD-10   International Classification of Diseases. ICD-10 is the latest edition (1994) of the international standard for diagnosis of disease with origins in the 1850s. The World Health Organization (WHO) is responsible for maintaining and updating this classification. In the USA, the American Hospital Association (AHA) serves as a clearing house for all ICD-9 issues. The USA is moving towards adoption of the ICD-10 standard.

in silico biology   The use of computational algorithms to create virtual systems that emulate molecular pathways, entire cells, or more complex living systems. The use of computers to simulate or analyze a biological experiment.

in vivo   Inside the living organism.

in vitro   In the laboratory or outside the organism.

indication   An "indication" for a drug or device refers to the particular disease or stage of that disease that the drug or device is intended to treat.

incidence	The incidence of a disease is defined as the number of new cases of disease occurring in a population during a defined time interval (see also prevalence).
IPPS	Inpatient Payment System – Medicare's payment system for reimbursing hospitals for inpatient services and products provided.
IRB	Institutional Review Board – a committee that is required to review ethical principles of biomedical studies and approve any protocol that involves human subjects. The role of the IRB is to protect the safety and privacy of clinical trial subjects.
IVD	In vitro diagnostics – products used to diagnose disease by analyzing or reacting with samples of human tissues, blood or extracts thereof.
KOLs	Key opinion leaders – these are the key practicing physicians or scientists whose papers and presentations are highly regarded by their peers. These KOLs are typically more aggressive in the treatment of their patients and test many leading new therapies, continuing to establish their reputation as leaders in the field. Identifying and engaging these KOLs is an important step in the product development process, with particular relevance to the marketing functions.
label	The FDA-approved label is the official description of a drug product,: it includes indication (what the product is to be used for); who should take it; adverse events (side effects); instructions for uses in pregnancy, children, and other populations; and safety information for the patient. It defines the specific market for the product. Labels are often found inside drug product packaging. Labels are also used for devices and diagnostics, and similarly define the market application that has been approved.
LCD; NCD	Local coverage decision (made by local Medicare contractors for each region); national coverage decision (made by CMS; applies to all local providers).
lead	These are typically leading compounds that are being developed towards a drug candidate. The next development step is to optimize the lead compound with respect to multiple product characteristics.
microbiology	A branch of biology dealing especially with microscopic forms of life.

monoclonal antibody (mAB)	Highly specific, purified antibody that is derived from only one clone of cells and recognizes only one antigen.
MSL	A Medical Science Liaison (MSL) is typically a trained physician or scientist, hired to engage thought leaders by a pharmaceutical company for marketing purposes. An MSL is hired to explain the benefits of the new drug by discussing the data and clinical relevance, usage, patient concerns, etc. with the practicing physician at a scientific and practical level.
novel chemical entity (NCE)	A compound not previously described in the literature; any new molecular compound not previously approved for human use, excluding diagnostic agents, vaccines, and other biologic compounds not approved by the FDA's Centers for Drug Evaluation and Research (CDER). Also excluded are new salts, esters, and dosage forms of previously approved compounds. (Tufts Center for the Study of Drug Development, Glossary, 2004.)
New molecular entity (NME)	A new molecular entity is an active pharmaceutical ingredient that has never before been marketed in the United States in any form. (The terms NME and NCE are used interchangeably).
NIH	National Institutes of Health – NIH is the world's premier medical research organization, supporting over 38 000 research projects nationwide in diseases including cancer, Alzheimer's, diabetes, arthritis, heart ailments, and AIDS. Includes 27 separate health institutes and centers (www.nih.gov). NIH had a $28.6 billion budget in 2005 with 17 543 employees.
NCD; LCD	National coverage decision (made by CMS; applies to all local providers); local coverage decision (made by local Medicare contractors for each region).
NPD	New product development.
off-label	Off-label use is the practice of prescribing drugs for a purpose outside the scope of the drug's approved label.
OPPS	Outpatient Payment System – Medicare's payment system to reimburse hospitals for outpatient procedures.
pass-through codes	Section 1833(t)(6) of the Social Security Act provides for temporary additional payments or "transitional pass-through payments" for certain innovative medical devices, drugs, and biologics for Medicare beneficiaries, even if prices for these new and innovative items exceed

Medicare's regular scheduled OPPS payment amounts. For drugs and biologicals, the pass-through payment is the amount by which 95% of the average wholesale price exceeds the applicable fee schedule amount associated with the drug or biologic. For devices, the pass-through payment equals the amount by which the hospital's charges, adjusted to cost, exceeds the OPPS payment rate associated with the device.

PBM   Pharmaceutical benefit managers (PBMs) manage pharmacy benefits, maintain formularies, and obtain discounts for bulk purchases of drugs for their clients – employers, insurance companies, and unions. A handful of large national companies and many small regional PBMs influence more than 80% of prescription drug coverage. The original purpose of PBMs was to offer cost-effective services, such as reliable claims information and issuance of drug cards for easy ID and account tracking. Over time, however, PBM's functions have evolved to include large-scale "block purchases" of drugs and medical products that dramatically lower their wholesale costs.

PCT   Patent Cooperation Treaty – originally formed in 1970 (and modified several times). Over 130 states are signatories to the PCT. The Treaty makes it possible to seek patent protection for an invention simultaneously in each of a large number of countries by filing an "international" patent application.

pharmacogenomic test Pharmacogenomics is the study of the stratification of the pharmacological response to a drug by a population based on the genetic variation of that population. This assay is intended to study inter-individual variations in whole-genome or candidate gene, single-nucleotide polymorphism (SNP) maps, haplotype markers, or alterations in gene expression or inactivation that may be correlated with pharmacological function and therapeutic response. In some cases, the pattern or profile of change is the relevant biomarker, rather than changes in individual markers.

PhRMA   The Pharmaceutical Research and Manufacturers of America is an organization that represents the country's leading pharmaceutical research and biotechnology companies (www.phrma.org).

pharmacokinetics (PK) The study of the process by which a drug is absorbed, distributed, metabolized, and eliminated by the body over time. Pharmacokinetics is often called the study of what the body does to the drug, whereas pharmacodynamics is the study of what the drug does to the body (from www.wikipedia.org).

pharmacodynamics (PD)
Pharmacodynamics is the study of the biochemical and physiological effects of drugs and the mechanisms of drug action and the relationship between drug concentration and effect. Pharmacodynamics is often called the study of what the drug does to the body, whereas PK is the study of what the body does to the drug (from www.wikipedia.org).

Phase I
Clinical testing phase for new drugs with the main aim to determine drug safety. Drugs are typically tested in a small group of healthy volunteers (note: cancer drugs are usually tested in cancer patients in Phase I studies).

Phase II
Clinical testing phase for new drugs that is aimed at identifying the optimal dose to be used in Phase III trials and tests for proof of efficacy of the drug with statistically significant results on the endpoint. Typically, Phase II trials are double blinded and have placebo controls.

Phase III
Clinical testing phase for new drugs that is aimed at definitively determining the drug's effectiveness and its side-effect profiles in significantly large (hundreds of thousands of patients) trials. These studies are also typically double blinded and placebo controlled. After the study is closed and while data are being prepared for presentation, a Phase IIIb may allow continued "compassionate use" of the drug by patients who have been in the Phase III study.

Phase IV
After a drug has been approved, pharmaceutical companies may conduct further studies of its performance, often examining long-term safety or expansion to other indications.

prevalence
The number of cases of a disease at a specified time divided by the number of individuals in the population at that specified time. The prevalence may be reported as a percentage of the population or as the prevalence per 100 000 people (see also incidence).

proteomics
The study of gene expression at the protein level, by the identification and characterization of proteins present in a biological sample.

QSR
Quality system requirements. A biomedical product development and production system is regulated by the QSR guidelines, encompassing environmental, management and other factors to ensure high quality, consistent products.

RBRVS and RVUs	Resource-Based Relative Value Scale (RBRVS) and Relative Value Units (RVUs). A relative value system that is used for calculating national fee schedules for reimbursement of physicians' services provided to Medicare patients. Physicians are paid on relative value units (RVUs) for procedures and services. The three components of each established value are: work RVU, practice expense RVU, and malpractice expense RVU.
Recombinant DNA (rDNA)	A combination of DNA molecules of different origin or chromosomal location that are joined using recombinant DNA technologies.
SOP	Standard operating procedure – documented procedures so that the SOP document reflects actual practice of procedures in various manufacturing, design review, testing, assays, laboratory procedures, etc. Standard operating procedures are an integral part of cGMP, GLP and QSR.
siRNA	Silencing or short interfering RNA (ribonucleic acid); control mechanism for controlling production of specific proteins by interfering with gene transcription.
sNDA	A supplemental NDA (sNDA) is typically submitted for additional indications for a marketed drug and adds information to a previously filed NDA.
surrogate endpoint	A surrogate endpoint is a marker – a laboratory measurement or physical sign – that is used in clinical trials as an indirect or substitute measurement that represents a clinically meaningful outcome, such as survival or symptom improvement. The use of a surrogate endpoint can considerably shorten the time required prior to receiving FDA approval. Approval of a drug based on such endpoints is given on the condition that post-marketing clinical trials verify the anticipated clinical benefit. The FDA bases its decision on whether to accept the proposed surrogate endpoint on the scientific support for that endpoint. The studies that demonstrate the effect of the drug on the surrogate endpoint must be "adequate and well controlled" studies; the only basis under law for a finding that a drug is effective.
(drug) target	Usually a protein, an enzyme, or a receptor in a cell or tissue that has been discovered to play a central role in the development or diagnosis of a disease.
USC	The United States Code is the codification by subject matter of the general and permanent laws of the United

States. The latest text (updated every six years) is available at www.gpoaccess.gov/uscode.

wholesale acquisition cost (WAC)
The price paid by a wholesaler for drugs purchased from the wholesaler's supplier, typically the manufacturer of the drug. On financial statements, the total of these amounts equals the wholesaler's cost of goods sold. Publicly disclosed or listed WAC amounts may not reflect all available discounts (text from HRSA website).

wholesaler
A wholesaler is a company that serves as a bridge between a drug manufacturer and a covered entity. This means any entity (including a pharmacy or chain of pharmacies) to which the labeler sells the covered outpatient drug, but that does not relabel or repackage the outpatient drug (Text from HRSA website, www.hrsa.gov/opa/glossary.htm).

Index

CPSIA information can be obtained at www.ICGtesting.com
Printed in the USA
243634LV00002B/2/P